Normality, Abnormality, and Pathology
in Merleau-Ponty

SUNY series in Contemporary Continental Philosophy

Dennis J. Schmidt, editor

Normality, Abnormality, and Pathology
in Merleau-Ponty

Edited by

Susan Bredlau *and* Talia Welsh

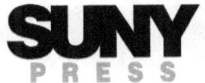

Published by State University of New York Press, Albany

© 2022 State University of New York

All rights reserved

Printed in the United States of America

No part of this book may be used or reproduced in any manner whatsoever without written permission. No part of this book may be stored in a retrieval system or transmitted in any form or by any means including electronic, electrostatic, magnetic tape, mechanical, photocopying, recording, or otherwise without the prior permission in writing of the publisher.

For information, contact State University of New York Press, Albany, NY
www.sunypress.edu

Library of Congress Cataloging-in-Publication Data

Names: Bredlau, Susan, editor. | Welsh, Talia, editor.
Title: Normality, abnormality, and pathology in Merleau-Ponty / edited by Susan Bredlau and Talia Welsh.
Description: Albany : State University of New York Press, [2022] | Series: SUNY series in contemporary continental philosophy | Includes bibliographical references and index.
Identifiers: LCCN 2021040611 (print) | LCCN 2021040612 (ebook) | ISBN 9781438486857 (hardcover : alk. paper) | ISBN 9781438486871 (ebook) | ISBN 9781438486864 (pbk. : alk. paper)
Subjects: LCSH: Public health—Philosophy. | Epidemiology—Philosophy.
Classification: LCC RA425 .N77 2022 (print) | LCC RA425 (ebook) | DDC 362.101—dc23/eng/20211005
LC record available at https://lccn.loc.gov/2021040611
LC ebook record available at https://lccn.loc.gov/2021040612

10 9 8 7 6 5 4 3 2 1

Contents

Acknowledgments   ix

Introduction
Normality, Abnormality, and Pathology in Merleau-Ponty's Work   1
   Susan Bredlau and Talia Welsh

Part I
Grounding a Phenomenology of Normality, Abnormality, and Pathology

Chapter 1
Toward a Phenomenology of Abnormality   19
   Jenny Slatman

Chapter 2
What Can We Learn about the Normal from the Pathological?
Merleau-Ponty, Goldstein, and Neuropsychology   41
   Gabrielle Jackson

Chapter 3
Merleau-Ponty and Ab/Normal Phenomenology: The Husserlian
Roots of Merleau-Ponty's Account of Expression   63
   Neal DeRoo

Chapter 4
The Abnormalcy of "Normalcy": Merleau-Ponty, Russon, and the Normativity of Experience 79
Susan Bredlau

Chapter 5
The Need for Merleau-Ponty in Foucault's Account of the Abnormal 97
Hannah Lyn Venable

Part II
Practical Phenomenological Applications of Merleau-Ponty's Theories of Normality, Abnormality, and Pathology

Chapter 6
Meandering Peripheries: A Ground without Figure for Relief 119
Adam Blair

Chapter 7
The Insight of Dispossession: Examining the Phenomenological and Political Significance of Merleau-Ponty's Account of the Spatial Level 141
Whitney Howell

Chapter 8
Moving without Movement: Merleau-Ponty's "I can" and the Memoirs of Bodily Immobility 165
James Rakoczi

Chapter 9
A Whole New World: Reimagining Divergent Sensory and Perceptual Experiences in Autism through Merleau-Ponty's *Phenomenology of Perception* 187
Jennifer E. Bradley

Chapter 10
Health and Other Reveries: Homo Curare, Homo Faber, and the Realization of Care 203
Joel Michael Reynolds

Chapter 11
The Desexualization of Disabled People as Existential Harm
and the Importance of Ambiguity 225
Christine Wieseler

Works Cited 249

Contributors 269

Index 273

Acknowledgments

"Through speech, then, there is a taking up of the other person's thought, a reflection in others, a power of thinking *according to others*, which enriches our own thoughts."[1]

This book was inspired by the 43rd annual meeting of the International Merleau-Ponty Circle, "The Normal and the Abnormal," held November 8 to 10, 2018, at the University of Tennessee at Chattanooga. We want to thank all the participants and celebrate all the spirited discussion that led us to think a special volume was needed to present to a larger audience the critical discussions the conference stimulated. We also want to thank the Vice-Chancellor of Research and the Graduate School, the College of Arts & Sciences, the Honors College, and the Department of Philosophy & Religion, who all graciously sponsored the conference. We deeply appreciate the work of Gail Weiss, the International Merleau-Ponty Circle's General Secretary, and David Morris, the Associate General Secretary, for all their work promoting Merleau-Ponty studies around the globe. Finally, we extend our warm thanks to Landon Everest Finke, Colton Greganti, and J. Wolfe Harris who aided us with editing and organizing the volume.

Introduction

Normality, Abnormality, and Pathology in Merleau-Ponty's Work

SUSAN BREDLAU and TALIA WELSH

We are living in a time when scientific research into human biology, psychology, and behavior advances daily, but also at a time when we hear an increasingly loud refusal to accept not just scientific research but any expert knowledge. From conspiracy theories that create alternate facts, to rejection of overwhelming evidence of climate change, to groundless dismissal of well-researched journalism, we seem to have become unhinged from the norms we followed before.[1] The catchphrase "the new normal" itself appears senseless because rather than entering into a perhaps dystopian yet stable set of "normal" behaviors, we seem instead to be standing on constantly shifting ground. Our shared community and obvious patterns of behavior with other humans is constantly tested. In the United States at the time of finishing this volume, we have already witnessed over 300,000 people die from COVID-19 due in part to the rejection of basic public health recommendations including mask wearing and social distancing. A study by Columbia University, published on October 21, 2020, estimates that 130,000 to 210,000 deaths were preventable, and since that publication we have seen the numbers of new cases and deaths skyrocket.[2] The reckless flaunting of factual information might instill a desire to return to a time when the assertions of knowledgeable people were recognized as authoritative.

In the academy, many of us—who have, likely for historically unjust reasons, achieved positions of relative security—are accustomed to having our expertise interrogated and challenged in the traditional pursuit of better knowledge and understanding and yet find ourselves speechless at the proliferation of worlds in which nothing is held as expert and everything is subject to possibly violent rejection. Thus a book that challenges our views of what is normal, abnormal, and pathological might seem inappropriate; perhaps we should, instead, turn our attention to reestablishing the firmer ground upon which we once stood. Yet while this book does not address all the manifold complex political, historical, and cultural reasons for our current condition, it does draw attention to how weakly grounded our sense of normality was all along and suggests that what our present condition calls for is not a return but a new path forward.

The Case of Schneider: Merleau-Ponty's Dynamic Conception of Embodiment

Maurice Merleau-Ponty's discussion of Johann Schneider in the *Phenomenology of Perception* serves as a rich opportunity for reflecting on the meaning of normality, abnormality, and pathology.[3] While serving as a soldier in the German army during World War I, Schneider was injured by shrapnel from an exploding mine. X-rays taken several years after the injury showed that Schneider still had some small metal shards in his brain.[4] Merleau-Ponty's attention to the injury's impact on Schneider's everyday life reveals his interest in thinking beyond the binaries that had dominated—and often still dominate—discussion of "abnormal" cases like that of Schneider, binaries that try to separate the diversity of human experience into categories such as well or sick, adjusted or ill-adjusted, normal or pathological. Moreover, while discussions of cases like Schneider's generally focus on identifying discrete behaviors or symptoms that distinguish the abnormal from the normal, Merleau-Ponty focuses on how Schneider's experience is, as a whole, structured differently from that of a "normal" subject. In this pursuit, he also provides a nuanced approach to discussions of normality, abnormality, and pathology that avoids blindly repeating culturally located normative assumptions.

Merleau-Ponty's description of Schneider's injuries and symptoms relies on the writings of the German neurologist Kurt Goldstein and the

German experimental psychologist Adhemar Gelb.[5] They first examined Schneider at a military hospital in Frankfurt, Germany, in 1916 and first published an article describing his injuries and symptoms in 1918.[6] Gelb and Goldstein reported that Schneider, whom they referred to as "Patient Schn.," had a number of unusual impairments, including alexia, visual form agnosia, loss of movement vision, loss of visual imagery, tactile agnosia, loss of body schema, loss of position sense, acalculia, and loss of abstract reasoning.[7] Yet they also reported that he was, with respect to a large number of everyday behaviors, seemingly unimpaired. For example, when Schneider was blindfolded in an experimental setting, he was unable to point to or grasp his nose;[8] in his daily life, however, he could easily blow his nose with a handkerchief.[9]

Some have accused Gelb and Goldstein of exaggerating or making up some of Schneider's symptoms and even of teaching Schneider to act in ways that would confirm their theories. When Carl Jung examined Schneider in the 1940s, for example, he found that Schneider, contrary to Gelb and Goldstein's reports, was able to see and recognize most objects.[10] Moreover, Jung thought that the abnormal behavior of making tracing movements with his hand or head, which Gelb and Goldstein reported that Schneider used to compensate for his visual impairments when asked to identify objects or letter objects, only seemed to be present in experimental situations, suggesting that Schneider was putting on a show for the scientists studying him.[11] The contemporary psychologist Georg Goldenberg even goes so far as to claim that "Schneider and Schn. were two different personalities. Schneider was an amiable, open-minded, vivid human being. Schn., by contrast, was a freak: speaking with an exalted, monotonous voice, shaking all over the body, exploring the world around him like an alien, he resembled a strange automaton more than a human being."[12] Nonetheless, others have defended Gelb and Goldstein's work. Another contemporary psychologist, Martha Farah, notes that if Jung did not observe many of the impairments that Gelb and Goldstein reported, this may have reflected that, 20 years after Gelb and Goldstein's initial reports, Schneider's brain had largely recovered from or adapted to its injuries.[13]

Gelb and Goldstein's first article about Schneider remains, Goldenberg writes, "a citation classic in neuropsychology."[14] He attributes this to the fact that "several of the symptoms that they claimed to find in Schn. were indeed detected in later patients";[15] these symptoms included agnosia, loss of movement vision, and loss of visual imagery. In a review of the impact that Schneider's case has had on the field of neuropsychology, Jonathan Marotta and Marlene Behrmann write that "the case of Schn. has significantly influenced the visual agnosia literature."[16] Cases of visual agnosia, which Marotta and Behrmann define as a "a disorder of visual recognition, in which a person cannot arrive at the meaning of some or all categories of visual stimuli, despite normal or near-normal visual perception and intact alertness, intelligence, and language,"[17] are often divided into two broad categories: apperceptive and associative. Someone with apperceptive agnosia is "unable to copy, match, or identify a drawing," while someone with associative agnosia is able to copy and match a drawing but unable to identify it.[18] While Gelb and Goldstein identified Schneider as having apperceptive visual agnosia, Marotta and Behrmann argue that Schneider had a form of integrative agnosia: "Patients with integrative agnosia appear to have available to them the basic features or elements in a display, but are unable to integrate all aspects into a meaningful whole."[19]

Contemporary psychology and neuroscience's focus on Schneider's visual agnosia raises a number of questions. Should Schneider be thought of as having a collection of relatively independent disorders—disorders with respect to vision, movement, and abstract reasoning, for example—or as having a single disorder that manifests itself in different, though dependent, aspects of his experience? That is, should we think of vision as operating quite independently of movement, abstract reasoning, and other functions, or should we think of all of these functions as contributing to a perceptual experience in which the whole is, so to speak, greater than the sum of its parts? This latter approach appears to be the one that Gelb and Goldstein advocated. With respect to the rehabilitation of those with brain injuries or diseases, Goldstein writes:

> If restoration is out of the question, the only goal of the physician is to provide the patient with the possibility of existing in spite of his defect. To do this one has to consider each single symptom in terms of its functional significance for the total personality of the patient. Thus it is absolutely necessary for the physician to know the organism as a whole, the total personality of the patient, and the change which the organism as a whole has suffered through disease. The whole organism, the individual human being, becomes the center of interest.[20]

Furthermore, contemporary psychology and neuroscience's focus on Schneider's visual agnosia contrasts sharply with the approach Merleau-Ponty takes in his discussions of Gelb and Goldstein's work on Schneider.[21]

Merleau-Ponty's focus is neither on Schneider's abnormal vision alone nor on his various impairments as unrelated to one another. Rather, Merleau-Ponty's focus, like Gelb and Goldstein's, is on Schneider's experience as a whole, and he understands Schneider's brain injuries as giving him a way of being-in-the-world with others that is very different from that of most other people. For Schneider, Merleau-Ponty argues, the meanings that once constituted his everyday experience of the world—and that do constitute the everyday experience of the world for most of us—are no longer operative and have been replaced by *new* meanings. Schneider's "abnormal" experience is thus not some damaged or deficient form of "normal" experience; rather, it is a unique experience in its own right.

Merleau-Ponty argues that attempts to understand Schneider's situation have generally drawn on one of two conceptual frameworks: empiricism and intellectualism. The empiricist framework, which is largely the framework of contemporary scientific research, understands a "normal" subject as one whose body possesses a set of physical properties or capacities that can be isolated by the natural sciences. A normal subject is, for example, one whose brain displays certain anatomical or functional features, while an "abnormal" subject is one whose brain does not display, or incompletely displays, these features, and, perhaps, displays other features. According to this naturalizing view, one answers the question of what is normal and what is abnormal by turning to the sciences and investigating humans and, in particular, human bodies as objects. The intellectualist framework, by contrast, understands a normal subject as one whose body is governed by explicit acts of consciousness. Normal subjects are, for example, conscious of the position of their bodies within objective space and direct the movements of the body within this space. Abnormal subjects, on the other hand, lack such consciousness of the body and world or, perhaps, simply deny that they have this consciousness.

Yet despite their differences, the empiricist and intellectualist frameworks share, Merleau-Ponty argues, the assumption that the body is merely an object; empiricism understands the body as a physical object, while intellectualism understands the body as an object of thought. Neither empiricism nor intellectualism recognizes, therefore, that the body is fundamentally a subject rather than an object; consciousness is embodied.

While both empiricism and intellectualism may be able to discover certain features of the human body or mind that are usually present and, therefore, identify situations in which these features are absent (and, perhaps, other features are present) as abnormal, these investigations leave unexamined the impact of such abnormality for the living subject. Any one illness or injury that can be reliably identified by the absence or presence of certain objective features is, nonetheless, lived by different people in different ways. Moreover, not all abnormalities are lived as pathological; indeed, some abnormalities may even be lived as beneficial.

Thus, throughout his discussion of Schneider, Merleau-Ponty argues that attending to Schneider's lived experience is critical for understanding his situation. Though the "cause" of his disorder is evident—he has metal shards in his brain—the precise character of his disorder only becomes evident if one accounts for Schneider's changed way of being-in-the-world. Merleau-Ponty thus lays the groundwork for a dynamic conception of abnormality and normality. Information from medical literature, so long as it focuses only on the body as an object and neglects the body as a subject, is insufficient for understanding a person's symptoms. Moreover, Merleau-Ponty provides the outline of the thesis, developed more fully in this volume, that one's embodiment is shaped by both personal experiences and social and cultural norms. Any attempt to identify or understand a pathological situation thus has to attend to matters that cannot be "seen" or quantified in standard medical testing. Despite the seeming obviousness of the origin of the pathological aspects of Schneider's situation, one cannot identify his situation as pathological without appealing to Schneider's experience, to his way of being-in-the-world.

Identifying the physical aspects of illness or injury, in other words, will be insufficient for understanding them since their meaning can be found only within the body as subject and not the body as object. Indeed, to be precise, the meaning of an illness is not so much within the body as subject but, instead, within the world that appears to this body as subject. Just as pointing out that our eyes are necessary for sight offers little or no insight into perceptual experience, pointing to a physical change offers little or no insight into the meaning of the injury for the injured person. So long as the lived experiences of those with illnesses and injuries are ignored or discounted, the illnesses and injuries will remain poorly understood. Though those with schizophrenia may all share a specific genetic profile, for example, their hallucinations often reflect their cultural situations.

Researchers have found that hallucinations vary widely in cultures, both in content as well as tone and perceived threat.[22] Likewise, researchers have noted that differences in socioeconomic status and how one experiences systemic racism is correlated with one's health outcomes even in the case when one's physical condition might seem "objectively" similar to those in different racial or socioeconomic groups.[23] Understanding symptoms, behaviors, and expressions of pathology requires going beyond accurate transcription of physical differences to a careful description of differences in lived experience. And such description, in turn, requires us to reflect on, and perhaps revise, our previous understandings of normality, abnormality, and pathology. After all, human experience—either individually or as a whole—is comprised of diverse—and even divergent—experiences.

Merleau-Ponty's references to and descriptions of a "normal" subject, whom he contrasts with Schneider, are not without controversy. As Gail Weiss notes, Iris Marion Young, Judith Butler, and others have criticized Merleau-Ponty for failing to recognize that his descriptions of "normal" experience do not actually "hold true for all individuals, regardless of gender, race, class, ethnicity, age, ability, etc.";[24] what Merleau-Ponty takes to be human experience may actually only be the experience of particular humans, humans who are, for example, white, male, and cisgender. Nonetheless, Weiss argues that even as Young

> offers a powerful critique of Merleau-Ponty insofar as he presents an allegedly neutral and universal experience of bodily transcendence, intentionality, and unity that is, in actuality, more frequently enacted by and associated with boys and men rather than girls and women . . . it is clear that the contradictory bodily modalities she is describing are problematic precisely because they fail to realize the possibilities for transcendence, intentionality, and unity that, like Merleau-Ponty, she believes that both male and female bodies are capable of achieving.[25]

Likewise, Weiss argues that while Butler, like Young, faults Merleau-Ponty for failing to adequately acknowledge "that the 'I can' is not merely an expression of embodied agency but also of cultural agency," she also praises Merleau-Ponty for "recognizing that the significance of our embodied experiences is always tied to a particular historical context . . . [thereby supporting] an understanding of gender as never purely natural but always naturalized."[26] Weiss draws our attention, therefore, to the "rich resources in Merleau-Ponty's own discussion that undermine a false view of the body schema as unaffected by the normative expectations of others, whether these latter are based on our race, our gender, our class, our religion, a particular ability or disability or on other aspects of our identities."[27] When Merleau-Ponty focuses on "allegedly abnormal experiences," Weiss argues, he does so "not as negative examples that reinforce the rigid boundaries of normality, but . . . to challenge our conceptions of what is normal, what is natural, and what can and should be normative."[28]

Drawing, then, on Merleau-Ponty's insight that a person's lived experience is critical to any account of the normal, abnormal, and pathological, and on the resources his work offers for recognizing how bodies that are differently gendered, raced, classed, and so forth will live the world differently, the chapters in this volume explore both the diversity of human experience and the possibility of whether, while acknowledging this diversity, there nonetheless remain good reasons for retaining a conception of normal experience. The questions addressed by these chapters include: Given the vast variety of forms that human experience takes, is it still worthwhile to search for universal features of human experience? Is it still legitimate to identify certain forms of experience or certain subjects as normal and others as abnormal? Since many abnormal kinds of embodiment, such as color blindness, do not impede an individual from having a healthy and happy life, should abnormality and pathology be distinguished from each other, and if they are distinguished, what is their relation? How does the fact that the definitions of normality, abnormality, and pathology have been different in different cultures and changed over time complicate our understanding of these concepts? Is it possible to assert some kind of natural, and thus universal, origin for these concepts or are they all inevitably overdetermined by our culturally specific, contemporary epistemologies?

The purpose of this volume is twofold. First, it will offer scholarly reflection on Merleau-Ponty's conception of embodiment and of the effects of pathology, disease, disorder, or social exclusion on embodiment. Second, it will contribute to the ongoing discussion within biomedical ethics, philosophy of medicine, philosophies of disability, and related fields of how we should, both theoretically and practically, take account of diverse forms of embodiment. Four interwoven themes drawn from Merleau-Ponty's work on normality, abnormality, and pathology are contained within: (1) Jenny Slatman, Gabrielle Jackson, and Christine Wieseler discuss and complicate Merleau-Ponty's description of Schneider; (2) Susan Bredlau, Hannah Lyn Venable, and Whitney Howell consider other pathological cases to further develop Merleau-Ponty's insights into normality, abnormality, and pathology; (3) Jenny Slatman, Adam Blair, James Rakoczi, Joel Michael Reynolds, and Christine Wieseler consider limitations of Merleau-Ponty's approach; and (4) Christine Wieseler, Whitney Howell, Adam Blair, and Joel Michael Reynolds argue that despite some limitations in Merleau-Ponty's work, rich resources remain for considering topics he did not speak extensively about, including gender, race, and disability. In the next section, we offer a short summary of the contents of this volume.

Part I—Grounding a Phenomenology of Normality, Abnormality, and Pathology

The first five chapters set the stage for the later chapters by explicating, refining, and examining the implications of Merleau-Ponty's conception of normality, abnormality, and pathology.

The first two chapters discuss the importance of Kurt Goldstein's work for Merleau-Ponty's by exploring the case of Schneider. In chapter 1, Jenny Slatman introduces the theme of the book, exploring Merleau-Ponty's conception of normality and abnormality. Merleau-Ponty, she argues, did not conceive of abnormality as the opposite of normality, but instead, following Goldstein, Merleau-Ponty recognized pathological states as distinguishably different from states of health. Moreover, Slatman asserts that phenomenology's focus on the body as lived tends to avoid consideration of mathematical models in its discussions of embodiment. However, she argues that the use of statistics complements phenomenological descriptions. The norms discovered by statistics often become normative; social and cultural attitudes and environments are often built upon these statistically generated norms, thereby limiting the possibilities of expression for those who merely fall toward either end of a standard distribution. In chapter 2, Gabrielle Jackson further analyzes the significance of Goldstein's work for Merleau-Ponty's philosophy. Attending first to Goldstein's general method, Jackson then carefully documents how Merleau-Ponty's articulation of the difference between the normal and the pathological draws upon and implicitly endorses Goldstein's own methodology. Thus, Jackson underlines the centrality of Goldstein's work for future phenomenological discussions that depart from Merleau-Ponty's.

In chapter 3, Neal DeRoo explores how expression functions in Edmund Husserl's and Merleau-Ponty's phenomenology, and, in so doing, complicates our understanding of what constitutes "normal" phenomenology. Merleau-Ponty's later work on expression takes up Husserl's idea that sense and being must be understood as having a reversible, asymmetrical relationship that is experienced as a phenomenal unity. In this approach, Merleau-Ponty works to end various kinds of dualism in phenomenology by seeing our primary mode of existence as a kind of interrogation. Merleau-Ponty thus continues the normal path of Husserlian phenomenology while also extending its scope, refusing to make consciousness central to his discussion of expression.

In chapter 4, Susan Bredlau draws on Merleau-Ponty's discussion of habit and hallucination in the *Phenomenology of Perception* and "psychological rigidity" in the lecture "The Child's Relations with Others," as well as on John Russon's discussion of the "ideal of normalcy," to argue for the inadequacy of a common conception of a "normal" self as one who freely chooses her behavior and is, as such, not compelled by her body, emotions, or relations with others. Rejecting this conception of a normal self does not mean, however, that we have no basis for identifying certain forms of experience as problematic. Rather, we must simply recognize that it is not the presence of compulsions as such that defines a situation as pathological, but instead the presence of compulsions that undermine, rather than support, a person's ability to acknowledge and flexibly navigate the multiple, often conflicting, aspects of her experience.

In the last chapter of part I, Hannah Lyn Venable, like Bredlau, discusses other pathological cases; in so doing, she explores how Merleau-Ponty's work provides essential clarification for Michel Foucault's discussion of abnormality in *History of Madness*. She points out that while Foucault explores the different forms that madness takes in different societies, his account suffers from two omissions. First, he never explores the origin of these different forms of madness and thus runs the risk that his account appears arbitrary since diversity in the experiences of the mad remains unclarified. Second, he takes no interest in better diagnosis or treatment and thus runs the risk that his account appears inapplicable to our present situation. Merleau-Ponty's phenomenology, she argues, allows us to explore and understand these different forms of madness as meaningful, and thus offers insight into why madness has taken the forms that it does and how it might be treated more effectively.

Part II—Practical Phenomenological Applications of Merleau-Ponty's Theories of Normality, Abnormality, and Pathology

The next five chapters examine the application of Merleau-Ponty's work to contemporary cases of abnormality and pathology and to the operation of the medical sciences. Phenomenological discussions of Morning Glory Syndrome, inverted perception, bodily immobility, and Autism Spectrum Disorder explore how the body's capacities are interwoven with its milieu, thus complicating our understanding of bodily differences. The last two chapters consider how the existence of narrow norms for healthy bodies limits our sense of what a life worth living is like and discuss the implications of these limitations for our use of genomic testing and our understanding of the sexuality of disabled persons.

Part II begins with Adam Blair's exploration of his own abnormal vision. Blair has Morning Glory Syndrome in his left eye. When using just his left eye, his perceptual experience does not conform to the standard phenomenological description of perceptual experience as having a figure/background structure. He describes what he sees with his left eye as only background with no possibility of a normal figure. The phenomenological description of his own perceptual experience, Blair argues, allows us to better understand Merleau-Ponty's conception of the constitution of sense and to better recognize the necessity of indeterminacy even within normal perception. By acknowledging a view of the world that is not driven by the contrast of figure-ground and that emphasizes indeterminacy and possibility over determinacy and particularity, we are better able to understand Merleau-Ponty's most important claims regarding perspective, sensation, and freedom.

In chapter 7, Whitney Howell also explores the implications of the phenomenological description of an "abnormal" experience for our understanding of experience more broadly. Howell focuses on how our sense of space is determined not simply by being in space but by personal, historical, cultural, and political affordances. Using examples from China Miéville, Simone Weil, and Sara Ahmed, Howell explores how space has normative dimensions that can go unrecognized in normal and normative forms of orientation. Particular spaces, in requiring a subject to have specific capacities if she is to belong to them "properly," both include certain individuals and exclude others depending on how closely these individuals adhere to the norms established by the particular space. Noting some limitations in Merleau-Ponty's account, Howell concludes by exploring the political implications of this account of spatial orientation and disorientation.

Chapter 8, by James Rakoczi, focuses on a little discussed but compelling body of literature on individuals who have lost much of their capacity for moving freely in the world. Rakoczi takes up these narratives and uses Merleau-Ponty's work on embodiment to point out that such accounts are not devoid of reference to movement, but instead, are saturated with references to movement; this calls for a more nuanced understanding of the role of movement, even for those whose movement is quite limited, in the constitution of sense and selfhood. In contrast to the phenomenon of extreme bodily immobility, autism has received significant scholarly attention in philosophy. Yet, as Jennifer E. Bradley argues in chapter 9, philosophical reflection on autism often focuses on the capacity of those individuals with autism spectrum disorder (ASD) to achieve certain intellectual tasks, such as recognizing the other person's mental state, or behaving in a particular controlled manner. Yet this approach, which implicitly assumes that abnormal behavior is necessarily pathological, overlooks the dynamic manners in which individuals with ASD make meaningful solutions to sensory disturbances. Drawing on Merleau-Ponty's work on space and on our relations with others, Bradley argues that a phenomenological approach offers a more adequate understanding of, and more effective therapies for, individuals with ASD.

The last two chapters reflect on how everyday identifications of what is, and what is not, "normal" often hide forms of privilege that deserve to be questioned—extending Merleau-Ponty's work to contemporary topics. In chapter 10, Joel Michael Reynolds discusses the contemporary case of pediatric whole genome sequencing tests, which are often used to predict a child's likelihood of developing serious, and sometimes terminal, illnesses. Using Merleau-Ponty's work on ambiguity, Reynolds explores how we tend to live the world both individually and with loved ones with a tacit expectation of control over "normal" circumstances. He argues that we tend to see humans through the medical lens as *homo faber*—a human that is in control and will continue in the same fashion over time—and *homo curare*—the human understood as connected to fate and to be cared for according to the human's particular individual situation. Reynolds argues for considering the latter more seriously and also exposes how the stance of the homo faber is often only possible for a small percentage of individuals—those who are white, cis-gendered, able-bodied, and upper-middle class. Given this, Reynolds argues, ethical discussions of tests such as pediatric whole genome sequencing should always take a larger social and political context into account. In the last chapter, Christine Wieseler explores how disabled people are often read as being inherently asexual due to their physical differences. She argues that ideals of normal sexuality constitute an existential harm to disabled persons, not just in contemporary popular thought but also in academic research. Returning to Merleau-Ponty's account of sexuality, she argues for a more ambiguous understanding of human existence and human sexuality outside the reification of normal and abnormal.

In this volume, we have endeavored to provide scholarly reflection on Merleau-Ponty's work on the topics of normality, abnormality, and pathology and to connect his work to contemporary research. Often as theorists we want to destabilize simple, biased understandings of what is normal and of what conclusions should be drawn from scientific research. Merleau-Ponty's work is exemplary in this regard, closely considering contemporary scientific research into the human condition while retaining a critical gaze toward it.

Even though many of us feel like observers of a disturbing shift toward nationalistic, racist, antiscientific, antiintellectual, and violent political regimes, we are never mere observers. In our state of trying to figure out how to live in this "new normal," we are always inextricably tied up in it. In *The Visible and the Invisible*, Merleau-Ponty famously writes, "Where are we to put the limit between the body and the world, since the world is flesh? . . . The world seen is not 'in' my body, and my body is not 'in' the visible world ultimately: as flesh applied to a flesh, the world neither surrounds nor is surrounded by it."[29] To think about normality, abnormality, and pathology is also to change and transform those terms. Yet the very freedom we have to investigate such ideas, expand our understanding of ourselves and the world, and appreciate more fully the experience of others also permits us to disengage from expertise, to follow conspiracies, and to refuse a common human bond. We hope that by complicating our view of normality, we can move beyond the alternatives of blindly trusting or utterly rejecting the work of experts and see how we ourselves are part of the process that constantly renews our understanding of the human condition.

Notes

1. Max Fisher, "Why Coronavirus Conspiracy Theories Flourish. And Why It Matters." *The New York Times*. April 8, 2020. www.nytimes.com/2020/04/08/world/europe/coronavirus-conspiracy-theories.html; David Hasemyer and Neela Banerjee, "Decades of Science Denial Related to Climate Change Has Led to Denial of the Coronavirus Pandemic." *Inside Climate News*. April 9, 2020. https://insideclimatenews.org/news/09042020/science-denial-coronavirus-covid-climate-change; Cary Funk and Meg Hefferon, "U.S. Public Views of Climate and Energy." *Pew Research Center: Science & Society*. November 25, 2019. www.pewresearch.org/science/2019/11/25/u-s-public-views-on-climate-and-energy

2. Irwin Redlener, MD, Jeffrey D. Sachs, PhD, Sean Hansen, MPA, Nathaniel Hupert, MD, MPH. "130,000–210,000 Avoidable COVID-19 Deaths and Counting in the U.S." October 21, 2020. https://ncdp.columbia.edu/custom-content/uploads/2020/10/Avoidable-COVID-19-Deaths-US-NCDP.pdf

As of this writing, the United States has had 16.5 million cases of COVID-19 and 301,006 deaths. Worldwide we stand at 73 million cases and 1.62 million deaths. We reference the Johns Hopkins Coronavirus Resource Center. https://coronavirus.jhu.edu/map.html

3. Merleau-Ponty's discussion of Schneider begins in Part One, Chapter Three of the *Phenomenology of Perception*, trans. Donald A. Landes (New York: Routledge, 2012), and continues in Part One, Chapters Five and Six.

4. J.J. Marotta and M. Behrmann, "Patient Schn: Has Goldstein and Gelb's Case Withstood the Test of Time?" *Neuropsychologia* 42 (2004): 633–638. Even this characterization of Schneider's injuries is, however, disputed. Marotta and Behrmann write that "Bay, Lauenstein and Cibis (1949) came to a different conclusion . . . They reported that there were many iron splinters in the soft parts of the left half of the skull and face but that all of them proved to be outside of the skull . . . [and] no evidence of a penetrating skull wound was found" (634). Goldenberg reports, "he was unconscious for 4 days. After healing from the wounds he suffered from vegetative and emotional lability, bradycardia, headache, and feelings of insecurity when standing or walking . . . . His mental capacities appeared normal apart from a slight reduction of the ability to memorize auditorily presented digits. He complained of rapid fatigue and of blurring of vision after prolonged reading" (G. Goldenberg, "Goldstein and Gelb's Case Schn: A

Classic Case in Neuropsychology?" In C. Code, C.W. Wallesch, Y. Joanette, and A.R. Lecours [eds.], *Classic Cases in Neuropsychology, Vol. II* [Hove: Psychology Press, 2003]: 281–300).

5. For a brief biography of Kurt Goldstein and a discussion of his collaboration with Adhemar Gelb, see Hans Teuber, "Kurt Goldstein's role in the development of neuropsychology." *Neuropsychologia* 4, no. 4 (1966): 299–310.

6. This article, "Psychologische Analysen hirnpathologischer Falle auf Grund von Untersuchungen Hirnverletzer," has, to our knowledge, never been translated into English.

7. Marotta and Behrmann, "Patient Schn," 633; Goldenberg, "Goldstein and Gelb's Case Schn," 282.

8. Rasmus Jensen. "Motor Intentionality and the Case of Schneider." *Phenomenology and the Cognitive Sciences* 8 (2009): 371–388.

9. Gelb and Goldstein argued that Schneider had apperceptive visual agnosia; their theory, Marotta and Behrmann write, "was that Schn lacked any visual experience of form (or Gestalt) but that he compensated for this deficit by tracing visually presented forms with movements of either the head or fingers, eventually recognizing the form by kinesthetic feedback" ("Patient Schn," 635).

10. Marotta and Behrmann, "Patient Schn," 635.

11. Marotta and Behrmann, "Patient Schn," 635.

12. Goldenberg, "Goldstein and Gelb's Case Schn," 295.

13. Martha Farah, *Visual Agnosia* (Cambridge, MA: MIT Press, 2004), 2. For further defense of Gelb and Goldstein, see also Jensen, "Motor Intentionality and the Case of Schneider," 374, footnote 6.

14. Goldenberg, "Goldstein and Gelb's Case Schn," 296.

15. Goldenberg, "Goldstein and Gelb's Case Schn," 296.

16. Marotta and Behrmann, "Patient Schn," 635.

17. Marotta and Behrmann, "Patient Schn," 633.

18. Marotta and Behrmann, "Patient Schn," 633.

19. Marotta and Behrmann, "Patient Schn," 636.

20. Kurt Goldstein, *Human Nature in the Light of Psychopathology* (Cambridge, MA: Harvard University Press, 1947), 6.

21. On the relation between Merleau-Ponty's work and that of Gelb and Goldstein, see Gabrielle Jackson's chapter in this volume.

22. Frank Larøi, Tanya Marie Luhrmann, Vaughan Bell, William A. Christian Jr., Smita Deshpande, Charles Fernyhough, Janis Jenkins, and Angela Woods, "Culture and Hallucinations: Overview and Future Directions." *Schizophrenia Bulletin* 40 (Suppl 4) (July 2014): S213–S220. doi: 10.1093/schbul/sbu012.

23. Tulay G. Soylu, Eman Elashkar, Fatemah Aloudah, Munir Ahmed, and Panagiota Kitsantas, "Racial/Ethnic Differences in Health Insurance Adequacy and Consistency among Children: Evidence from the 2011/12 National Survey

of Children's Health," *Journal of Public Health Research* 7, no. 1280 (2018): 56–62; Shervin Assari and Maryam Moghani Lankarani, "Poverty Status and Childhood Asthma in White and Black Families: National Survey of Children's Health," *Healthcare* 6, no. 62 (2018): doi:10.3390/healthcare602002; Shervin Assari, "Unequal Gain of Equal Resources across Racial Groups," *International Journal of Health Policy and Management* 7, no. 1 (2018): 1–9.

24. Gail Weiss, "The Normal, the Natural, and the Normative: A Merleau-Pontian Legacy to Feminist Theory, Critical Race Theory, and Disability Studies." *Continental Philosophy Review* 48 (2015): 80.

25. Weiss, "The Normal, the Natural, and the Normative," 84.

26. Weiss, "The Normal, the Natural, and the Normative," 84.

27. Weiss, "The Normal, the Natural, and the Normative," 89.

28. Weiss, "The Normal, the Natural, and the Normative," 93.

29. Maurice Merleau-Ponty, trans. Alphonso Lingis, *The Visible and the Invisible*. (Evanston, IL: Northwestern University, 1968).

Part I

Grounding a Phenomenology of Normality, Abnormality, and Pathology

Chapter 1

Toward a Phenomenology of Abnormality

JENNY SLATMAN

Introduction

The contrast between health and illness is often equated with the contrast between normal and abnormal, where health is seen as the normal state and illness as the abnormal one. In contemporary health care, what belongs to the domain of the normal is determined based on scientific insights, consensus within professional groups, and social and political norms. Against the background of current health policy that emphasizes a commitment to early and preventive treatment, it makes sense that the American Heart Association in November 2017 changed the standard for high blood pressure from 140/90 mmHg to 130/80 mmHg. The consequence of this adjustment is that 46 percent of the American population now suffers from hypertension.[1] This example shows how changeable standards or norms are, while at the same time making it clear that abnormality—not meeting the standard—is not necessarily equivalent to illness. Most people whose blood pressure is just above the new standard do not suffer from anything at all. Doctors may want to treat them, but if we label all these people as "ill," we end up with very few healthy people.

For most people, being ill or sick means suffering from something, experiencing pain or discomfort. If we limit ourselves here to somatic complaints, we could say that illness, as demonstrated by the blood pressure example, usually goes hand in hand with a certain form of bodily abnormality; however, bodily abnormality does not always go hand in hand with illness. In the same vein, having a genetic abnormality does not necessarily mean that you are currently ill, or will ever become ill. Other cases in which abnormality and illness do not always coincide include a range of physical limitations as well as visible physical abnormalities. If, after a diagnosis and successful treatment of cancer, you continue to live with one breast or without a nose, you are not sick, but you are abnormal. In addition, people with impairments can be said to deviate from the norm of normal functioning, but, very often, this is not seen as a disease but rather as a disability.[2] Perhaps even more importantly, a person with an impairment is often directly identified by others as abnormal. If you have only one leg, you are not sick, but you are abnormal.

In my previous research project *Bodily Integrity in Blemished Bodies*, I studied physical changes that occur as a result of cancer and cancer treatment and how people handled these changes.[3] Central to this research was the question of how people experience their visibly changed bodies. In order to understand these experiences, it was critical to see the individuals in their social context. These people did not only have to deal with a changed body but also with the fact that others might see them as abnormal because they are, for example, missing a breast, have a visible scar, or use a facial prosthesis. It will come as no surprise that the phenomenology of the body was at the heart of this research, for indeed, a phenomenological approach greatly facilitates the interpretation of embodied self-experiences. However, during this research project it also became clear that conventional phenomenology has its limitations.

Phenomenology is well suited for interpreting the phenomenon of illness, of being ill from a first-person perspective. Yet it provides far fewer tools for analyzing the phenomenon of bodily abnormality. Indeed, a sociological and/or social constructivist approach might seem more suitable for understanding abnormality. Yet, as I have suggested elsewhere, phenomenology can account for third-person perspectives on the body if it is developed in the direction of a sociophenomenology.[4] In this chapter I will elaborate on this suggestion and show how phenomenology can account for both illness and abnormality.

For my analysis, I will first return to the most important source text for contemporary phenomenology of health and illness: Maurice Merleau-Ponty's *Phenomenology of Perception*. In the first part of this chapter I will explain why, according to Merleau-Ponty, illness cannot be equated with abnormality. The distinction between illness and abnormality, I will explain, stems from the phenomenological methodological consideration of putting scientific knowledge and prejudices in parentheses. Merleau-Ponty was also profoundly inspired by the work of the German neurologist and psychiatrist Kurt Goldstein, who in *The Organism* writes, "It may be stated as certain that any disease is an abnormality, but not that every abnormality is a disease. No matter how we may define normality, there are certainly many digressions from the norm that do not mean being sick."[5] Merleau-Ponty's contemporary Georges Canguilhem also bases his main work, *The Normal and the Pathological,* on the work of Goldstein. Since Canguilhem discusses the distinction between the normal and the pathological much more explicitly than Merleau-Ponty, I will discuss their work in parallel.

From my analysis of these three authors, it will emerge that the use of statistics plays an important role in the distinction between illness and abnormality. According to phenomenology, statistics as a form of scientific knowledge must be bracketed. However, while following Merleau-Ponty's remark that the most important lesson to be learned from the phenomenological reduction is the impossibility of a total reduction,[6] I will, in the second part of this chapter, show that statistics should not be banned from our understanding of the lifeworld nor simply put in parentheses. I begin by reviewing Ian Hacking's analysis of how the rise of the concept of "normal" occurred at the same time as the rise of statistics in the nineteenth century.[7] Even though statistics is inherently descriptive in nature, Hacking asserts that it soon acquires a normative, prescriptive function. Our world is largely made up of "averages" that are considered to be normal *and* normative. Physical deviations from an average not only imply a statistical observation but also give rise to a judgment of some kind of failure. Thus, I will argue, physical deviation directly affects embodied subjectivity and agency.

Illness in the *Phenomenology of Perception*

In his philosophical analyses of the body, embodiment, and perception, Merleau-Ponty (1908–1961) makes extensive use of pathological cases. Let us first have a look at why he uses cases of illness within his philosophical analyses of embodiment. Since he contrasts the sick person (*le malade*) with the person who is normal (*le normal*), it seems that he uses illness to explain what is normal, that he understands normal embodiment or perception on the basis of pathological cases. Yet, this is too hasty a conclusion; his use of pathological cases needs to be placed in the context of his phenomenological approach. As Merleau-Ponty clearly describes in the preface to the *Phenomenology of Perception*, the phenomenological reduction and the eidetic reduction (or variation) are crucial methodological steps for phenomenology. The use of pathological cases fits within the design of the eidetic reduction; these cases serve as the variations necessary for finding the eidetic or the invariant of the embodied existence. In Edmund Husserl's view of the eidetic variation, intellectual imagination plays the most important role. In order to be able to determine the eidetic nature of something, we need to think up or imagine all possible forms of a particular phenomenon and then examine what cannot be omitted without the phenomenon ceasing to be the phenomenon in question.

For Merleau-Ponty, however, the eidetic variation is not just an intellectual exercise in which everything possible is first thought or fantasized to see what cannot be omitted. He uses factual variation and factual cases in order to arrive at something like the eidetic or the essential. In the preface, Merleau-Ponty describes this seemingly contradictory idea of a philosophy that focuses on the essential or essences while connecting to the factual as follows: "Phenomenology is the study of essences . . . [and yet it] is also a philosophy that places essences back within existence and thinks that the only way to understand man and the world is by beginning from their 'facticity.'"[8]

According to Merleau-Ponty, the normal cannot be derived from the pathological because illness is not the same as the loss of normal functions. Pathology and normality are different modalities of the same underlying phenomenon.[9] What the underlying phenomenon is becomes clear when we focus on the case of Schneider, first described by Gelb and Goldstein in 1920. This case plays a crucial role in Merleau-Ponty's conception of embodiment, and he describes it vividly in "The Spatiality of One's Own Body and Motricity" in the *Phenomenology of Perception*. Johann Schneider was a World War I veteran who suffered brain damage as a result of shrapnel. Due to this brain damage, his way of perceiving, orienting, and moving was considerably affected. Psychiatrists at the time classified his case as one of "psychic blindness."[10] Schneider was not blind, but with his eyes closed he was unable to perform so-called "abstract movements," movements that are artificially elicited. For example, when requested by his doctor, Schneider was not able to touch his nose (with his eyes closed) or to bend or stretch his limbs on command. However, if his nose was itchy, he could immediately touch his nose (with his eyes closed), and he could also find the handkerchief in his pocket to blow his nose. These kinds of movements are called "concrete movements;" though they are mechanically and physiologically the same as the abstract movements, they differ from abstract movements because they do not exceed a person's actual situation.

The fact that Schneider could not point to his nose on command should not be explained in terms of a defect in the sensory-motor system, as if something were wrong with a sense organ or a muscle. Pointing (*Zeigen*, abstract movement) and grasping (*Greifen*, concrete movement), although they have the same underlying anatomy and physiology, are two different intentional actions. The difference between the two forms of movement shows a variation in how we can relate to the world. Whereas concrete movement is primarily a way of dealing with our actual situation, abstract movement is about transcending that situation. The difference between the two forms of movement also shows a variation in the extent to which motor actions take place in a reflective or prereflective manner. Concrete movements generally take place without reflection or thought, whereas abstract movements require one's awareness of what one is doing. If you are asked to point to your nose on command, this is a movement that you think about for a moment; yet when your nose itches, you scratch it without reflection. It should be noted, however, that a concrete movement is not the same as a reflexive movement, such as moving one's lower leg when the knee is tapped with a reflex hammer. Whereas a reflex cannot be controlled, concrete movements can be controlled. You can become aware of concrete movements and reflect on them. Normally, though, this is not necessary, and the movement takes place in the flow of the situation.

Considering these two different forms of movement as possible variations of the phenomenon of embodied existence, we find motor intentionality as the invariant underlying both. According to Merleau-Ponty, motor intentionality is founded in what he calls the "intentional arc."[11] Our entire conscious life is underpinned by this arc, which contains a projection of our past, present, and future as well as of our social environment and our physical, moral, and ideological situation. This intentional arc allows us to situate ourselves somewhere and in a certain way(s). Yet in Schneider's case, Merleau-Ponty argues, his intentional arc is weakened (*se détend*) and its span into the future is diminished.[12] The metaphor of tensile strength and span refers to the possibilities, or the existential "I can" that people have. Our consciousness, says Merleau-Ponty, is not first of all an "I think," as Descartes and Kant said, but an "I can" (*je peux*).[13] The consequence of Schneider's injury, therefore, is not just a matter of his being unable to perform tasks because of his defects. It is also matter of what possibilities he experiences the world as offering him. Both the environment and the situation in which a person finds themselves and the physical functioning of that person determine together, as if in a dialogue, what that person's possibilities are. For Merleau-Ponty, having fewer possibilities, having a flaccid arc, is what is most characteristic of what we call illness. Schneider, the sick person, has fewer possibilities. The way he deals with his world and environment is characterized by a high degree of awkwardness. Illness, so we can say, affects his entire being, his existence.

In *Phenomenology of Perception*, Merleau-Ponty does not elaborate on how the dividing line between normality and illness is drawn. By taking a pathological case from clinical literature, he appears to assume unreservedly that medical literature defines where the line between the healthy and the pathological should be drawn. In addition, because he does not give a description of what is normal, he could be accused of a rather naive idea of normality: that normality is that which is not described in the clinical literature and is something that is given naturally. However, this is not the case. Merleau-Ponty describes illness as affecting a person's intentional arc. This description implies a dynamic understanding of both normality and pathology. In Merleau-Ponty's own work, this dynamic concept is not really made explicit—illness and normality are by no means the main themes in his work. In order to make it clear how we can interpret illness and normality as dynamic and as nonnaturalistic, I will now briefly discuss a number of elements from the work of Goldstein and Canguilhem.

The Normal and the Pathological According to Goldstein and Canguilhem

Kurt Goldstein (1878–1965) was an important inspiration for Merleau-Ponty's analyses of embodiment. From 1916 onward, he worked as a neurologist and psychiatrist in Frankfurt, where he saw many World War

I veterans with brain damage, including Johann Schneider. According to Goldstein, health represents the most adequate way in which the organism deals with its environment. Health, therefore, consists mainly of "preferred behavior" or "orderly behavior."[14] By this, he means that the way the human organism acts is based on all kinds of habits (and skills) that have been acquired through time, tradition, and education. From this, it immediately becomes clear that health or healthy action is not something universal but is instead always bound to a certain time and place in which preferences have been developed. Normality or health is therefore not based on a predetermined scientific or moral norm but is formed within a process of habituation. In other words, according to Goldstein, there is no such thing as a supra-individual norm that prescribes what normal or healthy physicality is. The norm that determines whether an individual is healthy or ill is formed by the individual organism while it relates and responds to its environment.

It is precisely this idea of health and normality that Canguilhem (1904–1995) further develops in his main work, *The Normal and the Pathological*. According to Canguilhem, the most important characteristic of health is a flexibility of standards or norms.[15] The healthy person or the normal person does not so much meet a predetermined standard of health; rather, the person's health consists of having the possibility to set new norms or standards over and over again. Therefore, he says that being healthy means "being normative," that is, being able to change and set norms. Whereas Goldstein states that normal physical action is based on a norm-producing process of habituation and adaptation, on an interaction between the organism and the environment, Canguilhem emphasizes that this is an open and infinite process in someone who is healthy.

According to Goldstein, illness or disease manifests itself in disturbed, disorderly behavior that goes hand in hand with a loss of skills (both cognitive and motor). His ideas about health and illness were crucially developed through the examination and treatment of many World War I veterans. These young soldiers suffered from all kinds of devastating health problems, including wound shock and shell shock. These symptoms typically could not be explained by the degree of the soldiers' physical injuries.[16] Goldstein, therefore, considered illness or disease not simply as a matter of organ or tissue failure but as a total body (or total organism) response. What he observed in injured veterans was that the loss of skills could trigger intense experiences of fear and uncertainty. He called this experience the "catastrophic reaction."[17] Merleau-Ponty and Canguilhem both take up Goldstein's idea of illness.[18] Illness manifests itself in a person's having fewer possibilities. Merleau-Ponty describes this in terms of a flaccid intentional arc or a reduced "I can." Canguilhem describes the pathological as an inferior norm of life (*norme de vie*). It is a norm but an inferior one "in the sense that it tolerates no deviation from the conditions in which it is valid, incapable as it is of changing itself into another norm."[19] According to Canguilhem, being ill is not the same as being non-normal or abnormal. The sick person is not ill because they deviate from a given norm; the sick person is ill because they "can admit of only one norm."[20] As he states, the sick person "is not abnormal because of the absence of a norm but because of [their] incapacity to be normative."[21] This means that they are not able to create other norms in other situations. A sick person is thus "normalized in well-defined conditions of existence and has lost their normative capacity, the capacity to establish other norms in other conditions."[22]

Health or normality, therefore, means that the organism is capable of more than just adapting to the environment. When an organism can only adapt to its environment, it only follows that specific situation and is not able to exceed the norm of the situation. It then remains bound to that specific environment and is not normative. Just being able to adapt indicates pathology.[23] We also saw this in the case of Schneider. Because he is capable of making concrete movements, Schneider is perfectly capable of coping with the given situation, but he is not able to play with or transcend the situation.

The Silence of Health

Goldstein, Canguilhem, and Merleau-Ponty all emphasize in their analysis of pathological cases the subjective illness experience, that is, the experience of illness from a first-person perspective. Referring to the then well-known statement of the French surgeon René Leriche (1879–1955) that "health is life lived in the silence of the organs," Canguilhem states that illness is always related to the *experience* of the sick person.[24] A person who only feels the silence of their organs is not sick in Canguilhem's opinion. This seems to be an easily refuted claim since diseases do not always go together with an experience of being ill: for example, early-stage cancer can still be categorized as being within the "silence of the organs." In such cases, people often do not feel anything is "wrong" or "abnormal" in their bodies. To diagnose a physical abnormality, physicians cannot trust patients' experiences but must rely on all kinds of medical diagnostic equipment. Canguilhem would reject this objection while claiming that contemporary medical knowledge and equipment that allows us to diagnose a disease without it having been "heard" by the patient can ultimately be traced back to patients' experiences. Medical knowledge, however disconnected it may now seem from patients' experiences, has been able to develop only on the basis of a rich history of patients who have shared their experiences with doctors. In other words, a device that measures blood sugar levels, even at a level where people have no symptoms, has been developed only because people with actual symptoms of low blood sugar went to their doctor. That is why Canguilhem writes: *"there is nothing in science that has not first appeared in the consciousness."*[25]

It is interesting to note that Canguilhem uses the terms "pathology" and "pathological" when he talks about the experiences of sick people. In contemporary parlance, pathology refers to "disease," and "disease," according to medical sociology, involves the biomedical perspective on an ailment, and should be distinguished from "illness" (the person's experience of that ailment) and "sickness" (the social meaning of being sick).[26] Canguilhem, by contrast, suggests that pathology is not necessarily the same as some localizable defect in the body (disease) but rather has its origin in the experience of illness. Only when doctors have developed all kinds of diagnostic tests to determine a possible somatic cause of those complaints does it become a disease. At the beginning of this chapter, I referred to high blood pressure and mentioned that even if people have an abnormal blood pressure value, they do not necessarily feel sick, and probably do not say they are sick. Symptomless high blood pressure is indeed not an illness, but it might be considered a disease or a precursor of disease since something is measured as being wrong or abnormal.

While Merleau-Ponty, Goldstein, and Canguilhem all emphasize the patient's first-person perspective, they criticize the prominence of the "disease-model" in contemporary medicine. This model, first developed in the eighteenth century and also described, for example, by Canguilhem's student, Michel Foucault, in his *Birth of the Clinic*, meant that doctors place increasing emphasis on research into underlying defects and abnormalities in anatomy and physiology for understanding, diagnosing, and treating patients' complaints. At the beginning of the nineteenth century, Bichat wrote that corpses had to be opened up in order to understand diseases better, thus creating a happy marriage between anatomy and pathology: anatomy becomes pathological while pathology is "anatomized."[27]

Before the eighteenth century, medicine focused more on the complaints and symptoms that patients reported to a doctor. In the modern era of medicine, the anatomical body became the focus. A disease, a pathology, is what you can locate somewhere in the body. Hence, as Drew Leder argues, the body that is central in modern medicine is actually the dead body, the corpse of pathological anatomy.[28] This emphasis on pathological disease, which in our time is increasingly reinforced by all kinds of diagnostic (imaging) technologies that make it possible to locate inconsistencies in the body without cutting it open, means that in clinical practice the patient's story disappears into the background. Goldstein, Merleau-Ponty, and Canguilhem, by contrast, want to centralize the patient's experience of illness.

Quantification of Pathology

In addition to the emergence of the so-called disease model in medicine, Canguilhem describes how in the nineteenth century a shift also occurred from a qualitative to a quantitative concept of disease. In his historical analysis, Canguilhem shows how the definition of health as "normal," introduced by the physician-physiologist François-Joseph-Victor Broussais (1772–1838), has led to the idea that the difference between disease and health is a quantitative difference.[29] According to Broussais, every organ has a "normal state." A deviation from this normal state implies illness, and this deviation occurs when an organ is, for example, too much or little stimulated by irritation or inflammation. In his time, Broussais was not taken that seriously and was even caricatured in Honoré de Balzac's work. Balzac ridiculed Broussais because, at the beginning of the nineteenth century, Broussais was still a fervent advocate of bloodletting. Balzaz wrote that just as much blood had been shed under Broussais' hands as during the Napoleonic battles.[30] Hacking states that it is because of Balzac's parodies of Broussais that the term "normal" appears in the French language.[31] And Canguilhem claims that it is mainly due to August Comte (1798–1857) that the idea of health as a "normal state" eventually became a widespread idea. Based on the "eminent philosophical principle" of Broussais, Comte argues that the pathological and the normal state do not differ substantially, or qualitatively, from each other. The pathological state is nothing more than too much or too little compared to the normal state.[32] This idea of disease is by no means foreign to us. Just think of the examples of normal and abnormal blood sugar levels or blood pressure. More sugar in the blood indicates a problem with an organ, and thus, a disease. With hypertension, or high blood pressure, the pressure of the blood on the wall of the blood vessel is so high that over time it can cause damage to the blood vessel wall.

In his analysis, Canguilhem criticizes this quantification of disease. First of all, he shows that both Broussais' and Comte's reasoning is not entirely consistent and that their determinations of "too much" or "too little" call for a qualitative, normative perspective: "To define the abnormal as too much or too little is to recognize the normative character of the so-called normal state."[33] For Canguilhem (and also for Goldstein), the pathological cannot be seen as a condition that differs only quantitatively from the normal condition. When your blood pressure is higher than 130/80 mmHg, you are not necessarily ill. Illness implies a *qualitatively* different state than health: you feel different; you are no longer able to do things the way you did before.

Canguilhem and Goldstein's criticism of the idea of disease as a quantitative difference also goes hand in hand with their view that a statistical perspective does not contribute to the understanding of whether an individual is ill or healthy.[34] A norm based on a statistical average does not do justice to the experience of the individual; such a norm cannot determine whether an individual is ill or healthy.[35] At forty beats per minute, Napoleon's pulse, compared to the average of seventy, is far too low, but the man was in good health. Apparently, those forty beats of his heart were sufficient to cope with the demands of life.[36]

Merleau-Ponty's work does not provide a comprehensive analysis of the meaning of statistics, but it is clear that, for him, a statistical perspective on the body is associated with the idea of the body as an object, the objective body. Such a perspective is not compatible with what he calls one's own body (*corps propre*), lived body (*corps vécu*), or the body as a subject (*corps sujet*). The bodily subject experiences themselves as embodied from the first-person perspective, which involves experiences of the body through localized sensations such as touch, pain, proprioception, kinesthetic sensations, warmth, and cold. Statistical measures of the body, like the medical gaze of a doctor, form an external perspective, a third-person perspective that concerns the objective body (*corps objectif*). Because Merleau-Ponty is not explicitly interested in the question of what is normal (and what is not), as Canguilhem and Goldstein are, he does not spend many words on statistics. It is, therefore, even more interesting to focus on a passage in which he mentions the statistical perspective in relation to human characteristics.

At the beginning of the chapter on freedom in the *Phenomenology* (in which he enters into a discussion with Jean-Paul Sartre), Merleau-Ponty explains that one cannot have an awareness of one's own qualities such as being jealous or being hunchbacked when one is restricted to a first-person perspective, a perspective *pour soi*. Let us consider here the reference to the hunchback (*le bossu*). The figure of the hunchback is an interesting one because—certainly after Victor Hugo's novel *Notre Dame de Paris* (1831) in which the hunchback Quasimodo plays the leading role—it is exemplary of abnormal embodiment in European culture. Merleau-Ponty describes the hunchbacked person as becoming aware of being hunchbacked only by comparing themselves with others, by seeing themselves through the eyes of someone else with whom they then take on a statistical or objective perspective on themselves.[37] Statistically, most people have a fairly straight back and no hunchback. The hunchback is, therefore, a statistical deviation from the average.

What is interesting about this incidental remark about the hunchback is Merleau-Ponty's claim that it is partly due to statistics that people become aware that they deviate from the norm, that they are abnormal. Yet, this is not the same as an awareness of illness. Like Goldstein and Canguilhem, Merleau-Ponty assumes that statistics—which set supra-individual norms—do not help to determine whether an individual is ill or not. For all three of them, awareness of illness is based on the patient's own experience, on the first-person perspective. This means that being hunchbacked is not really considered an illness because the person who is hunchbacked does not experience it from their first-person perspective as such. Here it becomes clear how we can interpret the difference between illness on the one hand and abnormality on the other hand in Goldstein, Canguilhem, and Merleau-Ponty. Illness is the lived experience of having fewer opportunities to deal with the situation and environment. Abnormality can exist without being "heard," whereby it remains hidden under the "silence of the organs," as long as it is not confronted with others and thus with a comparison with others.

Statistics and Abnormality

Abnormality, or abnormal embodiment, therefore, appears only within a framework of comparison. In medicine and public health, this framework is formed by large-scale biomedical, epidemiological, and statistical measurements. Goldstein and Canguilhem were both trained as clinicians, and their criticism of the statistical approach should thus be seen in the light of their view that this approach does not do justice to the experiences and stories of their (individual) patients. This is, of course, different for Merleau-Ponty. He was not a physician, and his criticism of a statistical approach to the body was not inspired by the wish to improve clinical practice. His criticism is philosophical in nature. Putting the statistical perspective on the body in parentheses in order to gain a better understanding of the embodied existence fits within the phenomenological exercise of "returning to the things themselves." The proposal for such a return implies that we should bracket our science-formed knowledge and prejudices as much as possible. Since the term "abnormal embodiment" is a result of statistics, it must be bracketed in the phenomenological interpretation of the embodied existence. In that sense, a phenomenology of abnormality seems to be a contradiction in terms. It is, therefore, no wonder that Merleau-Ponty does not use the term "abnormal" in his analysis of Schneider. Schneider, the patient (*le malade*), is contrasted with the normal (*le normal*). Nowhere is the normal (*le normal*) contrasted with the abnormal (*l'anormal*).[38]

In the remainder of this chapter, I want to show, however, that it is also possible to develop a phenomenological approach to abnormal embodiment. I will explain that the statistics of abnormality are not just a neutral form of scientific knowledge that exists peacefully and independently of the way people experience their bodies. Even though we intend to bracket statistical knowledge for our phenomenological analysis of lived experiences from a first-person perspective, such a bracketing, or such a phenomenological reduction, can never be complete. Our world is permeated with statistics. Most of our daily activities are dictated by statistical norms. In order to clarify how statistical knowledge infiltrates the lived experience of people, I will now take a trip outside phenomenology to discuss Hacking's analysis of statistics. In his historical analysis of nineteenth-century statistics in *The Taming of Chance*, Hacking establishes a direct link between the development of statistics and the emergence of the concept of "normal." According to Hacking, the concept of "normal" in the sense of "usual," "ordinary," and "common" originated in the nineteenth century.[39] Before that time, when it came to people or bodies, one did not speak of something like a normal person or a normal body but of "human nature."[40] The term "normal"—derived from the Latin *norma* and Greek *ortho*, which means "right angle"—takes on the meaning of "usual" through developments in statistics.

One of the most important statistical ideas is that most characteristics or properties are "normally distributed" within a population. The term "normal distribution," expressing this symmetrical distribution of properties, was introduced by Francis Galton (1822–1911) at the end of the nineteenth century, but before that it was already thought of in terms of the so-called Gaussian curve, which was used in the calculation of probability and named after the German mathematician Carl Friedrich Gauss (1777–1855). If properties are normally distributed, this means that the mean or average coincides with the median (the value that is in the middle) and the mode (the value that occurs most often). A normal distribution curve looks like a so-called bell curve that is completely symmetrical.

Typical examples of normally distributed properties include biometric properties (weight, height) and also students' grades. A typical normal distribution emerges only when the statistical calculation of mean, median, and mode is based on a large sample. The normal distribution and the mean are descriptive models that give us insight into the variation of properties within a certain population. Hacking, however, shows that as soon as the normal distribution appears on stage as a descriptive model, it also immediately acquires a normative function. The work of the Belgian statistician Alphonse Quetelet (1796–1874)—according to Hacking, the "greatest regularity salesman" of the nineteenth century—is exemplary in this respect.[41] Quetelet, who was very interested in all kinds of measures and calculations of the human body—thanks to him we also have the still widely used Body Mass Index (BMI) or Quetelet Index—managed to obtain a biometric dataset from the Scottish army that was remarkably rich for the nineteenth century. The chest size of about 5,000 soldiers was measured, probably to determine measurements for new uniforms. According to Quetelet's calculations, the chest size values are "normally" distributed. He did not yet call it a normal distribution—since that term was only later on introduced by Galton—but used the term "error curve," which Gauss used to represent the values of measurement errors in astronomy.

According to Gauss, the error curve showed that the values that occur most frequently and are concentrated in the middle are the least false values. The measured values further from the center and that occur less frequently are—most probably—erroneous. By means of this curve, Gauss could indicate, based on many measurements, which measurement of a certain planet was most likely correct. When Quetelet uses this error curve—which has the same graphical form as the normal distribution—to calculate the average chest size of the Scottish soldier, something remarkable happens, as Hacking indicates. Whereas Gauss based the average or mean and, therefore, the most correct measurement on multiple measurements of one and the same planet, Quetelet calculates the average size of the chest on the basis of measurements of many different soldiers. Quetelet seems to see the measurements of many different thoraxes as a multitude of measurements of one and the same body—the "average body." Quetelet thus approximates the average chest, or the average body, in the same way that Gauss considers a planet. Whereas a planet is a real entity, an average is not. Therefore, as Hacking writes: "Quetelet changed the game. He applied the same curve to biological and social phenomena where the mean is not a real quantity at all, or rather: he transformed the mean into a real quantity."[42]

This specific interpretation of the mean implies that values that lie (far) from the mean are considered to be errors, as actual deviations and not just as a statistical deviation. This means that if the average chest size is thirty-nine inches, then someone with a chest size of forty-seven inches is abnormal, a deviant. From the idea of the error curve, the average is equated with a standard or norm. A soldier with a chest size of forty-seven inches does not meet the standard. What we see in these analyses by Quetelet is that the average is not *only* a descriptive model of how the biometric values of chest size are distributed. The average itself becomes normative or prescriptive in the sense that it indicates how the chest of a Scottish soldier *should be*. For Quetelet, the statistical average is ideal. Based on his conviction that the natural and social world is structured and organized according to certain laws of regularity, he assumes that the statistical average is the expression of the ideal type within a given population. Quetelet, therefore, like most of his colleagues, agrees that statistics are of great importance to identify and improve the qualities of a population. Statistics were indeed considered an important tool for what Galton called "eugenics": the theory that a population could be enhanced through the elimination of inferior (hereditary) characteristics while embracing one specific (racist) idea of humankind. Interestingly, whereas most eugenicists considered the above-average person (i.e., the person endowed with exceptional strength or intelligence) as ideal, Quetelet considers the average person—*l'homme moyen*—as ideal. The average person is not only a statistical construct according to Quetelet, but also an actual entity. He does not see the average person as a mediocre person (as Galton did after him). No, for him the average is the ideal. He literally says: "An individual who epitomized in himself, at a given time, all the qualities of the average man, would represent at once all the greatness, beauty and goodness of that being."[43]

Hacking's analysis of Quetelet's work shows how the seemingly neutral and descriptive statistical mean becomes directly normative. Although nowadays we do not directly link mediocrity to the greatness of mankind, even in our time the ideal of the average is often embraced when it comes to appearance. In the 1990s, psychologists established that a beautiful face is nothing more than an average face.[44] Kathy Davis, who researched the motives of women who undergo cosmetic surgery, also observes that averages are more important than diversity.[45] Most women who underwent cosmetic surgery indicated that they wanted to be "ordinary" or normal in the sense of ordinary. They did not necessarily want to be more beautiful; they wanted to be more normal. So here we can clearly see how the idea of an average can easily ensure that individuals who, outside the scope of the statistically normal, regard themselves as different in a negative sense, and, therefore, even feel the pressure to adapt more to the norm, to normalize themselves, to belong more to the average, to be within the scope of the normal.[46] When you are average or normal in a certain population, you do not stand out, and you do not attract attention. However, if you are not average, then you stand out and are confronted with the comparative views of others that may hinder you. In addition, our entire living environment is geared to averages: architects, designers, and tailors use sizes that suit the majority of the population. If you fall outside the bell curve of the normal, most things do not happen automatically. This point can help us to integrate the abnormal into phenomenology.

A Phenomenology of the Abnormal

Merleau-Ponty argues that the hunchback needs the third-person perspective if they are to become aware of the fact that they are "different" from others. This is true, but this third-person perspective, which is fed by ideas about averages, is also part of our living environment. When Merleau-Ponty indicates that someone is not aware of their own characteristics, such as being hunchbacked, it means that this form of being embodied for that person, without the gaze of the other, has something in itself that is self-evident. We can also say that when the hunchback is not aware of their hump and experiences their body as a matter of course, their body forms the obvious zero point of action and orientation. This zero point coincides with the above-mentioned "I can." Therefore, we can say that the "I can" of the hunchback who is not aware of their hunchback is not diminished.

Based on his analysis of Schneider, Merleau-Ponty defines illness as a disruption or reduction of the "I can." This is also in line with Goldstein's view on disease in terms of a total body response resulting in "disordered behavior" and sometimes a "catastrophic reaction," and Canguilhem's idea that pathology goes hand in hand with the loss of normativity, that is, the capacity of setting norms. What I want to add here is that disturbances of the "I can" are not only provoked by illness or pathology. As Merleau-Ponty points out, there is a disturbance of the "I can" when the natural way to deal with your environment and situation is disturbed. But this disruption of the "I can" also occurs when people feel that their embodiment, their way of being embodied, is not self-evident within a specific social group. In his chapter "The Lived Experience of the Black (*le Noir*)," in his book *Black Skin, White Masks*, Frantz Fanon states that being black in white France in the 1950s has a direct impact on his body schema and thus on his physical subjectivity. According to Fanon, the body schema—which for Merleau-Ponty forms the basis of the "I can"—must be exchanged for a "racial epidermal schema" (*schéma épidermique racial*).[47] In *Queer Phenomenology*, Sara Ahmed elaborates on this: "For bodies that are not extended by the skin of the social, bodily movement is not so easy. Such bodies are stopped."[48] Being black in a white world means that you stand out, that your being embodied as "black" is never self-evident, that instead of being a zero point of orientation, you often become a point of attention for others. In this sense, being black in a white world leads to an inhibition of intentionality and possibilities; it leads to being arrested both figuratively and literally.

Merleau-Ponty, as we all know, makes no reference to skin color and argues that physical characteristics that are noticed from a third-person perspective belong, phenomenologically speaking, to the "objective body" and not to the lived body, the body as subject. Fanon and Ahmed show that skin color and racial characteristics have an enormous impact on the body as a subject, the body as the incarnation of the "I can." This observation can be extended to the domain of abnormal embodiment, that is, embodiment that statistically differs from what is considered normal within a social group, such as that of the hunchback. Because not being average within a social group often goes hand in hand with being different in a negative sense, it makes you stand out in this group, protruding so that you cannot pass for normal.[49] If that is the case, being nonaverage can have an impact on the lived body.

When Merleau-Ponty talks about the hunchback, he states that this person will experience themselves as different only from the perspective of the other. Perhaps it is true that a hunchback who lives in total social isolation or in a community with only hunchbacked people does not experience their hunchback as something different. In real life, however, this is never the case. In real life, we are always confronted with the comparative views of others. This gaze can affect someone's embodiment by transforming the self-evidently embodied zero point of action and orientation into a body that stands out to others. The gaze, therefore, directly affects the lived body because it breaks the self-evidence of it. Those whose physical appearance is statistically different can, therefore, experience a disturbance of their "I can" without any pathology as described by Merleau-Ponty, Canguilhem, or Goldstein.

Goldstein wrote that pathology always goes hand in hand with abnormality, but that abnormality does not always go hand in hand with pathology.[50] We can agree with this viewpoint of Goldstein if we think back to the example of high blood pressure. Blood pressure higher than 130/80 mmHg is currently considered abnormal in the United States, but, as mentioned above, most people with such blood pressure do not feel ill and would probably not say they are ill. Goldstein would indeed say these people are not ill. We could, therefore, say that Goldstein's distinction between disease and abnormality can very well be used to counteract contemporary medicalization.[51]

The norms and standards that Goldstein and Canguilhem are talking about are mainly physiological standards, standards that, according to Broussais, indicate the normal state of an organ or tissue. In this chapter, however, I am talking about norms or standards of how bodies appear. As I indicated above, standards of what a body should look like often correspond to average values within a population. Based on my explanation of the effect statistical reasoning can have in today's societies, I have put forward the suggestion that the mere fact of being physically abnormal can also lead to a distortion of the zero point of action and, therefore, to a reduction in possibilities. This applies to any physical characteristics that can be observed by others; it applies if you are black in a white society, you have a hump in a society where the majority do not, you are much taller or smaller than most, you are missing a limb, your breast is amputated, or your face is damaged.

In the phenomenology of the body, this variation in physical characteristics is very often considered to be characteristic of only the objective body and, as such, is usually bracketed and kept out of the analysis. What I have just shown is that perceptible physical differences—abnormality according to statistics—do not necessarily mean that someone is ill, but they should be included in the phenomenological analysis because they also concern the lived body. A phenomenology of abnormality integrates the third-person perspective, the perspective from the outside, into the first-person perspective. A phenomenology of abnormality can thus help us to describe and interpret how being physically different is experienced.

Notes

1. George Bakris and Matthew Sorrentino, "Redefining Hypertension—Assessing the New Blood-Pressure Guidelines," *New England Journal of Medicine* 378, no. 6 (2018): 497–499.

2. Jackie Leach Scully, "What Is a Disease? Disease, Disability and their Definitions," *EMBO Reports* 5, no. 7 (2004): 650–653.

3. This project was funded by the Dutch Research Council (NWO). For a summary and the results of this project, see www.nwo.nl/en/research-and-results/research-projects/i/85/6485.html

4. Jenny Slatman, "Multiple Dimensions of Embodiment in Medical Practices," *Medicine, Health Care and Philosophy* 17, no. 4 (2014): 556.

5. Kurt Goldstein, *The Organism: A Holistic Approach to Biology Derived from Pathological Data in Man* (New York: Zone Books, 1995), 326.
6. Maurice Merleau-Ponty, *Phenomenology of Perception*, trans. Donald A. Landes (New York: Routledge, 2012), 34.
7. Ian Hacking, *The Taming of Chance* (Cambridge: Cambridge University Press, 1990), 169.
8. Merleau-Ponty, *Phenomenology of Perception*, 7.
9. Merleau-Ponty, *Phenomenology of Perception*, 138.
10. Merleau-Ponty, *Phenomenology of Perception*, 147.
11. Merleau-Ponty, *Phenomenology of Perception*, 170.
12. Merleau-Ponty, *Phenomenology of Perception*, 172.
13. Merleau-Ponty, *Phenomenology of Perception*, 171.
14. Goldstein, *The Organism*, 48.
15. Georges Canguilhem, *The Normal and the Pathological*, trans. Carolyn R. Fawcett and Robert S. Cohen (New York: Zone Books, 1991), 182.
16. Stefanos Geroulanos and Todd Meyers. *The Human Body in the Age of Catastrophe: Brittleness, Integration, Science and the Great War* (Chicago: University of Chicago Press, 2018), 34–77.
17. Goldstein, *The Organism*, 49.
18. Marie Gérard, "Canguilhem, Erwin Straus et la phénoménologie: la question de l'organisme vivant," *Bulletin D'Analyse* 6, no. 2 (2010); Bernhard Waldenfels, "Normalité et normativité," *Revue de métaphysique et de morale* 45, no. 1 (2005).
19. Canguilhem, *The Normal and the Pathological*, 183.
20. Canguilhem, *The Normal and the Pathological*, 186.
21. Canguilhem, *The Normal and the Pathological*, 186.
22. Canguilhem, *The Normal and the Pathological*, 183.
23. Maria Muhle, "From the Vital to the Social: Canguilhem and Foucault—Reflections on Vital and Social Norms," *Republics of Letters: A Journal for the Study of Knowledge, Politics, and the Arts* 3, no. 2 (2014): 1–12.
24. Canguilhem, *The Normal and the Pathological*, 91.
25. Canguilhem, *The Normal and the Pathological*, 92–93.
26. Andrew C. Twaddle, "Illness and Deviance," *Social Science & Medicine* (1967) 7, no. 10 (1973): 751–762.
27. Michel Foucault, *Birth of the Clinic*, trans. A.M. Sheridan (London: Routledge, 1973), 131.
28. Drew Leder, "A Tale of Two Bodies: The Cartesian Corpse and the Lived Body," in *The Body in Medical Thought and Practice*, ed. D. Leder (Dordrecht: Kluwer Academic Publishers, 1992).
29. Canguilhem, *The Normal and the Pathological*, 47–64.
30. Hacking, *Taming of Chance*, 82–83.
31. Hacking, *Taming of Chance*, 166.

32. Canguilhem, *The Normal and the Pathological*, 51.
33. Canguilhem, *The Normal and the Pathological*, 56.
34. Canguilhem, *The Normal and the Pathological*, 181.
35. Goldstein, *The Organism*, 326.
36. Canguilhem, *The Normal and the Pathological*, 181.
37. Merleau-Ponty, *Phenomenology of Perception*, 497.
38. Merleau-Ponty uses the term "abnormal" in the *Phenomenology of Perception* only when he refers to the experiments by Stratton which incite "abnormal perception" in the chapter, "Space" (p. 248, note 4).
39. Hacking, *Taming of Chance*, 162.
40. Hacking, *Taming of Chance*, 161.
41. Hacking, *Taming of Chance*, 105.
42. Hacking, *Taming of Chance*, 107.
43. Theodore M. Porter, *The Rise of Statistical Thinking, 1820–1900* (Princeton, NJ: Princeton University Press, 1986), 102.
44. Judith H. Langlois and Lori A. Roggman, "Attractive Faces Are Only Average" *Psychological Science* 1, no. 2 (1990): 115–121.
45. Kathy Davis, *Reshaping the Female Body: The Dilemma of Cosmetic Surgery* (London: Routledge, 1995).
46. Here we see how statistics contributes to what Foucault has called "normalizing power." As a student of Canguilhem, Foucault developed an equally critical perspective to statistics and quantification in the human sciences. Whereas Canguilhem criticized the statistical approach for its clinical shortcomings, Foucault revealed how statistics and numbers turn people into objects that can be manipulated without exercising power in a blatant way. Indeed, as described by Hacking, who was greatly influenced by Foucault's early work, the descriptive statistical average or "normal" is often conflated with a normative "normal," which leads to a powerful normative language of normality and abnormality. Hacking, *Taming of Chance*, 169.
47. Frantz Fanon, *Peau Noire, Masques Blancs* (Paris: Seuil, 1952), 90.
48. Sara Ahmed, *Queer Phenomenology: Orientations, Objects, Others* (London: Duke University Press, 2006), 139.
49. Erwin Goffman, *Stigma: Notes on the Management of Spoiled Identity* (London: Penguin, 1963).
50. Goldstein, *The Organism*, 326.
51. Waldenfels, "Normalité et normativité," 63.

Chapter 2

What Can We Learn about the Normal from the Pathological?

Merleau-Ponty, Goldstein, and Neuropsychology

GABRIELLE JACKSON

Introduction

By the turn of the twentieth century, an influx of patients, many of them soldiers, were being admitted to hospitals and clinics. Injured in war by bullets and shrapnel but miraculously kept alive due to advances in battlefield medicine, many had varying degrees of neurological damage. Clinicians documented their behavioral disturbances, drew on the reported peculiarities of their inner experiences, and collated these with evidence of physical damage to the brain in order to guess the origins and processes of successful everyday existence. What they discovered would usher in a new epoch in the sciences of the mind.

Many of these patients suffered damage to the central nervous system. They were diagnosed with forms of language loss, or *aphasias*; loss of vision, or *agnosias*; changes in motor control, or *apraxias*; loss of memory, or *amnesias*; and also, curiously, *amusias*, the loss of the ability to recognize or produce music. Other patients with damage to the spine or nerves were diagnosed with various forms of neuropathy—with, for example, *phantom limb syndrome*, the feeling of the presence of a missing part of the body, often after its loss. Patient presentations were delivered to prestigious scientific societies, new journals with names like *Lesion* were established, and academic departments and labs were created in attempt to pinpoint what was normal but had gone missing in these patients.

Some scientists grew famous from their pioneering research. Paul Broca and Carl Wernicke, for example, became namesakes of the brain regions they investigated. Others, such as A.R. Luria and Oliver Sacks, became successful popularizers, reminding us in the most vivid ways that, in the case of the mind, the distinction between "normal" and "pathological" is not a simple matter of physical explanation. Even the staunchest physicalist admits that understanding the brain requires reference to experience in a way fundamentally different from clinical presentations of, for instance, the liver. It should be no surprise, then, that philosophers joined in too. Rare syndromes and disorders continue to be pressed into philosophical service as a means of disclosing truths about our "deeper selves," the "mysteries of consciousness," our "human uniqueness," and our "place in the world." Conditions such as *split-brains*, *blindsight*, and *walking corpse syndrome* seem "made to order for philosophers' thought experiments," as Daniel Dennett has quipped.[1]

Today *neuropsychology* takes as its domain of inquiry the study of mental processes—for instance, perception, cognition, memory, action, and emotion. In this respect, it is like psychology, psychiatry, neurology, and neuroscience. But unlike these fields, the primary data of neuropsychology comes almost exclusively from *lesion studies*, the observed patterns of ability and debility found in neurologically damaged patients.[2] Analysis of lesion studies generates claims not just about the functioning of intact neural tissues but also, importantly, about the normal mental processes damaged, modified, or undone by the lesion.

It is widely acknowledged—not least by scientists working within neuropsychology, who argue fiercely about the correct interpretation of each new empirical discovery—that lesion studies, done naïvely, are open to grave errors of inference. Scientists must proceed carefully when building theories of normal existence out of the observed effects of brain trauma because they run the risk of mischaracterizing *both* the pathological and the normal.

Maurice Merleau-Ponty discussed many lesion studies in his two early works, *The Structure of Behavior* and the *Phenomenology of Perception*. His analyses of human patients with neuropsychological syndromes and disorders were intended to reveal the invariant structures of intentionality.[3]

Merleau-Ponty was clear, however, that we cannot infer the normal from the pathological *directly*. When analyzing lesion studies, he stated that the key to understanding the contours of intentionality is found in the extraordinary role that *adaptions* play in the pathological situation. For a philosopher who rarely issued decrees, this prescription stands out. But what exactly are these adaptations? And, how do they reveal the normal? You would think the answers could be found in Merleau-Ponty's work. To a certain extent, they can be puzzled out—but not without a significant amount of guesswork, leaving the reader with a distinct sense that key details are being glossed over.

The reason for this, I propose, is that Merleau-Ponty was *summarizing* someone else's ideas. He actually was relating a story about the normal and the pathological first told by another theorist to whom he was deeply intellectually indebted: the German neurologist and psychiatrist Kurt Goldstein (1878–1965). Readers familiar with Merleau-Ponty will recognize Goldstein as the oft-cited source of information about "Schneider," a patient with whom Goldstein worked at his *Institute for Research on the Aftereffects of Brain Injury* in Frankfurt.[4]

It was Goldstein who offered a fully articulated method for how the pathological makes the normal intelligible—a formulation that we find *nearly verbatim* in Merleau-Ponty's writings. To understand what it was that so captivated Merleau-Ponty, to the extent that he would transpose Goldstein's approach into his own work, we must read Merleau-Ponty's words through Goldstein's texts, which is what I propose to do in this chapter.

Kurt Goldstein[5]

Goldstein was born in 1878, in Kattowitz, Germany (what is now Katowice, Poland). His family moved to Breslau around the time that he entered high school. He began university in Breslau but later transferred to the University of Heidelberg in order to study philosophy and literature. After a year in Heidelberg, Goldstein made an abrupt shift, returning to Breslau and changing his focus to medicine. He received his medical degree in 1903 at age twenty-five.

Goldstein trained under Carl Wernicke (1848–1905) and Alfred Schaper (1863–1905) at the University of Breslau in the newly created Department of Neurology and Psychiatry. In this era of medicine, patients with brain damage and disease were typically traded between medical and psychiatric departments. But Wernicke and Schaper both were convinced that neurological traumas had psychological symptoms. Goldstein learned about brain structures and functions and about how damage to neural tissues correlated with clinical symptoms.

Then, around 1909, Ludwig Edinger (1855–1918), the first German professor of Neurology, invited Goldstein to join him at the University of Frankfurt a/M in order to assist in creating a small outpatient treatment center for patients with brain injury and illness. This complex was, by all accounts, one of the first of its kind. Even in the early twentieth century, brain trauma was effectively the end of normal life. Patients were considered beyond repair; their care was mainly custodial. However, under the tutelage of Edinger, Goldstein came to believe that the aftereffects of brain damage and disease could be managed, if not overcome, if patients were given the proper attention and assistance. At first, the medical community treated this idea with deep skepticism, yet news of the center's early successes spread. The timing could not have been better, as hospitals across the country were absorbing exponential numbers of brain injured soldiers into their wards.

It is no surprise, then, that the German government became interested in the outpatient center. In 1914, Goldstein was tasked (under military authority) to expand the clinic into what became the *Institute for Research on the Aftereffects of Brain Injury* in Frankfurt. When Edinger died in 1918, Goldstein took over as professor of Neurology and became the director of the institute he had helped to create.

Goldstein gathered an even larger staff, consisting of medical doctors (psychiatrists and neurologists), orthopedists, psychologists, physical and occupational therapists, schoolteachers and craftsmen, who worked in teams to assist in the total rehabilitation of their patients. They developed intricate tests to pinpoint the exact contours of their patients' symptomology, and offered speech therapy, gait analysis, prosthetics and other assistive devices, and even vocational instruction.[6] Goldstein collaborated with Eva Rothman (1898–1960), a talented psychiatrist in her own right, who later became his wife. Goldstein also worked with psychologist Martin Scheerer (1900–1961), with whom he reunited again later in America. But the most significant professional relationship Goldstein developed was with psychologist Adhémar Gelb (1887–1936), who was Goldstein's most gifted and closest collaborator and dearest friend.

During Goldstein's tenure, thousands of patients passed through the *Institute*. These patients had all varieties of head wounds; some had small penetrations into the brain, while others had massive destruction of the lobes. It was in this period, sometime between 1909 and 1927, when Goldstein and Gelb first encountered the brain-injured patient Johann Schneider, whose lesion study is still presented in major textbooks as one of only a handful of classic cases in neuropsychology. Goldstein and Gelb's engagement with Schneider led to the development of key concepts still in use today: concrete and abstract movements, adaptive behavior, catastrophic reaction, and self-actualization (popularized in Abraham Maslow's work).[7]

As news of the *Institute* spread, Goldstein was offered a prestigious position at the Moabit Hospital in Berlin and invited to create an institute like the one in Frankfurt. This occurred at a pivotal moment in the twentieth-century sciences of the mind when *holism* was still competing with *localization* for dominance. Goldstein, both as a clinician and as a theorist, was playing an increasingly large role in shaping this debate and strongly advocated holism. Creating a second Institute in Berlin would greatly expand the reach of his ideas. The position itself was also quite prestigious, and Goldstein eagerly accepted. He arrived at Moabit Hospital in 1927 with many of his colleagues, whom he had asked to join him in setting up the new institute.

Goldstein's time in Berlin was cut short: "I could not enjoy this very interesting and, I think, promising work for longer than a few years because I was one of the first professors at the University to be arrested by the Nazis, and I had to leave Germany."[8] Indeed, Goldstein was professionally powerful, politically liberal, and proudly Jewish—an alarming combination to the National Socialists. And, although I can find no mention of it specifically in relation to Goldstein's work, the Nazis were, given what we know about their horrific treatment of the disabled under the Nazi regime, surely uncomfortable with the idea of "damaged" persons, even if they were their own soldiers, and perhaps even more uncomfortable with the thought of reintegrating them into the general population.

In 1933, Goldstein was arrested at his work, imprisoned, and tortured by the Nazis. He would have likely died in Europe but for a remarkable bit of luck. Rothman somehow found an audience with Hermann Goering and argued for Goldstein's release, which was granted on the condition that Goldstein and the rest of his Jewish colleagues leave Germany immediately. Goldstein fled to Amsterdam with Rothman, Gelb, and a handful of others who he had brought with him from Frankfurt or met in Berlin.

Remarkably, amid this chaos, while waiting for their American visas in Amsterdam and with a temporary appointment and support from the Rockefeller Foundation, Goldstein composed his most famous book, *Der Aufbau des Organismus* (later translated into English as *The Organism*). First published in 1934, this work offered a nonmechanistic, holistic theory of human biological life (what he called "organismic biology") based primarily on the study of brain-injured patients he encountered at the *Institute*. Unfortunately, another terrible turn of events occurred. Gelb contracted tuberculosis, and his visa was denied. In 1935, while Goldstein and Rothman boarded a ship for America, Gelb left for the Black Forest and died from his illness within the year. In under ten years, Goldstein had left behind his family, friends, title, and country. By most accounts, he was never quite the same.

This is not to say that Goldstein did not find a meaningful life in America. His daughter joined him two years later. He received his license to practice medicine in the United States and worked at major teaching hospitals in New York (Columbia) and Massachusetts (Tufts). He also had a private practice. He continued to publish his work, attend conferences, and deliver lectures, including the lecture "Human Nature in Light of Psychopathology" given as the *William James Lecture on Philosophy and Psychology* at Harvard in 1938–1939. He worked, he taught, he had an active professional life. But the sciences of the mind were headed down a radically different path in America than they had been in Europe.[9] Neurology was firmly committed to localization, and psychology was dominated by behaviorism. Both movements were aligned with modularity and nativism, and their conception of the organism was highly mechanistic. Although Goldstein was highly respected in the field, his organismic biology must have seemed "unscientific" if not downright bizarre. His ideas, explanations, and practices never quite caught hold in the New World.

Although we have few descriptions of Goldstein as a person, in a handful of short letters, biographies, and essays by the likes of Hans Jonas, Ernst Cassirer (Goldstein's cousin), Marianne Simmel, Karl Lashley, Hans-Lukas Teuber, and Aaron Gurwitsch, Goldstein was portrayed as serene, thoughtful, and attentive—"a philosophical scientist."[10] By the end of his life, Goldstein had written four major books and close to 200 articles, delivered countless lectures, taught neurology, and worked with thousands of patients. Goldstein and Rothman lived together in America until her untimely death in 1960 by suicide. Goldstein suffered a stroke (with aphasia) and, shortly thereafter, died in 1965.

The Prescription

In a single key paragraph in *The Phenomenology of Perception*, Merleau-Ponty offers us a prescription for what we can learn about the normal from the pathological. Well into the presentation of the behaviors exhibited by patient Johann Schneider, Merleau-Ponty wrote:

> How are we to make sense of this series of facts, and how should the function that exists for the normal person, but that is missing for the patient, be understood through them? It cannot be a question of simply transferring to the normal person what is missing in the patient and what he is trying to recover. Illness, like childhood or like the "primitive" state, is a complete form of existence, and the procedures that it employs in order to replace the normal functions that have been destroyed are themselves pathological phenomena. The normal cannot be deduced from the pathological, and deficiencies cannot be deduced from their substitutions, through a mere change of sign. The substitutions must be understood as substitutions, as allusions to a fundamental function that they attempt to replace, but of which they do not give us the direct image. The genuine inductive method is not a "method of differences," it consists in correctly reading phenomena, in grasping their sense, that is in treating them as modalities and variations of the subject's total being.[11]

This single paragraph contains the most detailed instructions offered in *Phenomenology of Perception* for determining the normal from the pathological. Yet, the prescription leaves open many questions. What is a "substitution" or, for that matter, a "fundamental function"? Why is illness a "complete form of existence"? Why should we prefer the "genuine inductive method" over a "method of differences"? Situating the above quotation within Goldstein's *oeuvre* provides the answers missing from Merleau-Ponty's text.[12] In what follows, I will work through this passage line by line, using principles and ideas found in Goldstein's work to give context to the passage and more fully reveal its meaning. This reading will also explain why Merleau-Ponty found Goldstein's method so appealing—namely, because it is well suited for uncovering the background structures of intentionality.

"How are we to make sense of this series of facts, and how should the function that exists for the normal person, but that is missing for the patient, be understood through them?"

In Goldstein's lifetime, clinicians had begun to think about the behaviors associated with brain lesions differently. Observers had long known that brain injury and illness produced changes in observable behavior and self-reported experience. The documentation of these correlations between brain damage and behavioral deficits dates back thousands of years. However, the relation between the pathological and the normal remained inscrutable.

Goldstein was among a small group of clinicians who held that the personal level effects of lesions were not "curiosa" or "oddities" resulting from the disease from which nothing about the normal could be understood.[13] Instead, Goldstein argued, overt reactions to a situation are "symptoms" of illness and injury if they are "abnormal"—that is, if they appear to the clinician or the patient as unexpected or inappropriate in some salient way.[14] Symptoms have an additional characteristic that makes them especially valuable. They are patterned by the particulars of the neurological trauma, with lineages traceable back to the normal functions they replaced. In Goldstein's words, "pathological phenomena can be recognized as an indication of lawful variations of the normal life process."[15]

Thus, the question "can we learn *anything* about the normal from the pathological?" was replaced with the question "*what* can we learn about the normal from the pathological?" The symptoms of pathology, if properly understood, will reveal normal function.[16]

"It cannot be a question of simply transferring to the normal person what is missing in the patient and what he is trying to recover."

If the pathological is indeed a lawful variation of the normal, then it may seem that the symptoms of brain damage and disease can disclose normal mental processes via a direct inference or deduction. But this thinking wrongly assumes that we already know what the "laws" are, and how damage and disease have "varied" them.[17] Goldstein repeatedly warned that we must proceed carefully when building theories out of observations of pathological phenomena—out of symptoms—because we run the risk of mischaracterizing normal existence by accidentally "transferring conceptions of one domain in the other, without regard to the peculiarities of the two."[18]

Admittedly, this risk is an unavoidable feature of neuropsychology itself. We do not know what is normal *imprimis*, so we turn to the pathological *per contra*. We intend to use the pathological to reveal the normal to us. But because we do not know in advance about the character of the normal that we were looking for and believe the pathological to have disturbed, we cannot be certain that our conclusions about the normal are correct. In other words, it is precisely because we do not know what the normal is that we look to the pathological to tell us. Again, Goldstein cautions that it is precisely because we do not know what the normal is that we cannot be sure if what the pathological exhibits is indeed the normal. I call this the "paradox of neuropsychology."

"Illness, like childhood or like the 'primitive' state, is a complete form of existence, and the procedures that it employs in order to replace the normal functions that have been destroyed are themselves pathological phenomena."

Goldstein's holism was multifaceted, encompassing a family of related ideas that includes dynamic equilibrium within the organism and between the organism and its environment, plasticity of the nervous system, an essential drive for good form, and forces that organize whole systems out of parts.[19] Goldstein supported all of these claims, at least in part, with empirical evidence. One of his strongest arguments concerned the idea that organisms are whole forms of existence and are not, therefore, composed out of functionally isolatable or articulable parts. Even the most basic reflex in a seemingly closed sensorimotor circuit, he argued, is part of a unified system, capable of being affected by slight alterations elsewhere in the organism or in the environment.[20]

In Goldstein's work, this analysis applied to the normal *as well as* the pathological. That is, if the normal is a complete form of existence, in which any change (anywhere) alters the entire system, then so, too, is the pathological a complete form of existence in which brain disease and damage have modified the whole system. "Disordered behavior in any field coincides always with more or less disordered behavior of the whole organism."[21] Everything is affected—"modified" or "altered"—to a greater or lesser degree.[22]

"The normal cannot be deduced from the pathological, and deficiencies cannot be deduced from their substitutions, through a mere change of sign."

It is hard to convince people today that there is anything odd *at all* about deducing normal function from brain disease and damage. Even the question of what we can learn about the normal from the pathological has, at least for neuropsychology, seemingly obvious answers; these answers are generated by what I call an "either-or" analysis. Either, having isolated what the patient *cannot* do, we learn about what we *can* do. It is from a striking absence—the patient's debility—that we deduce normal ability. Or, having isolated what the patient can *still* do, we learn about what we can do *too*. It is from the patient's retained capacity in spite of other losses that we posit normal capacity. The basic assumption in neuropsychology (and it is often quite explicit) is that *the pathological directly discloses the normal through either a reversal or an equivalence of sign.*

However, if patients have "morbid modifications" in their being, creating new forms of complete existence, *pace* Goldstein, then there are no easy transfers between the pathological and the normal because the precise nature of these shifts are not given in advance.[23] It is possible that what the patient can no longer do seems, on purely behavioral or even experiential grounds, like what we can do. But Goldstein acknowledged that an "imperfect or incomplete reaction," even an "actual failure," does not always signify a definitive incapacity.[24] The patient may be perfectly capable of a proper reaction but is far more concerned with the potential risk of failure, or of having no reaction at all, and thus displays a deficiency. Goldstein cautioned, too, that even the most surprising symptoms are not necessarily the most important ones. Unusual reactions may be what brought the patient to the hospital or drew the clinician to the bedside, and the clinician may be right in identifying certain behaviors as pathological. But there is no real reason that the first or the most striking symptom must be the dominant, essential, or fundamental one. Certain behaviors might appear highly unusual and declared pathological, yet those behaviors might be compensatory strategies for a totally different loss. In fact, Goldstein warned that fixating on the most striking symptom often carries the potential to obscure a more basic debility.[25]

It is also possible that what the patient can still do seems, again on behavioral or experiential grounds, like what we can do too. But Goldstein observed that even "correct reactions" may still be pathological.[26] At a minimum, the patient could put a preexisting capacity to an entirely new use. At a maximum, the patient could develop a capacity *de novo* that did not exist before the trauma. Either way, the patient "reached this reaction in a way quite different from the normal way."[27] In other words, pathologies can produce capacities and abilities so seemingly normal that they lead us to reading those dysfunctions back into normal life.

The conclusions drawn about what is normal from investigating brain injury and illness may differ dramatically depending on how we interpret observed behaviors and reported experiences. When everything has been shifted, disturbed, or even undone in ways that are not immediately obvious, they cannot be traced *directly* back to their original state. The "either-or" analysis becomes completely inadequate, and Goldstein detailed a viable alternative.

"The substitutions must be understood as substitutions . . ."

Goldstein urged us to pay more attention to how patients have productive and meaningful lives in spite of the significant impairments that brain injury and illness produce. We must pay attention to the "substitutions" and "detours" that patients use to carry out their tasks.[28] Goldstein described two main kinds of substitutions and detours. He referred to patterns of behavior in which patients circumvent situations that expose their pathology.[29] These behaviors are most like *detours* in our ordinary sense of the word. Avoiding situations that expose debility might itself seem awkward or disagreeable. But Goldstein reported that most patients are significantly less disturbed by these detours (and their associated drawbacks) than by failures to meet the demands of the situation, which call further attention to their pathology. This is especially so, Goldstein noted, if the failure would result in a "catastrophic reaction"—when truly disordered performances result in persistent negative effects for the patients—after which they may become depressed, unresponsive, distracted, or unable to perform tasks easily met under other circumstances.[30] It is no wonder patients avoid situations that would produce these consequences. Further, it calls into question the ethics of testing patients by putting them in situations where a catastrophic reaction may be likely. In this context, *anosognosia*, or the refusal to recognize one's own illness or injury, ceases to seem like a diagnosable syndrome and seems more like a genuine coping mechanism—a detour taken to avoid catastrophe.[31]

Yet, sometimes avoidance is not an option. Even in cases of severe brain disease and damage, patients are constantly responding to the demands of their situations, whether these are problems posed by the natural or social environment, experiments set before them in the lab, or tasks given by the therapist in the rehabilitation center. Indeed, sometimes patients must be pushed to uncomfortable limits for recovery to take hold. When pathology blocks what was once the "preferred behavior," we find the second kind of adaptation that interested Goldstein.[32] These behaviors are most like *substitutions* in our ordinary sense of the term. They manifest as compensations, strategies, tricks, cues, or shortcuts that allow patients to achieve, or nearly achieve, the same results as in the normal case but through different means. Substitutions are clever, generally robust but sometimes fragile, highly context dependent, and fallible. The power of substitutions is found throughout the literature in neuropsychology, where experimenters describe needing to design increasingly shrewd tests to outsmart their patients, who keep doing well (unexpectedly) despite their pathology. It is often when scientists successfully block substitutions that the anticipated dysfunctions emerge.

One remarkable feature of detours and substitutions is how careful observers often fail to recognize them. Clinicians who work with patients for years might not recognize a substitution until some odd experimental result. Relatedly, patients might not know they are on detours, even after the details are brought to their attention. For example, Goldstein described a patient with mind-blindness (recognizable as Schneider), unable to identify even the simplest visual forms—for example, straight *versus* curved lines. Within this optic chaos, the patient learned to use the contrast between light and dark *to read* with speed and accuracy. In Goldstein's words:

> He read by tracing stepwise along the light-dark margins, by making the macula, so to speak, glide over them. The experienced movement constituted, to him, a letter in the same sense as, for us, the seen letter. It is no question that he had achieved this kind of reading all by himself, really knowing neither how he developed it nor what he was actually doing.[33]

Making the absolute most of his remaining ability, Schneider engaged his ocular muscles, wiggling his macula back and forth over the borders of the characters, where the contrast between light and dark was most stark. Schneider treated written words like a braille text, but instead of palpating them with his fingertips, he quite literally palpated them with his look. Neither the patient himself nor those who worked closely with him over the years knew when or how he developed this remarkable adaptation. We might have initially thought that detours and substitutions (like Schneider's described here) are designed and effected within central consciousness, the result of a dedicated therapist working in coordination with an eager patient. However, they are just as likely to be developed and executed on the borders and fringes of consciousness, at the prepersonal level, and in the background of a modified pathological milieu, unknown even to the patient.

". . . as allusions to a fundamental function that they attempt to replace . . ."

Goldstein claimed that substitutions and detours are not random or haphazard. They are *systematically disordered*.[34] "Individual premorbid skills are necessary for the formation of substitutes. Therefore, the type of the respective substitute formation is not arbitrary."[35] In other words, substitutions and detours have common purposes, preserved values, or shared structures with the original performances they replaced. In various places, Goldstein referred to this connection between pathological performances and the normal ones they replaced as a "basic law," "basic function," and even "the 'essence' of the organism."[36]

The concept of a basic function may sound odd, but it surfaces frequently in Goldstein's work. The idea is that within every organism there are laws that guide it through life—ways that perception, action, affect, memory, and other activities are structured in coordination with the environment, and thereby directed toward various ends. Holists like Goldstein were drawn to this notion, but each had different ways of articulating what these ends are. The telos of such a function might be good form (Gestalt psychology), being well suited for and properly geared into the world (ecological psychology), the self-preserving functions of ego (Freudian psychoanalysis), or a basic level of organismic organization (equipotentiality). We find different terms for this basic function in the work of Goldstein's contemporaries. Willem van Woerkom wrote of a *representational function*.[37] Henry Head referred to *symbolic expression*.[38]

And in Goldstein's collaborations with Gelb there was *categorical (abstract) behavior*.[39] There is good reason to believe that, in Merleau-Ponty's work, this fundamental function took the form of "*motor intentionality*."[40]

Goldstein was never quite satisfied with his own articulation of this basic law. Unlike the named capacities we already have the concepts to identify, basic functions are harder to articulate. They operate beneath or before consciousness and thus are akin to drives. They are relational and dynamic. They are embodied and embedded, in the phenomenological sense. They are generic and versatile, allowing them to be put to many different (even highly specialized) uses, depending on the real-time and situation-specific needs of the organism. Fundamental functions seem to be structured in such a way so as to perform multiple functions without being composed of many functions. No wonder Goldstein struggled with their positive explication.

In the realm of neuropsychology, where brain disease and damage disturbed these basic functions, Goldstein was able to offer a negative characterization—that of a "Grundstörung" or "basic disturbance."[41] He allowed that basic functions could be realized in localized areas of the brain, but that they are more likely to be distributed across multiple brain regions. This means that lesions in different locations of the brain could disrupt *the same* basic function.[42] Thus, when faced with a collection of symptoms, even an apparent double dissociation between patients, Goldstein understood that the substitutions and detours might be the mutable expressions of the same, more basic, loss—the same pervasive modification of the organism.[43] Therein lies the key to understanding the normal through the pathological, the positing of a quasi-lawful connection between substitute and original, between detour and route.

"The genuine inductive method is not a 'method of differences,' it consists in correctly reading phenomena, in grasping their sense, that is in treating them as modalities and variations of the subject's total being."

Putting these points together, a relation emerges between the pathological and the normal that is not a naïve transferal, direct deduction, reversal, or equivalence of sign. These methods of difference, this either-or analysis, does not work. We can formulate Goldstein's method for how the normal is disclosed through the pathological in the following way. Neurological damage and disease create ripple effects by disrupting basic functions, placing patients in an entirely new domain of life. From within this altered milieu, all symptoms (even the absence of reactions) become substitutions or detours. These symptoms are not random; their disorder has a hidden order. To discover it, we must work our way from pathological phenomena down to some basic function that has become disturbed and back up again to ordinary performance, which reveals the undisrupted essence of the organism. For what we can learn about the normal from the pathological, this is "the value and importance for the possibilities of existence of the modified organism."[44] Merleau-Ponty referred to Goldstein's idea as "the genuine inductive method"—an appellation taken directly from *The Organism*.[45] It stands in stark contrast to the method of differences, as it is applied to lesion studies in neuropsychology, in both Goldstein's time and now.

Phenomenological Reduction-by-Proxy

At the start of this chapter, I claimed that by reading Merleau-Ponty's words through Goldstein's text, we might come to know what it was that so captivated Merleau-Ponty about the genuine inductive method, so much so that he absorbed Goldstein's ideas and presented them as if they were his own. I believe the reason for this is that Goldstein's approach is particularly effective at disclosing *the background* of intentional life, a focus of Merleau-Ponty's early works.

Merleau-Ponty wanted to describe the structures of intentionality that present the world to us without themselves showing up directly or determinately—what is called "the background." He acknowledged that the background (in principle, *qua* background) does not accommodate direct reflection—"it hides behind the objective world that it contributes to constituting."[46] As recent commentator Dan Zahavi paraphrases Merleau-Ponty's predicament, "our intentional rapport with the world . . . is so pervasive and tight, that we normally fail to notice it."[47] Taylor Carman makes a similar observation on Merleau-Ponty's behalf: the background is "so basic and so familiar that we are normally unaware of it, so inconspicuous and so transparent to our ordinary perceptual sense of ourselves as to be invisible."[48] In other words, because the background is so elemental and common, it is transparent to us and thus difficult to characterize.

In the preface of *The Phenomenology of Perception*, Merleau-Ponty declared that the only way to disclose these recessive structures of intentionality is to become estranged from them. In his words, "we must—precisely in order to see the world and to grasp it as a paradox—rupture our familiarity with it."[49] Yet we cannot do this because we are not able to separate ourselves entirely from our own intentionality, a point Merleau-Ponty acknowledged when he wrote, "the most important lesson of the reduction is the impossibility of a complete reduction."[50] It may seem, then, that Merleau-Ponty was back again to the original problem of how to uncover the background. Except for one thing. Even if we ourselves cannot become completely estranged from the background, then *maybe someone else can*. When Merleau-Ponty wrote about a kind of reflection that "loosens the intentional threads that connect us to the world in order to make them appear," he might not have been referring to our own contemplative relation to the background. Instead, or in addition, he may have been alluding to a variety of patients, known from famous case studies in the history of psychopathology and neuropsychology.[51] When their intentional ties to the world go slack, we observe their situation, which in turn discloses intentionality. These case studies have the potential to reveal the background by relating states of illness in which patients' familiarity with the world is ruptured, to our own states of health in which we are woven into the world. It is *phenomenological reduction-by-proxy*.[52]

Most scholars recognize some version of this point, that Merleau-Ponty's empirically informed phenomenology was his way of disclosing intentionality. But, why did Merleau-Ponty believe lesion studies (specifically) were so effective at revealing the background (in particular)?

The *details* of the lesion studies he chose certainly were significant in their own right. The most-discussed patients in Merleau-Ponty's work, Schneider as well as patients with phantom limbs and various forms of apraxia and ataxia, suffered a very specific basic disturbance manifested in and through their bodies—a weakening of motor intentionality. Insofar as Merleau-Ponty held that the living body is the background of intentionality, he was right to pursue disorders of embodiment in order to disclose it. But, the success of Merleau-Ponty's phenomenological reduction-by-proxy did not solely rest on the content of those well-chosen lesion studies.

The *methodology* he followed was equally crucial, because Goldstein's inductive method is particularly well suited for uncovering the background. Recall that substitutions and detours are formed out of the premorbid behaviors they replace, and yet each performance—whether pathological or normal—is a manifestation of the basic function of the organism. Merleau-Ponty treated both the prepersonal performances of the body and the pathological variations on those performances as manifestations of motor intentionality. This permitted a kind of "triangulation."[53] By gathering substitutions and detours from the pathological cases and following the contours of motor intentionality, Merleau-Ponty was able to reconstruct the features of the living body—notably its habits and skills—that constitute the background of intentional life. Thus, we find articulated in Goldstein's work a series of steps to make sense of series of facts—facts about what has changed for patients but is preserved (though hidden) in us—and a prescription for a methodology that Merleau-Ponty followed, to great effect, in his own work.

Notes

1. Daniel Dennett, *Consciousness Explained* (Boston: Bay Books, 1991), 322.

2. *Psychopathology* focuses on the classification, causes, and treatment of mental disorders (e.g., schizophrenia). Their neurophysiological origins or effects may or may not be important to any given clinician. *Neuropsychology* also focuses on personal level disturbances of behavior and experience. But, in contrast to psychopathology, their origins in brain damage or disease are of central importance.

3. Phenomenologists will be familiar with the notion of *intentionality*, or consciousness of something or other, a directedness or orientation of the subject toward something.

4. Merleau-Ponty directed the first French translation of Goldstein's book, *Der Aufbau des Organismus*, for Gallimard in 1952. But I was hard pressed to find other forays into the relationship between these two men. One exception is Theodore Geraets's examination of the similarities in Merleau-Ponty's critique of gestalt psychology in *The Structure of Behavior* and Goldstein's critique of the gestalt psychology in *The Organism*. Theodore Geraets, *Vers Une Nouvelle Philosophie Transcendantale: La Genèse de La Philosophie de Maurice Merleau-Ponty Jusqu' à La Phénoménologie de La Perception* (La Haye: Springer, 1971).

5. This abridged biography relies on the work of historians, biographers, and friends of Goldstein. Hans Jonas, "Kurt Goldstein and Philosophy," *American Journal of Psychoanalysis* 19 (1959): 161–164; Hans Jonas "In Memoriam: Kurt Goldstein, 1878–1965," *Social Research* 32, no. 4 (1965): 351–356; David Shakow, "Kurt Goldstein: 1878–1965," *American Journal of Psychology* 79, no. 1 (1966): 150–154; Hans Teuber, "Kurt Goldstein's Role in the Development of Neuropsychology," *Neuropsychologia* 4, no. 4 (1966): 299–310; Kurt Goldstein, "Kurt Goldstein," *A History of Psychology in Autobiography* 5, ed. Walther Riese (New York: Appleton-Century-Crofts, 1967): 147–166; Marianne Simmel, "Foreword," *The Reach of Mind*, ed. Marianne Simmel (New York: Springer, 1968): v–x; Marianne Simmel, "Kurt Goldstein 1878–1965," *The Reach of Mind*, ed. Marianne

Simmel (New York: Springer, 1968): 3–12; Oliver Sacks, "Foreword," *The Organism* (New York: Zone Books, 1995): 7–14; Anne Harrington, "Kurt Goldstein's Neurology of Healing and Wholeness," *Greater Than the Parts*, ed. Christopher Lawrence and George Weisz (New York: Oxford University Press, 1998) 25–45; Frank Stahnisch and Thomas Hoffman, "Kurt Goldstein and the Neurology of Movement during the Interwar Years," *Was Bewegt Uns?* ed. Christian Hoffstadt, Andreas Schulz-Buchta, and Franz Peschke (Freiburg: Verlag, 2010): 283–312.

6. Goldstein wanted to rehabilitate patients by modifying their bodies and their environments. Today, some theorists and activists might consider this goal controversial. In the early twentieth century, however, it was truly radical, and a major advance over treating brain damaged or diseased patients as futile.

7. Abraham Maslow, "A Theory of Human Motivation," *Psychological Review* 50 (1943): 382.

8. Goldstein, "Kurt Goldstein," 149–150.

9. There is a well-documented sociological and historical story to tell about how European intellectuals (many of them Jewish) were scattered across the Western world during the war years, graciously invited but never fully absorbed into the intellectual cultures that predated their arrival into their newfound homes. Goldstein is clearly part of this narrative.

10. Ernst Cassirer, "Two Letters to Kurt Goldstein," *Science in Context* 12, no. 4 (1999/1925): 661–667; Aaron Gurwitsch, "Gelb-Goldstein's Concept of 'Concrete' and 'Categorial' Attitude and the Phenomenology of Ideation," *Philosophy and Phenomenological Research* 10 (1949): 172–196; Simmel, "Foreword," v–x; Simmel, "Kurt Goldstein 1878–1965," 3–12; Teuber, "Kurt Goldstein's Role in the Development of Neuropsychology," 299–310; Karl Lashley, "Foreword," *The Organism* (Boston: Back Bay Books, 1963): xii–xiii.

11. Maurice Merleau-Ponty, *Phenomenology of Perception*, trans. Donald A. Landes (New York: Routledge, 1945), 110. In Merleau-Ponty's *The Structure of Behavior* we find a similar quotation: "The conduct of the patient is not deduced from the conduct of the normal person by simple subtraction of parts; it represents a *qualitative* alteration; and it is to the extent that certain actions demand an attitude of which the subject is no longer capable that they are electively disordered. There appears here a new kind of analysis which no longer consists in isolating elements but in understanding the character of a whole and its immanent law. Sickness is no longer, according to the common representation, like a thing or a power from which certain effects follow; nor is pathological functioning, according to a too wide-spread idea, homogeneous with normal functioning. It is a new *signification* of behavior, common to the multitude of symptoms; and the relation of the essential disorder to the symptoms is no longer that of cause to effect but rather the logical relation of principle to consequence or of signification to sign" (Maurice Merleau-Ponty, *Structure of Behavior*, trans. Alden Fischer [Boston: Beacon Press, 1963], 64–65).

12. Merleau-Ponty's understanding of the normal–pathological dyad was also likely influenced by Edmund Husserl who had an account of normality as concordance and optimality in the lifeworld. Edmund Husserl, Ms. D 13 XII; Edmund Husserl, Ms. D 13 XIV; Edmund Husserl, *The Crisis of European Sciences and Transcendental Phenomenology: An Introduction to Phenomenological Philosophy*, trans. David Carr (Evanston, IL: Northwestern University Press, 1970). See also Anthony Steinbock, "Phenomenological Concepts of Normality and Abnormality," *Man and World* 28, no. 3 (1995): 241–260; Joona Taipale, "Twofold Normality: Husserl and the Normative Relevance of Primordial Constitution," *Husserl Studies* 28, no. 1 (2012): 49–60; Sara Heinämaa, "Transcendental Intersubjectivity and Normality: Constitution by Mortals," *The Phenomenology of Embodied Subjectivity*, ed. Rasmus Thybo Jensen and Dermot Moran (New York: Springer International Publishing, 2013): 83–103; Maren Wehrle, "'There Is a Crack in Everything.' Fragile Normality: Husserl's Account of Normality Re-Visited," *Phaenomenon* 28 (2019): 49–75.

13. Kurt Goldstein, *The Organism: A Holistic Approach to Biology Derived from Pathological Data in Man* (New York: Zone Books, 1995), 29; Goldstein, "L'Analyse de L'Aphasia et L'Étude de L'Essence du Langage," 430; Kurt Goldstein, "L'Analyse de L'Aphasia et L'Étude de L'Essence du Langage," *Journal de Psychologie* 30 (1933): 430–496.

14. Goldstein, *The Organism*, 35. According to Goldstein, all reactions, whether normal or pathological, are performances, where a performance is "any kind of behavior, activity, or operation as a whole or in part that expresses itself overtly and bears reference to the environment. Hence physiological processes, events within the nervous system, mental activities, attitudes, and affectivities are not performances so long as they do not manifest themselves in some overt action" (Goldstein, *The Organism*, 42).

15. Goldstein, *The Organism*, 30.

16. At this point, it is important to recognize that the concepts *normal*, *typical*, and *average* as well as their supposed counterparts *pathological*, *abnormal*, *atypical*, *divergent*, and *deviant* have been rightly criticized in disability studies. The argument is that diverse modes of life, all potentially good, are *turned into disabilities* by historical and social structures (discursive and institutional) that fail to accommodate those deficits—*not* by the effects of brain trauma. Neuropsychology, in virtue of its focus on damage and deficits, reinforces a norm of bodily integrity (and its phantasmatic superiority), when in fact no one is ever truly whole, independent, or well-integrated. To this end, many disability theorists and activists reject labels like "normal" and "pathological" in favor of other *self-chosen* identities. Why, then, continue to use the normal–pathological dyad? Because this was and is the language of neuropsychology. But more important, within Goldstein's organismic biology, these concepts were freed from their dubious normativity. Goldstein's direct intellectual heirs, like Georg Canguilhem and Michel Foucault,

were directly influenced by his emendations to the normal and the pathological, theorists who in turn influenced the field of disability studies. Georges Canguilhem, *The Normal and the Pathological* (New York: Zone Books, 1989); Michel Foucault, *Discipline and Punish: The Birth of the Prison*, trans. Alan Sheridan (New York: Vintage Books, 1995); Simi Linton, *Claiming Disability: Knowledge and Identity* (New York: New York University Press, 1998); Ian Hacking, *The Taming of Chance* (New York: Cambridge Press, 1990); Lennard Davis, *Enforcing Normalcy: Disability, Deafness, and the Body* (New York: Verso, 1995); Rosemarie Garland-Thomson, *Extraordinary Bodies* (New York: Columbia Press, 1997); Eva Kittay, *Love's Labor: Essays on Women, Equality, and Dependency* (New York: Routledge, 1999); Robert McRuer, *Crip Theory: Cultural Signs of Queerness and Disability* (New York: New York University Press, 2006); Thomas Shakespeare, "Review of Oliver Sacks' *An Anthropologist on Mars*," *Disability & Society* 11 (1996): 137–139.

17. Goldstein, *The Organism*, 30.

18. Goldstein, "L'Analyse de L'Aphasia et L'Étude de L'Essence du Langage," 431.

19. Merleau-Ponty's analyses of lesion studies in both *Structure of Behavior* and *Phenomenology of Perception* relied on the detailed notes of clinicians, most of whom were holists of a sort: in Germany, Goldstein (clearly) and Adhemar Gelb, Kurt Koffka, Paul Schilder, Max Wertheimer, Wolgang Köhler, Edward Tolman, Christian von Ehrenfels, Viktor von Weizsächer; in Holland, F.J. Buytendijk, Helmuth Plessner; in France, Pierre Marie, Henri Piéron, Paul Guillaume, Jacques Chevalier, Jean Lhermitte, Willem von Woerkhom; in England, Hughlings Jackson, Henry Head and Karl Lashley.

20. For example, Goldstein argued that even the most paradigmatic of reflexes—the patellar tendon—resists a purely isolatable mechanical characterization. He wrote, "the patellar reflex has proved to be by no means invariably constant in the same individual. It varies, depending, among other things, on the position of the limb, on the behavior of the rest of the organism, and on whether or not attention is paid to it . . . a certain kind of attention diminishes the response, another kind exaggerates it . . . intensified by lesions of the pyramidal tract . . . this shows that, even under normal conditions, the reflex cannot be properly understood in terms of the isolated mechanism alone" (Goldstein, *The Organism*, 70–71). See also Goldstein, *The Organism*, 80.

21. Goldstein, *The Organism*, 329. See also Goldstein, *The Organism*, 322.

22. Goldstein, *The Organism*, 30, 51, 85. Goldstein preferred terms like "modified" and "altered" to refer to the ways the total organism is affected by pathology, which Merleau-Ponty also used, in a similar vein (Merleau-Ponty, *Phenomenology of Perception*, 119, 158, 357; Merleau-Ponty, *Structure of Behavior*, 65, 96, 123).

23. Goldstein, "L'Analyse de L'Aphasia et L'Étude de L'Essence du Langage," 435.

24. Goldstein, "L'Analyse de L'Aphasia et L'Étude de L'Essence du Langage," 433. See also Goldstein, *The Organism*, 162.

25. Goldstein, *The Organism*, 35. The full quotation from Goldstein reads: "Phenomena, more striking than others, are registered first and thus give the impression of being the dominant symptom. Most likely to attract attention, of course, are the atypical reactions to a normal situation and, in particular, the complete absence of any reaction when one is expected . . . in this way complete loss of a special function tends to be the outstanding symptom and conceals the real or basic defect" (Goldstein, *The Organism*, 35).

26. Goldstein, ""L'Analyse de L'Aphasia et L'Étude de L'Essence du Langage," 433. See also Goldstein, *The Organism*, 35.

27. Goldstein, "L'Analyse de L'Aphasia et L'Étude de L'Essence du Langage," 433.

28. Goldstein, *The Organism*, 52, 195–197; Goldstein, "L'Analyse de L'Aphasia et L'Étude de L'Essence du Langage," 433–434, 438; When describing patients, Merleau-Ponty also used Goldstein's terminology of "substitution" (Merleau-Ponty, *Phenomenology of Perception*, 80, 110, 129; Merleau-Ponty, *Structure of Behavior*, 67, 70, 110) and "detour" (Merleau-Ponty, *Phenomenology of Perception*, 129; Merleau-Ponty, *Structure of Behavior*, 37, 40, 70).

29. Goldstein, *The Organism*, 51–52, 55; Goldstein, "L'Analyse de L'Aphasia et L'Étude de L'Essence du Langage," 432, 438.

30. Goldstein, *The Organism*, 48–49; Goldstein, "L'Analyse de L'Aphasia et L'Étude de L'Essence du Langage," 438.

31. Merleau-Ponty discussed "anosognosia" in relation to phantom limbs (Merleau-Ponty, *Phenomenology of Perception*, 82–83, 149–150).

32. Goldstein, *The Organism*, 48–50, 265–282. Preferred behaviors adhere to principles of good Gestalten—ordered, promptness, smoothness, self-assurance, minimal expenditure of energy (economy), adequacy, success. They are accompanied by "feeling of smooth functioning, unconstraint, well-being, adjustment to the world, and satisfaction" (Goldstein, *The Organism*, 48–49).

33. Goldstein, *The Organism*, 196.

34. Merleau-Ponty used the term "electively disordered" (Merleau-Ponty, *Structure of Behavior*, 64).

35. Goldstein, *The Organism*, 195. See also Goldstein, *The Organism*, 105.

36. Goldstein, *The Organism*, 27, 104, 105.

37. Willem van Woerkom, "Sur La Notion de L'Espace (Le Sense Géométrique), Sur La Notion Du Temps et Du Nombre," *Revue Neurologique* 35 (1919): 113–119.

38. Henry Head, "Disorders of Symbolic Thinking and Expression," *British Journal of Psychology* 11, no. 2 (1921): 179–193.

39. Adhémar Gelb and Kurt Goldstein, *Psychologische Analysen Hirnpathologischer Fälle* (Leipzig: Barth, 1920). See also Aaron Gurwitsch, "Gelb-Goldstein's

Concept of 'Concrete' and 'Categorical' Attitude and the Phenomenology of Ideation," 172–196; Kurt Goldstein, "Notes on the Development of My Concepts," *Selected Papers/Ausgewählte Schriften*, ed. by Aaron Gurwitsch, Else Goldstein, and William Haudek (The Hague: Martinus Nijhoff, 1971): 1–12.

40. "Motor intentionality" is Merleau-Ponty's term for a *bodily* consciousness of something or other, a *mobile* directedness or orientation of the subject towards something (Merleau-Ponty, *Phenomenology of Perception*, 113, 137, 139). See also Gabrielle Jackson, "Maurice Merleau-Ponty's Concept of Motor Intentionality: Unifying Two Kinds of Bodily Agency," *European Journal of Philosophy* 26, no. 2 (2018): 773–774.

41. Goldstein, *The Organism*, 44, 105.

42. For this reason, Goldstein argued that "a localized defect and a defect in performance" does not imply "a relationship between the concerned area and a definite performance." Kurt Goldstein, "Remarks on Localisation," *Stereotactic and Functional Neurosurgery* 7, no. 1–2 (1946): 25. A specialized performance might depend on a basic function that is itself distributed across the brain.

43. In neuropsychology, a double dissociation of symptoms refers to the situation in which there is damage at one cerebral location leading to impaired performance on a sufficiently specific task (but no others) in one patient, *and* damage at another cerebral location leading to impaired performance on a different sufficiently specific task (but no others) in another patient. This imposition of pure case over pure case implies that *in healthy individuals* these task-specific performances are the output of independent mental processes realized in their respective undamaged cerebral locations. Double dissociation is considered the single most powerful tool in neuropsychology.

44. Goldstein, "L'Analyse de L'Aphasia et L'Étude de L'Essence du Langage," 433.

45. Goldstein, *The Organism*, 306.

46. Merleau-Ponty, *Phenomenology of Perception*, 140n99.

47. Dan Zahavi, "Merleau-Ponty on Husserl," *Merleau-Ponty's Reading of Husserl*, ed. Ted Toadvine and Lester Embree (Boston: Springer, 2002), 7.

48. Taylor Carman, *Merleau-Ponty* (New York: Routledge, 2008), 101.

49. Merleau-Ponty, *Phenomenology of Perception*, lxxvii.

50. Merleau-Ponty, *Phenomenology of Perception*, lxxvii.

51. Merleau-Ponty, *Phenomenology of Perception*, lxxvii.

52. Phenomenology is a first-person science. Adding the "by-proxy" to the phenomenological reduction does not abandon this perspective, and may even broaden what counts as a phenomenon for investigation. My assertion is that Merleau-Ponty was conducting phenomenological reduction-by-proxy with lesion studies in neuropsychology. I am uncertain whether he was doing the same when discussing case studies in psychopathology.

53. Jackson, "Maurice Merleau-Ponty's Concept of Motor Intentionality," 763–779.

Chapter 3

Merleau-Ponty and Ab/Normal Phenomenology

The Husserlian Roots of Merleau-Ponty's Account of Expression

NEAL DEROO

Introduction

The importance and centrality of expression to Maurice Merleau-Ponty's thought cannot be doubted. Donald Landes,[1] for example, has argued convincingly that, for Merleau-Ponty, expression is either essential to, or can be equated with, human experience[2], phenomenological practice,[3] behavior,[4] life,[5] embodiment,[6] perception,[7] action,[8] and the chiasm.[9] Since all of these are vital to Merleau-Ponty's analyses at various stages of his work, we see here, briefly, that this notion of expression is central to Merleau-Ponty's work as a whole, and not merely to his early (some would say more obviously phenomenological) work.

But the same list that demonstrates the ubiquity of expression in Merleau-Ponty raises two simultaneous questions: (1) why Merleau-Ponty wants to refer to this wide variety of phenomena as "expression;" and (2) the extent to which his later work remains within the realm of "normal" phenomenology. For even if we grant that things like human experience, behavior, embodiment, perception, and the chiasm might all, in fact, be elements of one and the same phenomenon, we are left to wonder why Merleau-Ponty should want to call this ür-phenomenon expression and whether phenomenology is the best method to describe or explain that ür-phenomenon. What, precisely, is expression for Merleau-Ponty that he characterizes this broad variety of things by that name? And how, precisely, do Merleau-Ponty's reflections on expression fit (or not) the label "phenomenology?"

The question of the precise nature of the definition of expression in Merleau-Ponty is a longstanding problem, and one that might simply have no answer.[10] But I think something important is lost—in our understanding of Merleau-Ponty, our understanding of the "phenomenon" that he was trying to describe, and in our understanding of phenomenology—if we fail to clarify why "expression" is the word he uses to name the difficult knot he is trying to untangle. In what follows, I hope to show that Renaud Barbaras's claim that "an interpretation can claim to be faithful [to Merleau-Ponty] only if it clarifies [. . .] the area of the Husserlian edifice where Merleau-Ponty's reflection is inscribed"[11] is especially true when it comes to expression. That is, I hope to show that rooting Merleau-Ponty's reflections on expression in Edmund Husserl's account of expression not only helps us better understand expression but also helps us see how even the late Merleau-Ponty remains, in a way, faithful to phenomenology.

To do this, I will begin by briefly explaining Husserl's account of expression as the phenomenal unity between sense and being (section I). Then, I will show how Merleau-Ponty's account of expression[12] evidences precisely such a phenomenal unity between sense and being—but only if we reconceive of a broader understanding of sense, being, and the "phenomenal" nature of the unity between them (section II). I will end by briefly showing how this account of expression, because of the way it follows from Husserl's account without merely repeating that account, constitutes a genuine advance *within* phenomenology, and therefore ought to be considered "normal" phenomenology, even as it opens new questions concerning what, precisely, "normal" phenomenology is (section III).[13]

Husserl's Account of Expression

I must begin, then, with an explanation of Husserl's account of expression, so that we can properly understand its effect on Merleau-Ponty.

If we seek to distill the bare bones of Husserl's account of expression,[14] it is that expression names the "phenomenal unity" between an experience (usually of an ontological object of some kind) and what is "manifest" in that experience (usually something epistemological, such as sense or meaning).[15] For Husserl (at least in the *Logical Investigations*), expression is primarily a function that alters how the thing is presented to the intuition of the perceiver.[16] At this stage, then, expression is marked primarily by a change in intention: the physical appearance is no longer taken merely in its perceptual intuitive sense but rather is taken to mean something. And it is crucial to expression that this intentional shift occurs immediately in the intuitive presentation of the object and decidedly not as a distinct intuition requiring a distinct act of "fulfilling or illustrative intuition."[17] That is, there is not a perceptual-intention that leads us to a distinct meaning-intention (as is the case in indication); in expression, the two are given as one, in a phenomenal unity.

This "phenomenal unity" has two essential characteristics that help us better understand the nature of expression. First, the elements of the unity are asymmetrical: the (perceptual) experience of the expression is "lived through," but it is the sense that is manifest in the expression that is "lived in."[18] For example, when I say "cat," the phoneme and the meaning are not equally important in the attention[19] given to the experience; rather, one more or less ignores the perceptual elements of the phoneme and focuses almost entirely on the meaning of the word.

Second, this asymmetry is not experienced as asymmetrical—as A motivating one to live in or enact B—but rather as a unity: I do not experience the experience (e.g., the hearing of the phoneme) and the meaning or sense manifest in that experience as two parts, but rather precisely as one. That I can later, through reflection,[20] distinguish the parts is essential to the nature of this unity as a phenomenal (rather than ontological) unity—but so, too, is the fact that in my primary experience, I experience the two elements as one.[21] Taken together, these essential characteristics describe the phenomenal unity that is the essential characteristic of expression: in it, I encounter two parts (an experience and a sense or meaning manifest in that experience), but I encounter them in and as a single experience.

In expression, then, an *epistemological* object—sense—necessarily attaches to an *ontological* object without erasing entirely the difference between them. Instead, via expression, an ontological object comes to exist for which sense "belong[s] to [its] being itself."[22]

Merleau-Ponty's Account of Expression

These essential elements of Husserl's account of expression—sense forming a phenomenal unity with an ontological object—are not only present in Merleau-Ponty's account of expression but in many ways form the impetus behind the move toward Merleau-Ponty's mature work.

Merleau-Ponty's early work (e.g., in the *Phenomenology of Perception*) remains characterized by a certain dualism or duality. Though it strives to overcome this duality, Merleau-Ponty himself recognizes that "The problems posed in *Phenomenology of Perception* are insoluble because I start there from the 'consciousness-object' distinction."[23] This distinction echoes an inherent duality that maps on to a series of philosophical distinctions at work in Merleau-Ponty's early work: interiority-exteriority, intellectualism-realism, essence-fact, meanings-beings, universality-finitude, and so on. The task of Merleau-Ponty's phenomenology, as he conceives it, is to think a way beyond the "bad ambiguity" that is merely a "mixture" of the two elements of this duality,[24] and instead find a way of explicating the more primordial "soil"[25] out of which these two possibilities emerge as possibilities: "to elaborate a concept of being such that its contradictions, *neither accepted nor 'overcome,'* still have their place."[26]

Doing this, in turn, requires "thinking *together* the dimensions of fact and essence, without either sacrificing essence to an ineffable depth or absorbing existence back into the knowledge provided by the understanding."[27] To do this, Merleau-Ponty must cease to think of these two elements in oppositional terms, and instead come to see the necessity of a movement between them: "to grasp the passage to essence as proceeding from existence itself, and the passage to existence as proceeding from essence itself."[28] Both Husserlian phenomenology and Sartean dialectics, in Merleau-Ponty's mind, fail to achieve this goal: Husserlian phenomenology remains too much a philosophy of essence and therefore cannot adequately deal with the question of "facts," of existence; Jean-Paul Sartre, on the other hand, overemphasizes the "unity" between the two (as a dialectical identity of opposites), and therefore cannot adequately deal with the distinction between them.

What we need, if we are to overcome the problems faced by both Husserl's and Sartre's approaches,[29] is a way of conceiving fact and essence (as emblematic here of the broader duality) as each a passage into the other that does not reduce them to a pure unity. Here we see the centrality of Husserl's account of expression to Merleau-Ponty's later "ontology" emerge, for the "phenomenal unity" of sense and being provides such a connection or unity between the elements of the duality while still maintaining a difference between them. By making the unity precisely a phenomenal unity, the unity is not—contra Sartre—ultimately one of identity, such that the difference between them is erased as merely apparent. And by making this difference distinctly phenomenal (i.e., experienced) rather than either essential or ontological, Merleau-Ponty's philosophy is able to move forward without building itself on one side of the duality or the other, thus implicitly covering over precisely the phenomenon that gives rise to the distinction between them, as Merleau-Ponty acknowledges he had inadvertently done in the *Phenomenology of Perception*.[30] As such, the phenomenal unity of expression allows Merleau-Ponty to do all that he claims one could ask a philosopher to do: to "admit" and "reflect upon" the "ontological diplopia," "rather than merely suffering from it."[31]

However, if Merleau-Ponty draws from Husserl's account of expression, this does not mean that he simply repeats the essentialist phenomenology he critiques Husserl for employing. Rather, Merleau-Ponty takes up the Husserlian concept of expression only by altering the understanding of the phenomenal nature of the unity of expression. Recall that, in this unity, two elements must have an asymmetrical relation (A motivates one to "live in" B) that is not experienced as asymmetrical, but as a unity. For Husserl, this unity was (primarily)[32] accomplished by the constituting acts of consciousness. It is the ego that performs acts of expression, which is why he is able to consider the phenomenal unity of expression to be an alteration of intentionality: in expression, consciousness ceases to take the object merely in its perceptual intuitive sense, and instead approaches it with a meaning-intention. On Husserl's early account of expression, then, the phenomenal unity is the unity of an appearing phenomenon, a unity accomplished by the constituting power of consciousness that is able to "move through" the mundane "facts" of the empirical world so as to live in the "essential" truths found in sense and meaning.

Such an account is insufficient for Merleau-Ponty, as it would reintroduce all the problems that plague any work (including his own early work in the *Phenomenology of Perception*) that remains too tied to the "philosophy of consciousness."[33] Instead, he conceives of the phenomenal unity of expression as pertaining to phenomenality itself and not merely to distinct phenomena appearing to and before a consciousness: for Merleau-Ponty, whatever appears does so always already as a unity of fact and essence, of being and sense. As such, appearance to consciousness is always already expression, insofar as the phenomenal unity of sense and being characterizes the very mode of consciousness itself, of experience itself.[34] consciousness does not simply add sense to being through its own constituting power, but rather sense and being are always already intertwined, even "before" the constituting acts of consciousness. This intertwining is phenomenal (indeed, is the very possibility of phenomenality itself) rather than simply ontological (on the side of "fact" or existence) or epistemological (on the side of "essence" or sense) and hence opens up the possibility of conscious, phenomenal experience: we are conscious because of the phenomenal condition of the world, rather than (as the early Husserl would have claimed) the world having phenomenological reality because of consciousness.

In understanding this claim and its relation to expression, much rides on the understanding of this intertwining as a phenomenal unity. In describing it that way, I mean that it meets the essential characteristics of such a unity outlined above: it is both asymmetrical and experienced as a unity. The second essential characteristic is, I think, uncontroversially satisfied: it is common for us to experience the world as a "unity" of sense and being. But does this unity remain "asymmetrical?" Here we run into a problem, for if the phenomenal unity remains asymmetrical, we seem to slide back into one side of the duality or the other, and hence miss precisely that which Merleau-Ponty labors so hard to articulate: we slide back toward essentialism if we privilege the "living in" the realm of sense and meaning, and back toward naïve realism if we privilege the "living in" the realm of facts. But if the unity is not asymmetrical, it is not clear that it remains the phenomenal unity that Husserl's account of expression is concerned with and which is so important to a phenomenological understanding of the world.

Merleau-Ponty's innovation here is to maintain the asymmetrical nature without privileging one side or the other by suggesting that the asymmetry flows in both directions: A motivates one to "live in" B, and B motivates one to "live in" A. That is, he finds a way through the dilemma of asymmetry via the notion of reversibility. Insofar as the unity of sense and being is taken to be constitutive of experience itself on the primordial level of experience, sense and being cannot emerge or exist primarily as distinct experiences (i.e., as an experience of sense or an experience of being). Therefore, it is not necessary that the asymmetry occur only in one direction (i.e., from a distinct act, A, to a distinct act, B). Rather, this notion of experience itself, as Merleau-Ponty conceives of it, introduces a certain "slippage" or passage between sense and being: sense inevitably takes us toward Being,[35] and Being inevitably takes us toward sense.[36] Therefore, being and sense—experienced as a unity in our experiencing—motivate us to move from one to the other, but without privileging one over the other in a way that would lose the true nature of this complex relationship.

We can make sense of this claim only if we come to understand the new conceptions of sense and being that Merleau-Ponty provides. In conceiving of experience itself as a phenomenal unity, he complicates the relationship between sense and being. Sense comes to be understood as the movement out of which subjects (and the "world") are constituted.[37] This movement is sometimes simply called "Nature," understood as the "auto-production" of sense[38] rather than as a collection of objects. On this understanding, sense is understood primordially as a background or field[39] that provides the foundation for distinct acts of sense: sense is a sort of "pre-culture"[40] that provides the foundation for later cultural acts, and the mode of being of such a primordial sense, therefore, is *Stiftung*.[41]

If sense is a field that exists, that "is," in the mode of *Stiftung*, this is in part because the "is," that is, Being, comes to be understood as interrogation[42]: "The existing world exists in the interrogative mode."[43] Being is understood here in its verbal sense: to be is to interrogate, that is, to operate as a type of questioning, to open something that demands an answer even as it precludes giving a final and definitive answer that would close the question down entirely, and therefore enable us to stop interrogating. Such a project of interrogating is simply called "living,"[44] and it is the fundamental mode of Being of all living creatures.[45]

But what is interrogated in such an interrogation, in which existence is equated with an interrogative living? Nothing else than sense itself, the precultural "field" in which one finds oneself living. In other words, every subject always exists in the tradition or institution(s) in which it lives precisely as an interrogation of that tradition and institution:[46] the subject always takes up the tradition/institution's projects as its own, or alters them, or questions why it should take up these projects and not others. Regardless, the subject always takes up its living within the bounds of some *Stiftung*, and its whole life is then lived in and as an interrogation of "those events which sediment in me a sense, not just as survivals or residues, but as the invitation to a sequel, the requirement of a future."[47] In doing so, the subject's Being is always driving it to "live in" the sense of its *Stiftung*, even as that sense exists precisely to provide the subject an orientation that enables it to "live in" being. This "reversibility" of sense and being is therefore essential to Merleau-Ponty's late "ontology"—even as it circumscribes that "ontology" as phenomenal unity, that is, as phenomenality.

Merleau-Ponty as Ab/Normal Phenomenologist

The later "ontology" of flesh and its connected concepts of Nature and institution [*Stiftung*], then, all arise out of Merleau-Ponty's reconception of Husserl's account of expression. "Flesh" is the name for "the body of interrogation, the body *as* interrogation"[48] and "Nature" is the name for the "auto-production"[49] of sense understood as "an introduction to the definition of Being."[50] In the "flesh," Merleau-Ponty shows the (phenomenal) unity of sense and being such that the two are experienced as one (in and as experience), though later reflection enables us to distinguish between them, at least theoretically (though just barely, and only under the auspices of the phenomenological reduction which uniquely enables the particular type of reflection needed to make this particular theoretical distinction in this case). This unity is found in experience itself—the "phenomenal unity" of expression is here conceived primordially as the very unity of phenomenality that opens the possibility of (phenomenal or conscious) experience itself. And such experience must, of necessity, contain a "slippage" between sense and being, where sense finds its mode of being in *Stiftung*, and Being is nothing else than the interrogation of that *Stiftung* in and as flesh. As such, there is an asymmetrical unity of sense and being in which sense pushes us to "live in" Being, and Being "pushes us" to live in sense—though we remain able to later distinguish between beings (which give rise to facts, exteriority, and that set of philosophical tropes) and meanings (which give rise to essences, interiority, and that set of philosophical tropes).

The "ontological diplopia" or duality at work in Merleau-Ponty's early works is here reflected on and articulated, without merely giving in to one side or the other. Expression is the primary means of this articulation, and therefore we see that Merleau-Ponty's mature ontology of the flesh is premised on the development of his account of expression: "All the axes of Merleau-Ponty's ontology appear to be really the fulfillment of a consistent philosophy of expression, which is itself directed by the will to surmount the equivocations of the first works,"[51] where that equivocation is overcome through the phenomenal unity of sense and being characteristic of Husserl's account of expression, which Merleau-Ponty takes up and radicalizes.

Showing this continuity with Husserl's account of expression helps explicate more clearly Merleau-Ponty's otherwise quite enigmatic use of the term expression. On the one hand, it explains why expression in his particular usage of that term is so hard to define: insofar as it names the very relation between being and sense that is assumed in Merleau-Ponty's definitions of being and of sense,[52] providing a positive definition of expression (beyond a merely formal definition) is nearly impossible. And indeed, even providing a distinct phenomenology of expression may prove impossible for Merleau-Ponty, and for the same reason: insofar as expression names first of all the unity of experience itself, and therefore is essential to phenomenality, it does not clearly emerge (at least in its most primordial form)[53] as a distinct phenomenon or experience of which one could then perform a phenomenology.

But this difficulty in providing a positive definition is not the end of the story for Merleau-Ponty's account of expression. The recourse to Husserl helps us see more clearly a formal definition of expression at work in Merleau-Ponty: expression as the phenomenal unity between sense and being. And this formal definition helps us not only understand the motivation behind Merleau-Ponty's later, so-called ontological works, but it also helps us see why Merleau-Ponty is compelled to use the term expression to characterize the phenomenon (or ür-phenomenon) under consideration. It is not poetic license or some metaphorical gesture toward the arts that causes Merleau-Ponty to adopt the language of expression and to give it such pride of place in his later work. Rather, Merleau-Ponty is driven to expression in and by his fidelity to Husserlian phenomenology.

Of course, this fidelity to phenomenology is not a simple repetition of what Husserl had done. Instead, it is an interrogation of the *Stiftung* of Husserlian phenomenology, a reworking of it that both begins from Husserlian phenomenology but then moves it in a direction that Husserl himself (probably)[54] did not take it. In light of this, Merleau-Ponty, even in his later works, can still be considered a "normal" phenomenologist.

But affirming or proving that claim depends, of course, on what one considers normal phenomenology. If being a normal phenomenologist merely means remaining consistent with Husserl, then, as I have tried to show, because of the centrality it accords to expression, Merleau-Ponty's later work betrays a fundamental continuity with Husserl's insights into expression,[55] and therefore ought to be considered within the realm of normal phenomenology. If, however, normal phenomenology requires a certain method, one rooted in first-person reflection, the phenomenological reduction, and, ultimately, the constituting power of consciousness, then it is not clear whether Merleau-Ponty is a normal phenomenologist. To be sure, even his later reflections trade on first-person reflection, maintain a distinction that can only be properly accessed via the reduction, and maintain some element of the constituting power of consciousness, and as such, Merleau-Ponty seems to retain even some of the phenomenological method.

But this method is not unchanged by its use in and by Merleau-Ponty. What Merleau-Ponty makes clear—in large part through his use of the language of expression as he develops it—is that expression is a more primordial phenomenon than the constituting power of consciousness: "We must recognize prior to 'acts of meaning' of theoretical and thetic thought, 'expressive experiences;' as prior to the signified sense, the expressive sense; and finally as prior to any subsumption of content under the form, the symbolic 'pregnancy' of the form in the content."[56] On this score, he comes to realize that it is not enough merely to root consciousness in a body; rather, one must see that consciousness, via the body, is rooted always already in experience (*Erlebnis*), and as such, to be genuinely rigorous, phenomenology must clearly articulate or explain experience itself. And doing that will require a language and an articulation that goes beyond concrete experiences, toward the more primordial "soil" out of which those experiences grow. Merleau-Ponty discusses this primordial "soil" under the language of sense (especially in its mode of being as *Stiftung*) and "wild being" (understood as necessary interrogation). But it is not clear that "sense" or "being," in these particular senses, ever appear directly *to* consciousness, insofar as they are constitutive elements *of* consciousness. As such, reflection upon them seems to be "abnormal" phenomenology, at best: a "phenomenology of the inapparent" or a "phenomenology of the invisible," of that which is not, and perhaps cannot be, present to consciousness in a distinct experience.[57] And can there be phenomenology, as we normally speak of it, if there is not a clear *something* appearing to *someone*?[58]

At stake in the question of whether Merleau-Ponty should be considered a normal or abnormal phenomenologist, then, is much more than just our (historical) understanding of Merleau-Ponty. At stake is the question of our understanding of phenomenology itself: is it primarily a project[59] or primarily a method? Is it necessarily idealist, or can it include also a certain (transcendental) realism or empiricism?[60] Can it provide an account of phenomenality itself, or can it only ever reflect on—and therefore articulate—distinct phenomena?

These questions open us onto relevant questions in contemporary phenomenological research. The question of what, precisely, phenomenology is remains a fruitful—and open—question. Reading Merleau-Ponty's later ontological works through the lens of his understanding of expression, and rooting that understanding in Husserl's concept of expression, helps us make a case for a broader conception of phenomenology, one that sees it as a project—perhaps even as a *Stiftung*—that must be continually interrogated so as to better be or become what it has always promised to be.[61] On this account, one can only ever rigorously describe a phenomenon if one can clearly articulate its phenomenal nature.[62] And one can only articulate its phenomenal nature clearly through careful explication of phenomenality itself, an explication that requires a clear description of experience itself.

It is here that Merleau-Ponty's later work situates expression: the phenomenal unity of sense and being is nothing less than experience itself. As such, Merleau-Ponty shows us, as Husserl had done, that understanding phenomenology rigorously requires a careful explanation of expression. And Merleau-Ponty helps us see more clearly that such an explanation must examine expression, not merely as a phenomenon, but as phenomenality itself. Expression is therefore key to untying the knot at the core of our experience, of clarifying how, precisely, it is that we make sense of our world. Hence, expression can be understood as central, not just to Merleau-Ponty's thought (as we discussed at the beginning of the chapter), but to phenomenology as a whole.

But proving that thesis must wait for another time. My hope in this chapter is simply to have shown that (a) only by recourse to Husserl's understanding of expression can we properly understand why Merleau-Ponty is compelled to describe experience using the language of expression; (b) doing so helps us see that Merleau-Ponty, even in his later work, remains essentially a phenomenologist; and (c) this suggests that expression is central to understanding the promise of phenomenology in a broadened sense. Proving the truth of that latter claim will have to wait for another time.

Notes

1. Donald Landes, *Merleau-Ponty and the Paradoxes of Expression* (London & New York: Continuum, 2013).
2. Landes, *Paradoxes of Expression*, 16.
3. Landes, *Paradoxes of Expression*, 17.
4. Landes, *Paradoxes of Expression*, 60.
5. Landes, *Paradoxes of Expression*, 60.
6. Landes, *Paradoxes of Expression*, 80.
7. Landes, *Paradoxes of Expression*, 81.
8. Landes, *Paradoxes of Expression*, 149.
9. Landes, *Paradoxes of Expression*, 170.
10. Cf. Landes, *Paradoxes of Expression*, 16–22.
11. Renaud Barbaras, *The Being of the Phenomenon: Merleau-Ponty's Ontology*, trans. Ted Toadvine and Leonard Lawlor (Bloomington: Indiana University Press, 2004), 68.
12. Landes does a superb job of tracing the continuity of the theme of expression throughout Merleau-Ponty's oeuvre, so there is no need for me to do it again here. And because a secondary aim of this chapter is to demonstrate that even the later work remains importantly phenomenological, I will focus in this work especially (though not exclusively) on the later use of expression.
13. This latter point is significant in discussion with scholars who consider Merleau-Ponty's late interest in ontology to be a move away from phenomenology; cf., for example, Michael R. Kelly, "The Subject as Time: Merleau-Ponty's Transition from Phenomenology to Ontology," David Morris and Kym Maclaren (eds.), *Time, Memory, Institution: Merleau-Ponty's New Ontology of the Self* (Athens: Ohio University Press, 2015).
14. I offer a more detailed account of Husserl's theory of expression in Neal DeRoo, "Spiritual Expression and the Promise of Phenomenology," *The Subject(s) of Phenomenology: Re-Reading Husserl*, ed. Iulian Apostelescu (Springer, 2020).
15. Edumund Husserl, *Logical Investigations*, trans. J.N. Findlay (London & New York: Routledge, 2001): Investigation I, 188.
16. In Husserl's words: "what constitutes the object's appearing remains unchanged, [but] the intentional character of the experience alters." This alteration of experience "finds support" in how the thing gives itself, but the essential nature of the experience of expression is found in "the intention directed upon the word itself" (Husserl, *Logical Investigations*, I, 193–194).
17. Husserl, *Logical Investigations*, I, 193.
18. See also Edmund Husserl, *Ideen zu einer reinen Phänomenologie und Phänomenologischen Philosophie. Zweites Buch: Phänomenologische Untersuchungen zur Konstitution*, Husserliana Band IV (The Hague: Martinus Nijhoff, 1952), 236.

19. I mean "attention" here, not in the sense of conscious attention, but rather in the sense described by Husserl in *Experience and Judgment* and in the passive synthesis lectures: as a "tending of the ego" (Husserl, *Erfahrung und Urteil*, 85), a being-affected by the pull or allure [*Reiz*] that something exercises on the ego (Husserl, *Transcendental logic*, 148); cf. Edmund Husserl, *Erfahrung und Urteil. Untersuchungen zur Genealogie der Logik* ed. L. Landgrebe (Hamburg: Meiner, 1948) and Edmund Husserl, *Analyses Concerning Active and Passive Synthesis: Lectures on Transcendental Logic*, trans. A.J. Steinbock (Dordrecht & Boston & London: Kluwer Academic, 2001).

20. Though I will not have time to go into this in much more detail here, the phenomenological reduction can be understood as a type of this reflection, one that opens up for us a particular kind of distinction. Hence, Jean-Luc Marion's claim of various "types" of reduction: eidetic, ontological, dosological, etc.; cf. Jean-Luc Marion, *Reduction and Givenness: Investigations of Husserl, Heidegger and Phenomenology* trans. T.A. Carlson (Evanston, IL: Northwestern University Press, 1998). To anticipate what is yet to come: understanding the reduction as a particular type of reflection that enables us to perceive the difference between sense and being in the very appearing of phenomena in our experience would be central to making the claim that Merleau-Ponty's later work remains importantly phenomenological in a way that maintains a somewhat "normal" use of phenomenology.

21. This marks it as different from indications, which are characterized by a unity of judgment: in an indication, I have an experience (Husserl's example is the perception of the canals on Mars; cf. Husserl, *Logical Investigations*, I, 184); I then use a judgment to draw a conclusion about something else based on that experience (i.e., the likely existence of intelligent beings on that planet). Here, the experience and what is manifest in the experience are experienced as two distinct things: a perception of canals and the judgment that this implies the existence of life there.

22. Edmund Husserl, *Experience and Judgment: Investigations in a Genealogy of Logic*, ed. L. Landgrebe, trans. J.S. Churchill and K. Ameriks (Evanston, IL: Northwestern University Press, 1973): 268. Husserl develops this idea in a very "Merleau-Pontian" way in his later phenomenology of the lifeworld: while he always maintains that an expression occurs whenever this "phenomenal unity" occurs, in his later work he is more aware of the fact that the product of expression is not merely an intentional shift but that, through that intentional shift, a meaning-full thing is produced. Attempting to account for this production leads to Husserl's later "genetic" philosophy, ultimately reaching a zenith in his account of a "spiritual meaning" that is "embodied" in the environment of the lifeworld (Edmund Husserl, *Die Lebenswelt. Auslegungen der vorgegebenen Welt und ihrer Konstitution. Texte aus dem Nachlass (1916–1937)*, Husserliana Band XXXIX

(Dordrecht: Springer, 2008), 427. This meaning is embodied especially in cultural objects such as "houses, bridges, tools, works of art, and so on" (Edmund Husserl, *Erste Philosophie. Zweiter Teil: Theorie der phänomenologischen Reduktion*, Husserliana Band VIII [The Hague: Martinus Nijhoff, 1959], 151) that he sometimes calls "spiritual products" (Edmund Husserl, *The Crisis of European Sciences and Transcendental Phenomenology*, trans. David Carr [Evanston, IL: Northwestern University Press, 1970], 270). But Husserl is adamant that this sense, this "spiritual meaning," is "not externally associated, but internally fused within as a meaning belonging to [the cultural object] and as *expressed* in it" (Edmund Husserl, *Phänomenologische Psychologie. Vorlesungen Sommersemester 1925*, Husserliana Band IX [The Hague: Martinus Nijhoff, 1962], 112; emphasis added). This theme of a spiritual meaning being embodied in the lifeworld is examined at much greater length in Simo Pulkinnen, "Lifeworld as an Embodiment of Spiritual Meaning: The Constitutive Dynamics of Activity and Passivity in Husserl," R. T. Jensen and Dermot Moran (eds.), *The Phenomenology of Embodied Subjectivity* Contributions to Phenomenology 71 (Cham: Springer, 2013).

23. Maurice Merleau-Ponty, *The Visible and the Invisible* ed. Claude Lefort, trans. Alphonso Lingis (Evanston, IL: Northwestern University Press, 1968): 200.

24. Maurice Merleau-Ponty, "An Unpublished Text by Maurice Merleau-Ponty: A Prospectus of his Work," *The Primacy of Perception* trans. A.B. Dallery, ed. J.M. Edie (Evanston, IL: Northwestern University Press, 1964), 3–11.

25. Barbaras, *Merleau-Ponty's Ontology*, 84.

26. Maurice Merleau-Ponty, "Themes from the Lectures at the College de France, 1952–1960," trans. J. O'Neill in *In Praise of Philosophy and Other Essays* (Evanston, IL: Northwestern University Press, 1988), 159.

27. Barbaras, *Merleau-Ponty's Ontology*, 83.

28. Barbaras, *Merleau-Ponty's Ontology*, 84.

29. And the need to overcome these two approaches to the duality explains the long introductory chapters at the beginning of *The Visible and the Invisible* dealing with Husserl and Sartre.

30. "The problems that remain after this first description [i.e., in the *Phenomenology of Perception*]: they are due to the fact that in part I retained the philosophy of 'consciousness'" (Merleau-Ponty, *The Visible and the Invisible*, 183).

31. Merleau-Ponty, "Lectures at the College de France," 158.

32. This is true in the account of expression in *Logical Investigations*, but perhaps not in the later account of spiritual expression. Pursuing the question of the development of Husserl's account of expression would take us too far afield for our purposes today; those interested should consult Neal DeRoo, "Spiritual Expression and the Promise of Phenomenology."

33. Merleau-Ponty, *The Visible and the Invisible*, 183.

34. Cf. Barbaras: ". . . this unity of the thing is grasped in and as an experience" or "the sense of the essence is to be unable to be distinguished from the experience of which it is the essence" (Barbaras, *Merleau-Ponty's Ontology*, 94).

35. Cf.: sense is "inseparable from the directedness of being" itself; David Morris, "The Chirality of Being: Exploring a Merleau-Pontian Ontology of Sense," *Chiasmi International* 12 (2011): 165–182. 170.

36. Cf. Merleau-Ponty, *The Visible and the Invisible*, 107: "a Being that therefore is sense and sense of sense" (translation modified).

37. On sense as a movement of self-differentiation and auto-production, see Martina Ferrari, "Poietic Transpatiality: Merleau-Ponty and the Sense of Nature," *Chiasmi International* 20 (2018): 385–401.

38. Maurice Merleau-Ponty, *Nature: Course notes from the College de France*, ed. Dominique Seglard, trans. Robert Vallier (Evanston, IL: Northwestern University Press, 2003): 3.

39. Cf. Maurice Merleau-Ponty, *L'institution/ la passivité: Notes de cours au Collège de France (1954–1955)* (Paris: Editions Belin, 2003).

40. Merleau-Ponty, *Nature*, 176.

41. Barbaras, *Merleau-Ponty's Ontology*, 58. In all the complexity this term comes to have in Merleau-Ponty's later work, where it is usually translated as "institution," but also has resonances of "foundation" and "tradition."

42. Merleau-Ponty, *The Visible and the Invisible*, 121.

43. Merleau-Ponty, *The Visible and the Invisible*, 103.

44. Cf. Leonard Lawlor, *Thinking through French Philosophy: The Being of the Question* (Bloomington: Indiana University Press, 2003): 1–2.

45. This fundamental intertwining of Being and living is an underexplored nexus at the heart of phenomenology, as both Michel Henry (with his account of Life as auto-affection) and Jacques Derrida (with his account of life as differance) attest, though in seemingly different ways.

46. Landes speaks of this in terms of "metastable equilibriums" and "transduction" throughout *Paradoxes of Expression*; for his introduction of these terms, see Landes, *Paradoxes of Expression*, 22–27.

47. Merleau-Ponty, "Lectures at the College de France," 108–109.

48. Barbaras, *Merleau-Ponty's Ontology*, 144.

49. Merleau-Ponty, *Nature*, 3.

50. Merleau-Ponty, "Lectures at the College de France," 156.

51. Barbaras, *Merleau-Ponty's Ontology*, 65.

52. That is to say, on this account being is an expression of sense/*Stiftung*, and a *Stiftung* is always an expression of being.

53. Of course, we can still speak of distinct acts of, for example, "artistic expression" or "linguistic expression," and so we can conceive of doing a "phenomenology of linguistic expression" or a "phenomenology of artistic expression"—but none of these are yet "expression" itself, in its "primordial" form. If the term is not to be wholly equivocal, such varieties of "expression" must bear some essential relationship to expression itself, but they are not yet the same thing, either: a "phenomenology of artistic expression" might tell us something about expression, but it is not itself yet a "phenomenology of expression" proper.

54. Again, Husserl's later account of spiritual expression may prefigure many of Merleau-Ponty's later moves, as Merleau-Ponty himself suggests; cf. Merleau-Ponty, *The Visible and the Invisible*, 183.

55. Which itself is central to the project of Husserlian phenomenology, as I have argued in "Spiritual Expression and the Promise of Phenomenology."

56. Maurice Merleau-Ponty, *Phenomenology of Perception*, trans. C. Smith (London: Routledge and Kegan Paul, 1981): 291.

57. This obviously opens on to the (disputed) question of the phenomenological status of the so-called "theological" phenomenologists (cf. Dominique Janicaud, "The Theological Turn of French Phenomenology" trans. Bernard G. Prusak in *Phenomenology and the "Theological Turn": The French Debate* (New York: Fordham University Press, 2000): 16–103), but only within a broader phenomenological context of "the inapparent" or the "inconspicuous," a theme made explicit already in Heidegger (cf. Martin Heidegger, "Seminar in Zahringen" in *Seminare*, ed. Curd Ochwadt, GA 15 [Frankfurt am Main: Klostermann, 1986]). The debate on this "phenomenology of the inapparent" remains strong to this day; cf., for example, Jason Alvis, "Making sense of Heidegger's 'phenomenology of the inconspicuous' or inapparent," *Continental Philosophy Review* 51 (2018): 211–238; and Francois Raffoul, "Phenomenology of the Inapparent" in D. Legrand and D. Trigg (eds.), *Unconsciousness between Phenomenology and Psychoanalysis*, Contributions to Phenomenology (in cooperation with the Center for Advanced Research in Phenomenology), 88 (Cham: Springer, 2017).

58. A question taken up in Michael R. Kelly, *Phenomenology and the Problem of Time* (New York: Palgrave MacMillan, 2016).

59. I make the case for reading phenomenology as a project of rigorously explicating sense as what (in Fregean terms) connects "subjective conceptions" with "objective referents" in Neal DeRoo, "Spiritual Expression and the Promise of Phenomenology."

60. This question lies, in many ways, at the heart of any understanding of the relationship between Deleuze and phenomenology, but also, perhaps, between phenomenology and the so-called "object-oriented ontologies."

61. For more on the centrality of the promise to phenomenology and phenomenological method, cf. Neal DeRoo, *Futurity in Phenomenology: Promise and Method in Husserl, Levinas and Derrida* (New York: Fordham University Press, 2013).

62. Otherwise, one risks describing it either as a mere appearance (in "essentialist" phenomenology) or as mere fact (in "realist" philosophy).

Chapter 4

The Abnormalcy of "Normalcy"

Merleau-Ponty, Russon, and the
Normativity of Experience

SUSAN BREDLAU

Introduction

In his discussion of hallucination in the *Phenomenology of Perception*, Merleau-Ponty draws our attention to a situation that we would likely characterize as pathological and asks us to examine the basis upon which we make this characterization. When faced with a person with schizophrenia who is hallucinating, Merleau-Ponty writes:

> There is no question of taking him at his word, nor of reducing his experiences to mine, nor of coinciding with him, nor of holding myself to my point of view; rather it is a question of making explicit my experience and his experience, such as it is indicated in my own, or of making explicit his hallucinatory belief and my real belief, and of understanding them through each other.[1]

In this chapter, I will argue that Merleau-Ponty implicitly relies on a criterion that is internal—rather than external—to experience to identify situations like that of a person with schizophrenia as pathological. For

Merleau-Ponty, what defines a person's situation as pathological is not that she fails to meet a standard or norm established independently of her experience; a pathological situation is not, for example, one in which a person fails to exercise sufficient self-control and experiences her behavior as compelled rather than chosen. Instead, what defines a person's situation as pathological is her inability to answer adequately to the demands of her own experience; a pathological situation is one in which a person's capacity for behaviorally acknowledging and navigating differently compelling—or even conflicting—aspects of her experience is underdeveloped.

This chapter has three sections. In the first section, I draw on John Russon's discussion of the "ideal of normalcy" in *Human Experience* to criticize the common conception of a "normal" self as one who freely chooses her behavior and is, as such, not compelled by her body, emotions, or relations with others. The "ideal of normalcy," Russon argues, leaves us unable to account for neurosis—situations in which a person experiences herself as compelled to act in ways that are at odds with her present relations with other people and things. Indeed, Russon argues, the ideal of normalcy is itself a neurotic stance; rather than avoiding compulsion, the ideal of normalcy cultivates a compulsion for self-loathing that fundamentally conflicts with our relations to others and the world. In the second section, I argue that the phenomenon of "psychological rigidity" described by Merleau-Ponty in "The Child's Relations with Others" has much in common with the phenomenon of neurosis discussed by Russon. Moreover, Merleau-Ponty's reasons for identifying psychological rigidity as pathological are quite similar to Russon's reasons for identifying the ideal of normalcy as pathological: both privilege a single aspect of emotional experience at the expense of others and do so in a way that affects many—or even all—sectors of a person's life. In the third section, I return to Merleau-Ponty's discussion of hallucination and argue that what defines the experience of the person with schizophrenia as pathological for Merleau-Ponty is not that she is vulnerable to hallucination and compulsive behavior—a "normal subject," Merleau-Ponty argues, shares such a vulnerability—but, instead, that this vulnerability is lived in a way that denies the interpersonal aspects of her present experience.

Russon and the "Ideal of Normalcy"

In *Human Experience*, John Russon argues that we typically understand the self as "a discrete individual, separate from a world of things and other individuals upon which she passes judgment, and separate from her own embodiment, which is treated as a tool or a vehicle that she 'has' or 'uses.'"[2] Furthermore, we typically conceive of the relations between persons in terms of explicit laws that guarantee each person the freedom to pursue her own ends so long as this pursuit does not interfere with others' freedom to pursue their own ends.[3] This conception of the self and of interpersonal relations implies, Russon writes, an ideal of normalcy: "The ideal of normalcy pictures a self that is calm, cool, and collected—a self that is not immediately swept away by circumstances and can stand back in dispassionate contemplation of the situation and control its own decisions and actions."[4] A normal self, then, "is pictured as a self-contained choosing power that is not intrinsically compelled by its body, by its emotions, or by its family ties: these latter aspects can be subjects about which the normal self makes choices, but they cannot control its very choosing ability."[5] Russon argues that the ideal of normalcy offers an important insight into human experience; our bodies and emotions are not givens to which we must simply submit, and we are not defined absolutely by the community or communities in which we participate. More specifically, we are not defined absolutely by those familiar others—our families—through whom we developed our first sense of self. The ideal of normalcy is right, therefore, to recognize our individual irreducibility to any sense of self that has already been established in our previous experience.

Yet despite its important insight into the nature of the self, the ideal of normalcy is ultimately inadequate. Consider, for example, Russon's example of a woman who wants to eat healthier food and yet finds herself continuing to eat entire bags of candy. According to the ideal of normalcy, we should understand her as choosing to eat the candy and fault her for her choice. Yet the woman does not actually experience her eating as a matter of choice:

> The a priori claim that she must have been able to control herself is not accurate as a phenomenological description of her experience. No doubt the woman herself senses this to the extent that she really believes about herself that she *cannot* control her eating, that is, it is not true that she can simply and immediately change her behavior if she so desires.[6]

The very existence of situations like the woman's "give[s] the lie," Russon writes, "to the narrative of the normal self."[7] The ideal of normalcy simply does not offer the resources for understanding a self that is not, according to the ideal of normalcy, normal—that is, a self that experiences itself as not, in fact, freely choosing its behavior.

If we are to make sense of such situations, Russon argues, we must turn to our experience itself and, rather than imposing an external standard—like that of absolutely uninhibited free choice—on it, instead seek to articulate its basic structure. When we do so, we discover that our experience is fundamentally emotional and habitual: "The ideal of the normal self is an ideal of singular isolation but [. . .] our singular existence is never won in isolation but is, rather, won only through participation and absorption in our surroundings."[8] That we should experience our feelings and actions as, at least in certain respects, compelling is not an optional aspect of our experience. Moreover, as I will discuss in more detail shortly, this compelling aspect of our experience, far from being a hindrance to our capacity for choice, is actually its basis; as Russon writes, "It is true that we are beings who are capable of choosing and thinking and being self-reflective," but these capacities are "only available to us on the basis of the habitual relationships we have accomplished."[9]

Furthermore, Russon argues, in addition to being fundamentally emotional and habitual, our experience is also fundamentally defined by dissociation. Our understanding of the world, others, and ourselves—an understanding that, for the most part, is implicit in our behaviors rather than something of which we are explicitly aware—is accomplished through our engagement with particular places and people. Insofar as these particular places and people elicit different forms of engagement, we develop multiple different understandings of ourselves, others, and the world. Each of these understandings, while revealing our situation as significant in one way, simultaneously conceals our situation as significant in other ways; our engagement with a particular place or person is simultaneously our disengagement—our dissociation—from other particular places and people.[10] Thus, Russon writes, dissociation is "our original mode of being in a world, and is not a falling away from a prior state of self-unity."[11] This fundamentally dissociative character of our experience is particularly manifest in our different moods: "When we are angry with someone we cannot remember what it is like to feel tender toward that person, and, similarly, when we again become tender we cannot see how we could ever be angry with that person."[12]

Insofar as our different understandings of ourselves, others, and the world belong to relatively separate sectors of our lives, we may not experience the existence of these different understandings as problematic. Yet, Russon writes:

> Even if there is no immediate point of contact between two sectors, they implicitly interact with each other, for at a fundamental level each realm of contact operates with the view that it is the same "me" acting as in each other case, that is, each of these spheres of local contact rests on the premise that it can be an engagement with the world that coheres with the rest of my contacts.[13]

Because dissociation is inherent to our experience, we "automatically live in a state of implicit self-challenge."[14] When different sectors of our lives are developed in ways that bring them into contact, this implicit self-challenge can become explicit, and we can experience the different understandings that are constitutive of these different sectors as in conflict with each other. Such conflicts, Russon writes, are "often most manifest in the presence of other people": "Around some friends, for example, I can be confident, but around other people, perhaps my father, I think of myself as weak and incompetent."[15] Moreover, these conflicts reveal that the behaviors that enact our understanding of ourselves, others, and the world, even when they might seem to be private matters, are actually fundamentally intersubjective gestures. Our everyday behaviors, including our ways of walking, eating, and sleeping, "embody our care" for others.[16] Likewise, we recognize others' habits as embodying their concern—or lack of concern—for us.

Situations in which the understanding we have developed with respect to one aspect of our lives comes to be in conflict with the understanding we have developed in another aspect are, Russon writes, situations of neurosis: "We call it 'neurosis' when this dissociation is a problem, when some sector of a person's life cannot function compatibly with the demands of intersubjective life as developed in other sectors of that person's life."[17] Situations of neurosis reveal the emotional and habitual foundation of our behavior, and thus also reveal that our capacity for choice—for acting differently than we have before—is not simply given but is, instead, developed.[18] To be able to choose to act differently, we must first be able to act differently. Yet we will only be able to act differently if we have developed habits that support this different action. That our capacity for choice is dependent upon, rather than independent of, our habits and emotions is precisely what the ideal of normalcy fails to recognize; the ideal of normalcy "introduces the goal of free choice, but does not itself supply the means to realize this goal."[19] Thus, Russon argues, what defines a situation as neurotic is not—as the "ideal of normalcy" might have us believe—the existence of compulsion as such; compulsion, in the form of emotion and habit, is an escapable aspect of all experience. Instead, what defines a situation as neurotic is the existence of specific compulsions that, though they were empowering in a past situation, are disempowering in the present situation; "the neuroses are the ways in which a multiply figured situation of contact is at odds with itself, such that its inherent trajectory toward freedom in inhibited by its habitual realization of its potentiality."[20] Furthermore, when addressing a neurotic situation, the goal cannot be—as the "ideal of normalcy" might have us believe—to eliminate all habits but must, instead, be to develop "the habits of contact that support us as choosers."[21]

We should not, therefore, under the sway of the ideal of normalcy, respond to neurotic situations with self-condemnation and punishments; these responses assume a capacity for making different choices that simply does not yet exist and are, as such, self-defeating. Instead, we should respond to neurosis by, first, studying our actions to understand how they are "enacting intelligent patterns of behavior in response to the call of familiar situations"[22] and, second, rehabituating ourselves so that we become capable of responding differently.[23] Changing one's behavior is a matter of forming new habits rather than simply changing what one chooses. As such, a person's behavior often cannot change immediately; indeed, Russon writes, "making such changes is typically a long-term and difficult project."[24]

Insofar as the ideal of normalcy fails to recognize that our ability to choose is dependent upon rather than independent of "our embodied, intersubjective character,"[25] it is deeply problematic at a conceptual level. Yet, Russon argues, the ideal of normalcy is also deeply problematic at an existential level. Far from being the opposite of neurosis, the ideal of normalcy is actually, Russon argues, the neurotic stance "par excellence."[26] In valuing the capacity for deliberate choice above all else, the ideal of normalcy "sets itself up as an opponent to a life shaped and governed by emotion."[27] Yet, Russon writes, although:

> The stance of normalcy intends to get beyond being governed by emotion [. . .] in truth it is a position that simply elevates

one passion to a position of tyranny within its decision making. The appearance of dispassionate self-control in the normal self really rests on the fact that a brand of cruelty or self-hatred has become, in the normal self, the ruling passion.[28]

The self that the ideal of normalcy encourages us to attain, far from escaping all compulsion, simply enacts a specific kind of compulsion: a compulsion for self-abuse or self-denial. Furthermore, this compulsion, rather than affecting only certain sectors of a person's life, affects her life as a whole; "here the hindering emotion is not a periodic threat to the smooth functioning of the core of self-identity but is that core itself."[29] Thus far from avoiding the neurotic situations that, according to the ideal of normalcy, are pathological, the "normal" self creates a fundamentally neurotic situation.

As Russon notes, insofar as we have "defined the normal life as itself the hindering neurosis par excellence," we might wonder whether "we can still speak of the neuroses as a problem, that is, is there a criterion other than normalcy to which we can turn to evaluate the worth of neurotic behavior patterns?"[30] Yet even as we reject the ideal of normalcy as the criterion by which we identify a situation as pathological, we can still, Russon argues, identify neurotic situations as problematic: "If we stick to the need for an internal criterion of meaningfulness, we can find two related senses in which the notion of 'illness' can be applied to neurotic phenomena."[31] First, people may themselves identify the inflexible domination of one emotion over all others in a particular sector of their life as problematic. Consider, for example, a man who responds with extreme anger to anyone who offers him constructive criticism; if someone even suggests that something he has done might have been done better, this man lashes out, raising his voice and hurling insults. This person has a job he genuinely enjoys and coworkers whom he genuinely respects. Yet despite his satisfaction with his job and his admiration for his coworkers, he becomes enraged whenever his performance is reviewed. He is simply unable to behaviorally acknowledge or integrate the positive feelings he has toward his job and coworkers with the negative feelings aroused by criticism; his enraged response admits only of dissatisfaction and contempt. Insofar as this man does not want to jeopardize his continued employment, then, he is highly frustrated by his behavior and identifies it as pathological. He wants to respond differently to constructive criticism and experiences his inability to do so as problematic.

Second, even if people do not themselves recognize their inability to behaviorally acknowledge and integrate conflicting feelings as problematic, insofar as this inability results in behaviors that mistreat others, others can do so. Thus, for example, even if the person described above does not recognize his extreme anger toward constructive criticism as problematic, his coworkers would be right to identify it as such. His enraged response to their constructive criticism not only denies his own positive feelings toward his coworkers but also the relation of respect and admiration that has developed between them. His behavior effectively accuses his coworkers of being untrustworthy and uncaring. Yet insofar as there is little or no basis for such an accusation in the history of his interactions with his co-workers, it is he—and not his coworkers—who is being untrustworthy and uncaring. As a betrayal of the positive relationship that exists between him and his coworkers, his behavior is not only self-destructive but also harmful to others, and thus can be identified as pathological.[32]

Before continuing, I want to emphasize that although my focus has been on the individual at the center of a neurotic situation and his rehabituation, this individual could certainly benefit from other people's rehabituation and from the elimination or transformation of various social norms. Just as much as other people—either individually, as, for example, parents or friends, or collectively through, for example, social norms—can contribute to the creation of a neurotic situation, other people can also contribute to the overcoming of a neurotic situation. Furthermore, I want to emphasize that not all of the situations that a person experiences as problematic will be neurotic situations. For example, situations in which a person is stigmatized or persecuted by others, while they could certainly lead to the creation of a neurotic situation for this person, do not begin as such. Indeed, while such situations involve conflict, insofar as this conflict—as well as the impetus to resolve the conflict through behavioral change—does not originate in the person himself but, instead, in others, these situations demand the rehabituation of others rather than of the individual person.[33]

Our existence is fundamentally bodily, emotional, and interpersonal, and thus our actions will always be, in certain respects, compelled. Yet our habits, feelings, and relations with others, rather than essentially thwarting our free choice, are, instead, the essential foundation of our free choice. Our ability to freely choose our actions exists because of—and not in spite of—the compulsive aspects of our body, emotions and relations with others. Nonetheless, the foundation for choice established by our habits, feelings, and relations with others can be more or less supportive of our free choice. It is not, in other words, the presence of compulsions that defines a situation as neurotic but, instead, the presence of compulsions that undermine, rather than support, a person's ability to acknowledge and flexibly navigate the multiple, often conflicting, aspects of her experience.[34]

Merleau-Ponty and "Psychological Rigidity"

Having established that a common conception of a normal self—a self whose behavior is entirely a matter of choice and that is, therefore, free from the compulsions of the body, emotions, or interpersonal life—is inadequate, I turn now to Merleau-Ponty's discussion of "psychological rigidity." As described by Merleau-Ponty, the phenomenon of psychological rigidity has many similarities to the phenomenon of neurosis discussed by Russon. Moreover Merleau-Ponty argues, much as Russon argues with respect to neurosis, that what defines psychological rigidity as pathological is an inability to behaviorally acknowledge and flexibly respond to conflicting aspects of experience.

Merleau-Ponty's discussion of psychological rigidity draws on the work of Else Frenkel-Brunswik and, in particular, her article "Intolerance of Ambiguity as an Emotional and Perceptual Personality Variable."[35] "Psychological rigidity," Merleau-Ponty writes:

> is a notion that originated in psychoanalysis, although it is far from being an orthodox Freudian conception. It means the attitude of the subject who replies to any question with black-and-white answers; who gives replies that are curt and lacking in any shading; who also is generally ill disposed, when examining an object or a person, to recognize in them any clashing traits; and who continually tries, in his remarks, to arrive at a simple, categorical, and summary view.[36]

Children who exhibit psychological rigidity claim, for example, that their families are either absolutely good or absolutely bad: "Either the family is perfection itself—one could not wish for a better—or it is horrible. In any case there are never any nuances."[37]

Yet even as children who exhibit psychological rigidity claim to experience their families as, for example, absolutely good, there is evidence that their experience is actually much more complex. First, Merleau-Ponty writes, "when these subjects analyze and describe their parents, they always confine themselves to mentioning the inessential, external traits, as though they are afraid to enter into a more detailed analysis and to recognize imperfections in the persons around them."[38] According to Frenkel-Brunswik, "we find a preponderance of references to physical and other external characteristics rather than mention of more essential aspects of the parents' personalities."[39] Second, Merleau-Ponty writes, "each time one tries to catch them unawares and obtain responses whose real significance escapes them they are generally negative toward their parents."[40] When asked, for example, "to make a list of the people they would take along if they had to live for several years on a desert island," these children omit their parents from the list.[41] Finally, when these children are given the Thematic Apperception Test, a projective psychological test that asks subjects to tell stories about ambiguous pictures, "one notices that their descriptions of their parents emphasize their coercive, punitive aspects."[42]

Thus Merleau-Ponty, following Frenkel-Brunswik, argues that there is not a "psychological force or genuine conviction"[43] motivating the claims of a psychologically rigid person: "Rigid subjects are in reality, when more closely examined, likely to be profoundly divided in their personality dynamics."[44] The children's claims rather than reflecting their experience of their families as, for example, perfect, actually reflected their experience of their families as deeply imperfect: "In sum, the subjects who carry within themselves extremely strong conflicts are precisely those who reject, in their views of external things, the admission that there are particular situations that are ambiguous, full of conflicts, and mixed in value."[45] That is, these children expressed complete satisfaction with their families not because they were completely satisfied but because they experienced their dissatisfaction as inexpressible. Indeed, Frenkel-Brunswik notes, many of these children had good reasons for not expressing their conflicting feelings: "Some of the children live in a situation comparable to permanent physical danger, which leaves no time for finer discriminations and for attempts to get a fuller understanding of the factors involved but in which quick action leading to tangible concrete results is the only appropriate behavior."[46]

Merleau-Ponty recognizes that our experiences of particular persons or environments will always be complex and will often involve conflicting feelings. Few—if any—of the people and environments we experience are absolutely good or absolutely bad. We will likely always find our parents or others with whom we are close as, for example, praiseworthy in some respects and worthy of criticism in other respects. However, we can respond to these conflicting feelings either by denying them or by honestly acknowledging them. The former response reflects the attitude that Merleau-Ponty, following Melanie Klein, refers to as ambivalence: "Ambivalence consists in having two alternative images of the same object, the same person, without making any effort to connect them or to notice that in reality they relate to the same object and the same person. [. . .] What is lacking in rigid subjects is [. . . the] capacity to confront squarely the contradictions in their attitudes toward others."[47] The latter response reflects the attitude that Merleau-Ponty, following Klein, refers to as ambiguity: "ambiguity is an adult phenomenon, an attitude of maturity, which has nothing pathological about it. It consists in admitting that the same being who is good and generous can also be annoying and imperfect. Ambiguity is ambivalence that one dares to look at face to face."[48]

As with the neurotic situation, then, psychological rigidity involves a privileging of one aspect of experience at the expense of others. For children who exhibit psychological rigidity, their contentment with their parent, for example, dominates while their frustration and anger are denied. Thus, much as Russon argues with respect to neurosis, Merleau-Ponty argues that it is the inflexible denial of all but one aspect of an experience that marks psychological rigidity as pathological. It is not the presence of conflicting emotions but, rather, the *denial* of conflicting emotions that is pathological; a psychologically rigid person does not take into account or "interiorize" the "problems that arise on account of the discordant traits that are to be found in each and every individual."[49] In other words, a "normal" or nonpathological situation is not one in which a person has successfully eliminated all conflicting feelings from her experience. Rather, it is one in which a person confronts these conflicts directly, realizes that conflict as such cannot be altogether eliminated, and, nonetheless, finds a way to navigate them behaviorally:

> What characterizes a psychologically mature subject for Mrs. Frenkel-Brunswik is not that he does or does not have ambiguities; it is the *way in which he treats his ambiguities*. If he hides them from himself, if he flees them, if he does not confront them, he is psychologically rigid. If, on the contrary, he faces them squarely, he has arrived at maturity.[50]

Our experience will always involve a variety of—sometimes conflicting—bodily habits, emotions, and relations with others, and to claim otherwise is to practice a kind of self-rejection. Indeed, Merleau-Ponty recognizes that psychological rigidity, like the ideal of normalcy, often applies to all, rather than just one, sectors of a person's experience: "In a more general way, not only with their parents but with regard to all moral and social problems as well, these subjects proceed by dichotomizing."[51] With respect to various opposites—Frenkel-Brunswik identifies these as including "dominance-submission, cleanliness-dirtiness, badness-goodness, virtue-vice, masculinity-femininity"[52]—a person with psychological rigidity adheres to one and denies the other, displaying a "mania cleanliness," for example, or claiming that children must be absolutely obedient to their parents.[53]

The criterion by which Merleau-Ponty identifies psychological rigidity as pathological is not, then, external to experience; he is not claiming, for example, that experience should not include conflicting feelings. Instead, his criterion is internal to experience; he claims that conflicting feelings in experience should be acknowledged rather than denied. Thus Merleau-Ponty, like Russon, though he rejects one understanding of pathology, offers another: what is pathological is a stance that denies the diversity of feelings within a person's experience in favor of a single feeling and that promotes the inflexible domination of this feeling over her behavior. By contrast, a nonpathological stance acknowledges the diversity of feelings within a person's experience and allows for flexibility with respect to how these feelings are reflected in a person's behavior.

Schizophrenic Hallucination

Now that we have developed an understanding of a pathological situation as one in which a person is unable to acknowledge or behaviorally integrate conflicting aspects of her experience, let us turn to Merleau-Ponty's discussion of hallucination and consider how the understanding of pathology developed in the previous two sections might enrich our understanding of the hallucinations associated with schizophrenia. Merleau-Ponty rejects both empiricist/materialist and intellectualist/rationalist understandings of hallucination. The hallucinations associated with schizophrenia cannot, he argues, be understood as resulting simply from physiological abnormalities that produce perceptual experiences in the absence of the external stimuli usually coupled with perceptual experience. If these hallucinations were simply abnormally produced perceptual experiences, he asserts, then those with schizophrenia should be unable to distinguish their hallucinations from their perceptual experiences. Yet, Merleau-Ponty writes, "The most important fact is that patients distinguish, for the most part, between their hallucinations and their perceptions."[54] At the same time, however, these hallucinations cannot be understood as resulting simply from a failure of reason with respect to a content of experience that is imaginary rather than perceptual: "The hallucination is not a rash judgement or belief for the same reasons that prevent it from being a sensory content: judgment or belief could only consist in positing the hallucination as true, and this is precisely what the patients do not do."[55]

To understand Merleau-Ponty's own account of hallucination, then, I think we should take seriously his comment that "the most important fact" is that those with schizophrenia can distinguish, for the most part, between the hallucinatory and the perceptual aspects of their experience. By doing so, we can notice another, quite remarkable, aspect of his account. For a person with schizophrenia, Merleau-Ponty suggests, the hallucinatory aspects of experience are as, if not more, absorbing than the perceptual aspects of her experience *even after* these aspects have been explicitly identified as hallucinatory, that is, as experienced by her alone. The existence of a person with schizophrenia is centered on those aspects of experience unshared with others—that are hallucinatory rather than perceptual—and these hallucinatory aspects have, so to speak, taken the place of these perceptual aspects: "The perceived world has lost its expressive force, and the hallucinatory system has usurped this force."[56] By contrast, for a person who does not have schizophrenia, those aspects of experience experienced alone are largely relegated to the periphery of existence. Existence is centered, instead, on those aspects of experience that *are* shared with others, that *are* perceptual: "The normal subject does not revel in subjectivity, he flees from it, he is really in the world [. . .]."[57] When considering the hallucinations of a person with schizophrenia, Merleau-Ponty implies, it is the centrality of those aspects of her experience that are *not* shared with others and the peripherality of those aspects of experience that are shared with others that deserve our attention.

Thus Merleau-Ponty argues that empiricist and intellectualist conceptions of hallucination share the same—incorrect—assumption: "The two doctrines presuppose the priority of objective being, and attempt to introduce the hallucinatory phenomenon into it by force."[58] Rather than assuming that the world that appears to us first exists independently of us, we should, instead, recognize the world that appears to us *as appearing*. Perceptual experience, rather than being the representation of an already given world, is, instead, the presentation of a meaningful world. What we perceive is, therefore, always inextricable from who we are as perceivers. In other words, what we perceive is never simply "objective." It is also always irreducibly "subjective" and is, as such, always vulnerable to hallucination: "hallucination and perception are modalities of a single primordial function by which we arrange around ourselves a milieu with a definite structure, and by which we situate ourselves sometimes fully in the world and sometimes on the margin of the world."[59]

For Merleau-Ponty, then, what distinguishes the person who does not have schizophrenia from the person who does is not that the latter is vulnerable to hallucination and compulsive behavior while the former is not: "we only succeed in giving an account of the hallucinatory deception by stripping perception of its apodictic certainty and perceptual consciousness of its full self-possession."[60] If hallucinations can, Merleau-Ponty writes, "count as reality" for the person with schizophrenia, this is only "because reality itself is reached for the normal subject in an analogous operation. Insofar as he has sensory fields and a body, the normal subject himself also bears this gaping wound through which illusion can be introduced."[61]

As we have already noticed in section one with respect to both the person who wants to eat healthier food yet finds herself unable to do so and the person who wants to welcome constructive criticism and yet finds himself unable do so, our behavior does not necessarily reflect our explicit knowledge and desires. Moreover, even when our behavior does reflect our explicit knowledge and desires, we must recognize our ability to choose our actions as an achievement rather than a given. We are able to choose our actions only insofar as we have developed the habits that make these actions possible; that is, we are only able to choose our actions if these actions have, in a sense, become compelling.

What distinguishes the situation of a person with schizophrenia as pathological, then, is not that she, unlike a "normal" subject, is vulnerable to hallucination and compulsive behavior. If we think of the person who has schizophrenia as succumbing to hallucination, we should equally think of the person who does not have schizophrenia as succumbing to perception. Moreover, we should recognize that the behaviors of both have an element of compulsion and are not simply matters of choice.

That is, a person without schizophrenia no more chooses to center her existence on those aspects of her experience that are shared with others than the person with schizophrenia chooses to center her existence on those aspects of her experience that are not shared with others. As perceivers, our existence is always bodily, emotional, and interpersonal and hence is neither simply reflexive nor simply deliberately chosen, neither fully self-possessed nor fully self-dispossessed. The hallucinations of a person with schizophrenia, Merleau-Ponty suggests, are the result of a long-term process in which the perceptual aspects of her experience have—for reasons that could include troubled or problematic relations with others—been increasingly neglected and the nonperceptual aspects of her experience increasingly attended to. This process culminates in nonperceptual aspects of her experience becoming so central to her existence that they begin to be experienced as perceptual—as shared with others even when they are not.

In experiencing the hallucinatory aspects of her experience as almost solely worthy of her attention, a person with schizophrenia effectively denies the perceptual aspects of her experience and the interpersonal world inherent to these perceptual aspects.[62] Of course, there may be good reasons for a person with schizophrenia to turn away from or deny the interpersonal world; indeed, this person's earliest relations with others may have effectively driven her out of the interpersonal world by refusing to recognize her as a participant in this world.[63] Nonetheless, we can identify the situation of a person with schizophrenia as pathological insofar as it enacts a behavioral denial of the interpersonal world in a situation where those with whom she interacts *do* welcome her participation in this world.[64] That is, it is pathological insofar as it denies inherent aspects of her present experience.[65] Likewise, the situation of a person without schizophrenia may still be pathological if this person, while acknowledging the perceptual aspects of her experience, nonetheless denies other nonperceptual—imaginary or memorial, for example—aspects of her experience.

In his discussion of hallucination, then, as in his discussion of psychological rigidity, Merleau-Ponty defines a person's situation as pathological not because her behavior is compelled but, instead, because her behavior is compelled in ways that do not acknowledge the complexity of her present experience. Our experience is embodied, emotional, and interpersonal, and, as such, our behavior will always reflect our habits, feelings, and relations with others. Any attempt to resolve pathological situations like those discussed in this chapter, then, should aim not at eliminating the influence on our behavior of our body, emotions, and relations with others, but instead, at allowing these influences, through the development of new habits, to operate differently than before.

Notes

1. Maurice Merleau-Ponty, *Phenomenology of Perception*. Trans. Donald A. Landes (New York: Routledge, 2013), 354.

2. John Russon, *Human Experience* (Albany, NY: SUNY Press, 2003), 83.

3. Russon, *Human Experience*, 83–84.

4. Russon, *Human Experience*, 88.

5. Russon, *Human Experience*, 88.

6. Russon, *Human Experience*, 86.

7. Russon, *Human Experience*, 85.

8. Russon, *Human Experience*, 90.

9. Russon, *Human Experience*, 86.

10. For a richly developed discussion of this point, see Whitney Howell's chapter in this volume, "The Insight of Dispossession," especially the section entitled, "Dispossession."

11. Russon, *Human Experience*, 77.

12. Russon, *Human Experience*, 77.

13. Russon, *Human Experience*, 80.

14. Russon, *Human Experience*, 81.

15. Russon, *Human Experience*, 80.

16. Russon, *Human Experience*, 81.

17. Russon, *Human Experience*, 81.

18. Russon, *Human Experience*, 86.

19. Russon, *Human Experience*, 91.

20. Russon, *Human Experience*, 92.

21. Russon, *Human Experience*, 86.

22. Russon, *Human Experience*, 86.

23. Russon argues these familiar situations are often those established by family life; for further discussion of this point in Russon's work, see Kirsten Jacobson, "The Body as Family Narrative: Russon and the Education of the Soul." *Anekaant: A Journal of Polysemic Thought* 3 (2015): 49–57.

24. Russon, *Human Experience*, 87.

25. Russon, *Human Experience*, 84.

26. Russon, *Human Experience*, 90.

27. Russon, *Human Experience*, 89.

28. Russon, *Human Experience*, 89.
29. Russon, *Human Experience*, 90.
30. Russon, *Human Experience*, 91.
31. Russon, *Human Experience*, 92.
32. On the issue of betrayal in our relations with others, see John Russon, *Bearing Witness to Epiphany* (Albany, NY: SUNY Press, 2009), 88–94; and Susan Bredlau, *The Other in Perception* (Albany, NY: SUNY Press, 2018), 86–90.
33. See, for example, Helen Ngo's discussion of racism as primarily unfolding in the register of bodily habit (848) in "Racist Habits: A Phenomenological Analysis of Racism and the Habitual Body." *Philosophy and Social Criticism* 42, no. 9 (2016): 847–872.
34. Indeed, Russon argues elsewhere that conflict is inherent to our experience of home; see *Sites of Exposure*, (Albany, NY: SUNY Press, 2017), 35–60.
35. For further discussion of Merleau-Ponty's use of research on child psychology in his own writing and his own work as a professor of child psychology, see Talia Welsh, *The Child as Natural Phenomenologist* (Evanston, IL: Northwestern University Press, 2013).
36. Maurice Merleau-Ponty, "The Child's Relations with Others." Trans. William Cobb. In *The Primacy of Perception*, ed. James M. Edie (Evanston, IL: Northwestern University Press, 1964), 101.
37. Merleau-Ponty, "The Child's Relations with Others," 101.
38. Merleau-Ponty, "The Child's Relations with Others," 101.
39. Else Frenkel-Brunswik, "Intolerance of Ambiguity as an Emotional and Perceptual Personality Variable." *Journal of Personality* 18 (1949): 108–143.
40. Merleau-Ponty, "The Child's Relations with Others," 101.
41. Merleau-Ponty, "The Child's Relations with Others," 101.
42. Merleau-Ponty, "The Child's Relations with Others," 102.
43. Merleau-Ponty, "The Child's Relations with Others," 101.
44. Merleau-Ponty, "The Child's Relations with Others," 101.
45. Merleau-Ponty, "The Child's Relations with Others," 105.
46. Frenkel-Brunswik, "Intolerance of Ambiguity as an Emotional and Perceptual Personality Variable," 118.
47. Merleau-Ponty, "The Child's Relations with Others," 103.
48. Merleau-Ponty, "The Child's Relations with Others," 103.
49. Merleau-Ponty, "The Child's Relations with Others," 107.
50. Merleau-Ponty, "The Child's Relations with Others," 107, his italics.
51. Merleau-Ponty, "The Child's Relations with Others," 102.
52. Frenkel-Brunswik, "Intolerance of Ambiguity as an Emotional and Perceptual Personality Variable," 117.
53. Merleau-Ponty, "The Child's Relations with Others," 102.
54. Merleau-Ponty, *Phenomenology of Perception*, 349.
55. Merleau-Ponty, *Phenomenology of Perception*, 350.

56. Merleau-Ponty, *Phenomenology of Perception*, 358.
57. Merleau-Ponty, *Phenomenology of Perception*, 358.
58. Merleau-Ponty, *Phenomenology of Perception*, 351.
59. Merleau-Ponty, *Phenomenology of Perception*, 358.
60. Merleau-Ponty, *Phenomenology of Perception*, 359.
61. Merleau-Ponty, *Phenomenology of Perception*, 358. See also Hannah Venable's discussion of this passage in light of the relation between Merleau-Ponty's account of hallucination and the work of Foucault, in chapter 5 in this volume, "The Need for Merleau-Ponty in Foucault's Account of the Abnormal."
62. More recent work on schizophrenia, particularly work that offers serious consideration of the lived experience of a person with schizophrenia, also argues that for a person with schizophrenia the interpersonal world is experienced as threatening; see, for example, Paul Henry Lysaker, Jason K. Johannesen, and John Timothy Lysaker, "Schizophrenia and the experience of intersubjectivity as threat." *Phenomenology and the Cognitive Sciences* 4 (2005): 335–352.
63. See, for example, R.D. Laing, *The Divided Self* (New York: Penguin Books, 1990) and Gregory Bateson, *Steps to an Ecology of Mind* (Chicago: University of Chicago Press, 1990). Furthermore, just as a person's relations with others may play a role in the development of schizophrenia, so too may a person's relations with others play a role in mitigating the development of schizophrenia. See, for example, Jane E. Brody, "Interventions to Prevent Psychosis," *The New York Times*, September 2, 2019.
64. Nonetheless, as E.A. Belanger and colleagues document, the very health professionals who should offer the person with schizophrenia a more welcoming relation with others often have great difficulty doing so. See E.A. Belanger et al. "Negative Symptoms and Therapeutic Connection: A Qualitative Analysis in a Single Case Study with a Patient with First Episode Psychosis." *Journal of Psychotherapy Integration* 28, no. 2 (2018): 171–187.
65. If those with whom the person with schizophrenia interacts continue to drive her out of the interpersonal world, then we may need to consider these others' behavior as just as—and perhaps even far more—pathological than that of the person with schizophrenia.

Chapter 5

The Need for Merleau-Ponty in Foucault's Account of the Abnormal

HANNAH LYN VENABLE

Introduction

Whether with contempt or admiration, current writers on the history of psychiatry continue to acknowledge the work of Michel Foucault. His extensive survey on the history of the abnormal has clearly influenced how a history of psychiatry should be written by challenging historians to question the reasons behind shifting perspectives on mental health. Due to both his historical contribution as well as the simple persuasive power of his writing, many philosophers acknowledge the insights found in his unique account of the abnormal. I will argue, however, that we can successfully draw on Foucault's work on the abnormal only once we recognize that it is Maurice Merleau-Ponty's work in psychology that serves as its hidden foundation. In fact, I will go so far as to say that without claiming this foundation, Foucault's account of the abnormal will fall short and fail to accomplish even its own internal goals: in other words, his account cannot and should not stand on its own.

In order to uncover the hidden foundation of Foucault's account of the abnormal, we may turn to the biographical links between Merleau-Ponty and Foucault. Merleau-Ponty served as a teacher and model for many of the rising French philosophers, including Foucault, during the 1940s and 1950s. However, what is less well recognized, at least in the English scholarship, is that Foucault faithfully attended Merleau-Ponty's 1949–1952 *Child Psychology and Pedagogy* lectures.[1] At the same time as attending these lectures, Foucault pursued and obtained his *licence* in psychology, taught psychology classes, and worked at the Hôpital Sainte-Anne.[2] From this, there is no question that Foucault's early studies of the abnormal were under the direct influence of Merleau-Ponty.[3] Nonetheless, we still do not know if this formation is still in place when Foucault writes and publishes his *History of Madness* in 1961 as Foucault's work in other places has been highly critical of the phenomenological enterprise.

The proper way, then, to establish the foundation for Foucault's account of the abnormal is to look at the structural links between Merleau-Ponty and Foucault. While the biographical links reveal that Foucault received insights from a Merleau-Pontean psychology, it is only through an examination of the structural soundness of Foucault's account that we can discover its phenomenological roots. The historical structures presented by Foucault, while certainly powerful and helpful tools for understanding the experience of the abnormal, need more justification than historical data and analysis. Upon examining Foucault's account, we are still left asking: *why* are the historical structures shaped this way, and what is the *source* for these recurring patterns? We will find, however, that the historical structures are already manifest in the phenomenological patterns; in other words, the historical construction of the abnormal actually comes out of the existential experience of the abnormal. To illustrate the dependence of Foucault's historical account on Merleau-Ponty's phenomenological one, I will offer a brief overview of Foucault's concept of the abnormal and then present the problems or gaps that are found there. I conclude by demonstrating how Merleau-Ponty's method fills these gaps and provides the structural support needed to stabilize his historical account.

By arguing for the necessity of Merleau-Ponty in Foucault's account, I am not placing a priority on Merleau-Ponty over Foucault. In fact, I believe Merleau-Ponty's work requires Foucault's rich historical analysis and acute awareness of human brokenness; thus, there is also a need for Foucault in Merleau-Ponty's account of the abnormal.[4] For the purposes of this chapter, however, we will be focusing solely on the way that Merleau-Ponty specifically enriches and supports Foucault's account.

Foucault's Account of the Abnormal

To begin, I will give a brief summary of Foucault's account of the abnormal from his 1961 *History of Madness* and his 1974–1975 lectures entitled *Abnormal*. The abnormal, for Foucault, is a "modern" category given to people who struggle with mental disorders and who are not able to assimilate fully into present society as a result. By "modern," Foucault means something that originated in the nineteenth century and continues up to the present time.[5] Through his study, he shows how the definition of madness (*la folie*) changes over time because it is subject to the societal perceptions of reason and unreason or the rational and the nonrational.[6] The terms "rational" and "nonrational" are always historically contingent for Foucault, but his context will tell us whether he is referring only to a particular society's view, such as the modern understanding of the "rational" meaning "normal" or "knowable," or whether he wants to capture all the historical meanings under the term, such as the "overarching unreason" (*déraison*). These evolving perceptions, understood in both of these contexts, make up the consciousness of madness and are revealed in how institutions change in order to address the problem of madness.

The way we view madness today, or our modern consciousness of madness, has created the category of the *abnormal* and can be best understood by tracing the two previous types of consciousness found in the Renaissance and in the classical age.[7] During the Renaissance of Europe, Foucault cites historical texts and events to show that the consciousness of madness contained a "continuous dialectic" between madness and reason because of the recognition that the rational and nonrational were interconnected and in all parts of creation.[8] In this context, although the nonrational was to be feared, it was also a reminder of the necessary "dark" and "tragic" elements of human experience.[9] Foucault uses his famous example of the sixteenth-century Ship of Fools to show the privileging of the "dialectical experience of madness."[10] He argues that the mad were placed on these aimless ships not primarily for the purpose of exclusion but as a symbolic representation of the "senseless in search of their reason."[11] Just as the mad on the ships were searching for the light of reason, all humans, according to this mentality, are on a journey toward reason and truth. Yet there is still something to be feared in madness, as seen in the representative figure of the Renaissance: the *human monster*. This monster demonstrates "the spontaneous, brutal, but consequently natural form of the unnatural" and magnifies the irregularities and deviations inherent in the world.[12]

The great fear of the nonrational of the sixteenth century combined with the growing desire for a purified society brought about a more complicated consciousness of madness in the classical age. At this time, the concerns about madness retain some of the dialectic but also embrace practical, enunciatory and analytic perspectives as well.[13] Again, Foucault believes that the changes in the structures of institutions show the deeper shift in the consciousness of madness. He writes: "What happened between the end of the Renaissance and the height of the classical age was therefore not simply an evolution of the institutions: it was a change in the consciousness of madness, and thereafter it was the asylums, houses of confinement, gaols [jails] and prisons that illustrated that new conception."[14] During the Great Confinement of the seventeenth century in Europe, large numbers of people were labeled mad and locked away; for example, over 1 percent of the population of Paris was incarcerated over a period of just a few years.[15] European society needed places of confinement all the more during this time with the rise of the sequestering of the mad. This was motivated by the idea that madness, now equated with the nonrational, must be separated entirely from the rational because displays of the nonrational were considered displays of immorality. Foucault writes, "Madness was seen through an ethical condemnation of idleness" and other sins so much so that "madness found itself side by side with sin."[16] The push for confinement and correction is seen in the classical representative figure called the *"individual to be corrected [l'individu à corriger]"* or the "incorrigible."[17] The figure of the human monster faded to the background as institutions sought to remove and reshape these individuals according to this new ethical model.

With the suppression of the nonrational and the growing concern for correction, Foucault claims that the definition of madness changed again in the nineteenth and twentieth centuries into the modern notion of the abnormal. The mad are no longer a constructive reminder of the nonrational as in the fifteenth and sixteenth centuries, nor are they equated with the nonrational and hidden away as in the seventeenth and eighteenth centuries, but are now people who have deviated from the normal standards of society and need to be fixed, through both ethical and medical means, to be brought back into society. This mindset began in the Great Reform, which sought to improve the conditions of the mad in the given institutions in order to "cure" them.[18] Now, madness is no longer linked to the nonrational of previous ages but is "totally alienated from the forms of knowledge, no longer even made an object of division," as Frédéric Gros puts it.[19] Drawing only on the analytic perspective, madness is defined solely objectively and can no longer even be placed as an object in the division between the rational and the nonrational, as it was in the classical age. Just as the modern reformers "cured" the mad by returning them to reason, so madness having lost any link to the nonrational can be cured by a return to the rational.

The figure of the *onanist* or masturbator arises out of the classical age and then crosses over into the modern age becoming the last ancestor to the abnormal individual.[20] The onanist is seen as someone who secretly breaks the rules and must be made to conform to the "normal" standards of society, showing the priority placed on the categories of the normal and the abnormal. Lastly, we have the figure of the *abnormal individual* representing someone who needs to be fixed—no longer seen as a monster, no longer seen as incorrigible—but simply as someone not normal. But even with the emphasis on conformity, the nonrational can never be completely forgotten, Foucault argues, as it bursts forth unexpectedly in our world through the arts, seen in the works of Nietzsche, Van Gogh, Artaud, and others.[21]

In each age, Foucault uncovers how the treatment of the mad depends on the perception of the rational and nonrational, offering "not discoveries," as Jean Khalfa puts it, "but historical constructions of meaning."[22] To summarize these constructions in overly simplified terms, we found that during the Renaissance, the rational and the nonrational, seen as truth and darkness, had a mutually dependent dialectic relationship, and, thus, the mad were seen as connected to the world and represented the world as it was. During the classical age, a division between the rational and the nonrational, representing the moral and immoral, resulted in confinement of the mad in order to purge society of any nonrational elements. With the nonrational of the past hidden, it was eventually forgotten so that in the modern age the mad are seen as abnormal, not as tragic wanderers or immoral outsiders but as people in need of correction. And yet, even in recent times, there results certain eruptions of madness, particularly in the arts, that demonstrate the historical link to the nonrational. We turn now to see what gaps or problems arise from Foucault's historical account of the abnormal.

Questioning Foucault's Account

No doubt, we can see the persuasive power in Foucault's account due to the sense of unity that he brings to hundreds of years of complex historical records on madness and due to the way he uncovers the roots of our present understanding of the abnormal. And yet, upon reflection, we find gaps in Foucault's account that may cause us to question and even dismiss his claims. Although there are many critiques of Foucault's method, I will present two critical issues, the problem of arbitrariness and the lack of application, which apply directly to his account of the abnormal.[23]

Foucault is known for pulling away from his phenomenological training, and seen even as breaking free from what is claimed to be its "fixed and absolutist view of human subjectivity."[24] But in doing so, does Foucault then lose a reference point or a foundation for his claims? If the abnormal depends on the changing consciousness of madness, which in turn is based on the shifting perceptions of the rational and nonrational, then it seems that the abnormal is nothing at all in itself but whatever society at the moment decrees that it is. This leads us to ask whether the abnormal becomes arbitrary, subject to the whims of the historical forces of the time. Despite its cohesion, Foucault's account of the abnormal can feel arbitrary because of its lack of grounding for its claims and its inability to root the ideas of the rational and the nonrational in anything other than societal perceptions.

Partially due to this problem of arbitrariness, Foucault's work lacks a direct application to the current world of mental health. Foucault is often criticized, as Angelos Evangelou points out, for "having no real interest in the mad and for offering no hope and no alternative for their treatment."[25] Many have seen his work as unhelpful to individuals with mental disorders because of his aversion to the modern approach to mental health and his scathing critique of the psychiatric industry as a whole. I believe that these two problems, arbitrariness and impracticality, can be addressed through the aid of Merleau-Ponty.

Merleau-Ponty's Aid

As we have seen, Foucault needs a way of validating his historical account. I will argue that he can do this by turning to Merleau-Ponty's phenomenological understanding of common human experience. I justify this turn to Merleau-Ponty for two reasons. First, in a general sense, historical structures often arise from experiences already present in the perceptual world. Thus, we can better understand the historical structures when we see how they are grounded in bodily experience. For example, we can see the roots of the social desire to set up some form of government in the bodily experience of order, both in the organization of the body itself with all the organs functioning together and in the system for how the body relates to the outside world. In a similar way, the historical structures of madness are better supported when traced back to the bodily experiences of madness itself. A second reason for calling on the aid of Merleau-Ponty is found in the specific relation that Foucault has to phenomenology. Due to the major role that Merleau-Ponty played in Foucault's formation, Foucault's training in phenomenology spills over into his work on madness, as seen in his continued use of some phenomenological vocabulary in the *History of Madness*.[26] By looking to Merleau-Ponty, we are able to make explicit this hidden foundation already lurking behind the historical accounts.

In light of these reasons, we can give credence to Foucault's historical structures of the abnormal by rooting them in Merleau-Ponty's phenomenological patterns found in the abnormal experiences of the body. In doing so, we will also provide Foucault's account with hope of an application; by showing that the historical and existential can be matched, we are then better able to understand fully the nature of many disorders.

Rooting Historical Structures in Phenomenological Patterns

While keenly aware of the social-historical milieu of the human, Merleau-Ponty avoids the problem of arbitrariness by bringing us "some *general truths*," as Talia Welsh calls them, "about human development and intersubjective life."[27] Through his phenomenological-existential analysis, he demonstrates that the abnormal is best understood by revealing the general truths found in human experience, in experiences of both the rational and the nonrational. Merleau-Ponty consistently finds the Cartesian view of rationality unsatisfactory and states that we, along with others in Hegel's tradition, must continue to "explore the irrational and integrate it into an expanded reason."[28] Thus, in the study of the abnormal, Merleau-Ponty aims to explore the irrational (one type of the nonrational)—as seen in experiences typically ignored and rejected by modernism, such as hallucinations, hysteria, melancholy, and more—and then to enlarge the modern understanding of the rational accordingly.[29] He further describes how the nonrational is at the core of human experience and the source for anything that we call "reason." Through this expansion, Merleau-Ponty goes beyond the categories of the rational and the nonrational, showing us they are best understood in a dialectic, reversible relationship, later called the unity of the flesh. His phenomenological analysis, which exposes general truths of human experience and moves beyond the rational–nonrational dichotomy, provides the phenomenological patterns needed to root Foucault's historical structures. I will establish this phenomenological foundation for the abnormal by, first, describing how madness can be accessible and meaningful and, second, demonstrating the presence of these patterns in the disorder of schizophrenia.[30]

Beginning with the accessibility of madness, we should remember that Foucault uncovers the historical tendency to define madness according to the current understanding of the rational, but he does not offer a reason for this phenomenon: for example, in the classical age, the madness was equated with the nonrational in hopes of maintaining a rational and moral society; and more recently, in the modern age, madness is seen as something abnormal that needs to be fixed and cured in order to conform to the modern standard of the rational as the "normal" and "objective." This continual search to understand displays of the abnormal is not arbitrary but comes out of the phenomenological principle that madness is accessible to our understanding and is not devoid of meaning; madness is an integral part of human experience, arising out of it and being central to it. Merleau-Ponty writes that abnormal cases, as seen in madness, and normal experiences, as seen in perception, "despite all their differences, are not self-enclosed [*ne sont pas fermées sur elles-mêmes*]; they are not islands of experience without any communication and from which one cannot escape . . . [they open] onto a horizon of possible objectifications."[31] Although abnormal experiences are different from usual human experiences, they are not cut off from common human experience; *they are not closed on themselves* (as the French literally says). These experiences display a link among humans and make up a shared horizon of human experience.[32]

Reflecting on the experiences of homesickness and hallucinations can illustrate the shared horizon of nonobjective space. When we are homesick, we are far from something or someone that we love and feel we are not truly living in our actual objective space. My body may be in one place, "but this landscape is not necessarily the landscape of our life . . . and if I am kept far from what I love, I feel far from the center of real life."[33] While experiencing a hallucination is a more extreme form of feeling far from the center of real life, it is similar in that we feel as if we are somewhere else, although our body remains in objective space. Whether or not we distinguish between the objective and nonobjective spaces in the moment, both experiences of homesickness and hallucinations represent experiences of the nonrational because we feel the power of a space that is not actually there and can be rationally shown to be elsewhere.

To say that we can have rational access to experiences of the nonrational, such as those in hallucinations, is not to acquiesce to a rationalistic explanation of disorders nor to give into some kind of "irrational conversion," as Merleau-Ponty writes, but to perform an "intentional analysis" that reveals a sense of meaning in human behavior and points to the integration of the rational and the nonrational.[34] M.C. Dillon argues that ontology, as the "search for the logos or meaning of things," is at the heart of Merleau-Ponty's project.[35] Dillon writes, "Merleau-Ponty's ontology provides an explication of phenomena in the light of which phenomenology can understand itself—without being naïve or dogmatic—as inquiry whose subject matter is real."[36] Phenomenology explores what is real, and, while not boasting of complete comprehension, it does claim to reveal meaning and order in the real world. This is because, whether we as humans choose it or not, "we are condemned to meaning [*sens*]"; as Merleau-Ponty famously reminds us: we can relate to the world only in a meaningful way.[37] The capacity of the rational helps disclose the logic present in the world; as he writes: ". . . there is a logic of the world that my entire body merges with."[38] By understanding the patterns in abnormal behavior, as seen in the rational–nonrational relation, we can get a glimpse into the logic found in human experience, both existentially and historically. The logic present in the world is not an abstract logic, but a "lived logic" that gives meanings that can be grasped only by embodied humans.[39] Despite changes in the historical perspectives and in the representative historical figures (the monster, the incorrigible, and the masturbator), this lived logic is precisely what grounds the historical search for the meaning behind the abnormal, including the continual tie of the abnormal to the perceptions of the rational and the nonrational.

Due to the accessibility of the abnormal, Merleau-Ponty is then able to gain insight into the complexities found in many disorders in the *Phenomenology of Perception*. Here we will look at the disorder of schizophrenia as an example to illustrate the phenomenological patterns of the abnormal. For people with schizophrenia, a fragmentation occurs in their mental lives such that on top of reality is a layer of fantasy. This added layer does not replace objective reality, nor do the objects of the real world disappear, but it gives reality a new signification. When one experiences hallucinations, one can still cross a room, avoiding the furniture and objects on the floor, because the hallucinations are on top of the already perceived reality.[40] Merleau-Ponty concludes that "hallucination and perception are modalities of a single primordial function . . . *because reality itself is reached for by the normal subject in an analogous operation*" to the abnormal subject.[41] Both experiences, hallucinatory and perceptual, come from the same pattern of human experience because we perform an analogous task of drawing on the nonrational, primordial function of the human to engage with the world.

In terms of the rational and the nonrational, we find that the reliance on the nonrational is present in both cases of perception and hallucination, but that the patient with schizophrenia is not regulating the nonrational by the rational in the proper ways. This explanation still uses the terms "rational" and "nonrational" not to produce another division but to show the complexity of the experiences. Here, even in strange behaviors, the rational is still present for the patient because the experiences make sense and have valid reasons for the person. What differs is that application of the rational is broken because it is disconnected from the actual world: "The falsehoods of mentally disturbed individuals are not themselves deceiving; there is always something positive in their vision which serves to ground their actions."[42] There is always some structure of the world "around which the mentally ill organize their behavior," as Talia Welsh explains, for hallucinations are best understood as "'like' our perceptions but false" and as containing a similar meaning or sense in them.[43] It makes sense, for example, for patients to speak to someone who appears to them in a hallucination because the patient feels that the person is present at least in some way.[44]

Phenomenologically speaking, abnormal behavior found in a hallucination is an experience of a fantastical reality, as represented by the nonrational, which organizes itself around a positive structure, often represented by the rational. The best way to understand the behavior is in the way the rational and the nonrational are related to each other and manifest themselves as a relation within behavior. But, Merleau-Ponty does not stop here at the rational–nonrational relation, for, although it can be helpful to describe behavior in these terms, just as we often describe the body as an object in certain contexts and as a subject in others, he wants to move beyond these categories. In his famous hand-touching-hand example, he shows that the body can never only be an object because it is also always a subject experiencing the world.[45] The reversibility of the flesh, as it is later called, can be applied to abnormal behavior, showing that the deeper meaning can be seen only when we recognize the unity of the behavior. The behavior of a schizophrenic, for example, cannot fully be understood according to the rational and nonrational categories as we must know the intention and orientation of the person as a whole.[46] This reversibility also explains why Foucault has both the rational and the nonrational, even in their variations, present in each age because it is in their balance and unity that we find a meaning of the abnormal. Even in the contemporary times, where the priority is placed on the rational, this unity shows why elements of the nonrational cannot be forgotten but must still break through in "explosions" of madness, as Foucault describes.[47]

Therefore, Merleau-Ponty shows that the drive behind the historical structures to define madness is the existential reality that madness can be understood; there is a logic and meaning to madness because of the way it relates to human experience. Further, we found that the historical presence of the rational–nonrational relation was both confirmed and transcended in the phenomenological principles because abnormal behavior displays a unity and a sense due to the integration of the rational and nonrational capacities.

Hope of Application

In addition to providing a foundation for his historical structures, Merleau-Ponty offers Foucault the opportunity of applying his theory to the world of mental health. Merleau-Ponty's work in psychology has had a tremendous impact not only in philosophy but also in psychology because of Merleau-Ponty's analysis of real experiences and his willingness to employ some of the nosological language of psychology.[48] By using Merleau-Ponty's work as a point of entry, we can also make Foucault's work relevant to the current psychological world. Foucault speaks about many of the same conditions and disorders as Merleau-Ponty, and thus, by pairing the existential account with the historical account of a disorder, we can apply Foucault's work to specific situations.

Looking again at schizophrenia as an example, we can demonstrate the benefits of synthesizing Foucault and Merleau-Ponty's respective descriptions of the disorder (see table 5.1). In Merleau-Ponty's account of schizophrenia, as we saw above, he demonstrates how a hallucination is not an experience of an alternate reality, but an altered reality, where the objective world has a distorted subjective layer placed on top of it. Foucault's historical account of hallucinations adds another element to this feeling of distorted reality. He shows that since the classical age, hallucinations have often been intertwined with guilt because the person was seen as having an "error of mind," specifically due to an error in "physical truth."[49] Owing to the classical moral lens that we discussed earlier, the person exhibiting this error received an ethical condemnation by society. Yet even in present day, although we have hidden away this idea of moral failing, the feeling of guilt is often found in those who experience mental illness. Foucault writes:

> Psychopathology might feign surprise at finding feelings of guilt [*culpabilité*] mixed in with mental illness, but they had been placed there by the obscure groundwork of the classical age. It is still true today that our scientific and medical knowledge of madness rests implicitly on the prior constitution of an ethical experience of unreason.[50]

The feelings of guilt are not an accident but derive from the past historical judgment that the abnormal is rooted in an immoral relation to the nonrational. Condemnation continues to pervade the experiences of schizophrenia because, while the medical community would never speak of mental illness in ethical terms now, some of the methods still used today are designed to make the recipients feel a strong sense of culpability for their disorder.[51]

Although Foucault focuses on broad societal structures rather than individual experiences of schizophrenia, his description of the structures begins to make sense when they are linked to the individual. From the phenomenological descriptions, we already know the type of confusion that is felt due to the broken rational–nonrational relation evident in the behavior. With the basis of the confusion already present, we can then

Table 5.1. Schizophrenia in Merleau-Ponty and Foucault

Disorder	Brief Definition	Merleau-Ponty References	Foucault References	Present Equivalent
Schizophrenia (especially experiences of hallucinations)	A breakdown between thought, emotion, and behavior causing withdrawal from reality to fantasy; mental fragmentation, often accompanied by hallucinations	schizophrenia, PP 127, 294, 299–304, 309, 349–350, 355, 357, 359, 544n72, 551n94; hallucinations, PP 36, 150, 212, 231, 304, 308, 349–360, 551n84, 552n95, CPP 41–44, 177, 180–181, 359, 376–377	schizophrenia/psychosis, MIP 5 (including hebephrenia and catatonia), 7–8, 84, HM 201; hallucinations, MIP 48–49, HM 115–116, 132, 179, 193, 197, 201, 211–213, 239–241, 257, 277, 367–368, 619n	Related to schizophrenia spectrum disorders

Note. References refer to Merleau-Ponty's *Phenomenology of Perception* (PP) and *Child Psychology and Pedagogy* (CPP) and Foucault's *Mental Illness and Psychology* (MIP) and *History of Madness* (HM). The present equivalent is based on the 2013 *Diagnostic and Statistical Manual of Mental Disorders V* (DSM-5), the national guide for all psychopathological diagnoses in the United States.

further explain the disorder through the acknowledgment of the unspoken cultural structure that condemns it and sees a moral failure in errors of physical judgment. By starting with how an individual experiences the nonrational in a hallucination through the phenomenological, we can then connect that experience of the nonrational with the historical condemnation of that behavior. Here we find a deeper analysis for the experience of the nonrational exemplified both in a feeling of nonobjective space and in the feeling of guilt. On a practical level, the hope is that when we ground the historical in the phenomenological, we then have access to both perspectives on schizophrenia; this helps us better understand the experience of the disorder and better support the person struggling.[52]

Conclusion

To conclude, I have argued that Foucault's account of the abnormal, while persuasive, needs the phenomenological foundation of Merleau-Ponty. The societal perceptions of the abnormal are actually coming out of general truths found in human experience. The desire to define the abnormal according to our notion of the rational arises out of the existential reality that madness has meaning and connects to the logic of the lived world. The historical tension of the rational–nonrational derives from the reversibility of the flesh displayed even in disordered behavior. In other words, the phenomenological account tells us *why* abnormal behavior can be understood, while the historical account tells us *how* it plays out in present society. When we permit the phenomenological to ground the historical, we have an even greater understanding of the abnormal, which can allow us to care in better ways for those struggling with mental health.

One of the reasons that Merleau-Ponty's work offers ideal support for Foucault's account is because of the way it already opens itself up to further historical implications.[53] Foucault arguably fills a gap in Merleau-Ponty by offering historical accounts of the abnormal, but we must recognize that this type of exploration is already implied in Merleau-Ponty's method itself. Even at the end of the *Phenomenology of Perception*, Merleau-Ponty demonstrates the importance of history and writes rather movingly:

> I am a psychological and historical structure . . . And yet, I am free, not in spite of or beneath these motivations, but

rather by their means. For that meaningful life, that particular signification of nature and history that I am, does not restrict my access to the world; it is rather my means of communication with it. It is by being what I am at present, without any restrictions and without holding anything back, that I have a chance at progressing . . .⁵⁴

Merleau-Ponty accurately notes that it is through our awareness of being both a psychological and historical being that we can be free to be who we are, to push away the boundaries sometimes blocking our way and to progress toward greater freedom and greater understanding of the abnormal, as a shared aspect of human experience.

Notes

1. Philippe Sabot, "Entre psychologie et philosophie. Foucault à Lille, 1952–1955," in *Foucault à Münsterlingen. À l'origine de l'Histoire de la folie*, ed. Jean-Françoise Bert and Elisabetta Basso (Paris: EHESS, 2015), 110.

2. Didier Eribon, *Michel Foucault*, trans. Betsy Wing (Boston: Harvard University Press, 1992), 42, 48.

3. Jean-François Bert, "Retour à Münsterlingen," in Bert and Basso's *Foucault à Münsterlingen. À l'origine de l'Histoire de la folie*, 14.

4. To further investigate the way Foucault supports Merleau-Ponty, please see Judith Revel, *Foucault avec Merleau-Ponty* (Paris: Vrin, 2015) and Nick Crossley, *The Politics of Subjectivity: Between Foucault and Merleau-Ponty* (Aldershot: Avebury, 1994).

5. Michel Foucault, *Abnormal: Lectures at the Collège de France 1974–1975*, ed. Valerio Marchetti, Antonella Salomoni and Arnold I. Davidson, trans. Graham Burchell (New York: Picador, 2003), 325–326, 328. Although psychological practices have undergone changes, Foucault sees a consistent approach to mental health from the nineteenth century to contemporary times and calls it the "analytical consciousness of madness." See Michel Foucault, *History of Madness*, trans. Jonathan Murphy and Jean Khalfa (London: Routledge, 2006), 169–170.

6. In this chapter, I will be using the terms "rational" and "nonrational" for Foucault's terms "reason" and "unreason" (*déraison*) because it helps capture both Merleau-Ponty's and Foucault's understanding of the terms.

7. Foucault is also heavily influenced by Georges Canguilhem's account of the normal and the abnormal found in *The Normal and the Pathological* (Brooklyn: Zone Books, 1991). See the helpful exposition of Canguilhem in the section, "The Normal and the Pathological According to Goldstein and Canguilhem,"

in Jenny Slatman's chapter 1 of this volume, "Toward a Phenomenology of Abnormality," 24–26.

8. Foucault, *History of Madness*, 181.
9. Foucault, *History of Madness*, 28.
10. Foucault, *History of Madness*, 8–21, 169.
11. Foucault, *History of Madness*, 10, 13.
12. Foucault, *Abnormal*, 56.
13. Foucault, *History of Madness*, 164–174. The practical no longer speaks with the mad and physically excludes them from "rational" society. The enunciatory is seen in a quick pronouncement of madness without need for explanation. The analytic supports judgments of madness with supposed objective claims. These intertwining and contradictory perspectives create the complicated consciousness of madness of the classical age.
14. Foucault, *History of Madness*, 120.
15. Foucault, *History of Madness*, 47, 54.
16. Foucault, *History of Madness*, 72, 86.
17. Foucault, *Abnormal*, 57–58, 326, my italics.
18. Foucault, *History of Madness*, 475, 480, 509, 511.
19. Frédéric Gros, *Foucault et la folie* (Paris: Presses Universitaires de France, 1997), 39, my translation: "la folie, totalement aliénée dans les formes du savoir, ne fait même plus l'objet d'un partage."
20. Foucault, *Abnormal*, 60.
21. Foucault, *History of Madness*, 536.
22. Jean Khalfa, "Introduction," in Foucault's *History of Madness*, xiv.
23. One problem often discussed with Foucault's account is the issue of historical accuracy. We cannot address that here, but for an excellent overview and persuasive response to the debate on Foucault's historical validity in the *History of Madness*, see Colin Gordon, "Rewriting the History of Misreading," in *Rewriting the History of Madness: Studies in Foucault's 'Histoire de la folie,'* ed. Arthur Still and Irving Velody (London: Routledge, 1992), 167–184.
24. Tony Schirato, Geoff Danaher, and Jen Webb, *Understanding Foucault: A Critical Introduction*, 2nd ed. (London: Sage Publications, 2012), ix. For further thoughts on Foucault's relation to phenomenology, see Gros, *Foucault et la folie*, 125–126; Hubert L. Dreyfus and Paul Rabinow, *Michel Foucault: Beyond Structuralism and Hermeneutics*, 2nd ed., with an *Afterword by and an Interview with Michel Foucault* (Chicago: University of Chicago Press, 1983), 50, 161; and Todd May, "Foucault's Relation to Phenomenology," in *The Cambridge Companion to Foucault*, ed. Gary Gutting (Cambridge: Cambridge University Press, 2005), 284–311.
25. Angelos Evangelou, *Philosophizing Madness from Nietzsche to Derrida* (London: Palgrave Macmillan, 2017), 137. See also Peter Barham, "Foucault and the Psychiatric Practitioner," in Still and Velody's *Rewriting the History of Madness*, 47.

26. Words such as "perception" and "experience" are frequently used. See Jean Khalfa's comment on phenomenological vocabulary in his introduction: Jean Khalfa, "Introduction," in Foucault's *History of Madness*, xx.

27. Talia Welsh, "Translator's Introduction," in Maurice Merleau-Ponty, *Child Psychology and Pedagogy: The Sorbonne Lectures 1949–1952*, trans. Talia Welsh (Evanston, IL: Northwestern University Press, 2010), xiii, my italics.

28. Merleau-Ponty, "Hegel's Existentialism," in *Sense and Non-Sense*, trans. Hubert L. Dreyfus and Patricia Allen Dreyfus (Evanston, IL: Northwestern University Press, 1964), 63. This was originally published in *Les Temps modernes* in 1946.

29. I see the "irrational" as a type of the larger notion of the "nonrational." See my "At the Opening of Madness: An Exploration of the Nonrational with Merleau-Ponty, Foucault, and Kierkegaard," *Journal of Speculative Philosophy* 33, no. 3 (2019): 475–488.

30. Although Merleau-Ponty uses the term "abnormal" only a handful of times in *Phenomenology of Perception*, he does use the term "normal" quite often in order to show the contrast between the normal and the psychopathology. I employ "abnormal" in this contrasting sense to the "normal" and am especially concerned with its relation to experiences of madness.

31. Maurice Merleau-Ponty, *Phenomenology of Perception*, trans. Donald A. Landes (London: Routledge, 2012), 305, translation slightly altered; French: Merleau-Ponty, *Phénoménologie de la perception* (Paris: Gallimard, 1945), 345.

32. See William Hamrick's helpful article on Merleau-Ponty's use of normal and the abnormal: "Language and Abnormal Behavior: Merleau-Ponty, Hart and Laing," ed. Keith Hoeller, *Merleau-Ponty and Psychology, A Special Issue from the Review of Existential Psychology and Psychiatry* 18, nos. 1, 2 & 3 (1982–1983), 181–203.

33. Merleau-Ponty, *Phenomenology of Perception*, 299.

34. Merleau-Ponty, *Phenomenology of Perception*, 59.

35. M.C. Dillon, *Merleau-Ponty's Ontology* (Bloomington: Indiana Press University, 1988), 4.

36. Dillon, *Merleau-Ponty's Ontology*, 6.

37. Merleau-Ponty, *Phenomenology of Perception*, lxxxiv.

38. Merleau-Ponty, *Phenomenology of Perception*, 341.

39. Merleau-Ponty, *Phenomenology of Perception*, 50.

40. Talia Welsh, *The Child as Natural Phenomenologist: Primal and Primary Experience in Merleau-Ponty's Psychology* (Evanston, IL: Northwestern University Press, 2013), 43.

41. Merleau-Ponty, *Phenomenology of Perception*, 358, his italics, translation slightly modified; French: Merleau-Ponty, *Phénoménologie de la perception*, 400.

42. Merleau-Ponty, *Child Psychology and Pedagogy: The Sorbonne Lectures*, 177.

43. Welsh, *The Child as Natural Phenomenologist*, 43.

44. Patients can often distinguish between an actual person and an imaginary person, even if they continue to interact with the imaginary person in their hallucinations. See Susan Bredlau's excellent analysis of this phenomenon in the final section, "Schizophrenic Hallucination," of her chapter, "The Abnormalcy of 'Normalcy': Merleau-Ponty, Russon and the Normativity of Experience," in this volume (90–94). She explains, "For a person with schizophrenia . . . the hallucinatory aspects of experience are as, if not more, absorbing than the perceptual aspects of her experience even after these aspects have been explicitly identified as hallucinatory . . ." (91). Also, see Merleau-Ponty's discussion, *Phenomenology of Perception*, 349–360.

45. Merleau-Ponty, *Phenomenology of Perception*, 94.

46. One of the best examples of this is found in Merleau-Ponty's extended discussion on the disorders of the patient Schneider. It is only by recognizing how the dysfunction affects him as a whole that his behavior makes sense. See the excellent discussion on Schneider in the section, "The Case of Schneider: Merleau-Ponty's Dynamic Conception of Embodiment," in the Introduction to this volume by Talia Welsh and Susan Bredlau (2–9). For Merleau-Ponty's discussion, see *Phenomenology of Perception*, 105–140, 157–160, 174, 201–202.

47. Foucault has a notion of the flesh as well and, although it arises out of a different context than Merleau-Ponty's, it also aims to provide a unity to human experience. The complementarity between Merleau-Ponty and Foucault on the idea of the flesh is best seen in John Carvalho's article demonstrating how their two conceptions—Merleau-Ponty's ontology of the flesh and Foucault's genealogies of the flesh—are a folding over of one another, pointing to different aspects of the same reality. See John Carvahlo, "Folds in the Flesh: Merleau-Ponty/Foucault," in *Rereading Merleau-Ponty: Essays Beyond the Continental-Analytic Divide*, ed. Lawrence Hass and Dorothea Olkowski (Amherst, NY: Humanity Books, 2000), 308–309.

48. A sampling of the most recent work includes: Eric Matthews, *Body-Subjects and Disordered Minds: Treating the "Whole" Person in Psychiatry* (Oxford University Press, 2007); Shaun Gallagher, *How the Body Shapes the Mind* (Oxford: Oxford University Press, 2005), 244–246; Andrew J. Felder and Brent Dean Robbins, "A Cultural-Existential Approach to Therapy: Merleau-Ponty's Phenomenology of Embodiment and Its Implications for Practice," *Theory & Psychology* 21, no. 3 (2011); Matthew Broome et al., *The Maudsley Reader in Phenomenological Psychiatry* (Cambridge: Cambridge University Press, 2012); Louis A. Sass, Jennifer Whiting, and Josef Parnas, "Mind, Self and Psychopathology: Reflections on Philosophy, Theory and the Study of Mental Illness," *Theory & Psychology* 10, no. 1 (2000); Scott D. Churchill and Frederick J. Wertz, "An Introduction to Phenomenological Research in Psychology: Historical, Conceptual, and Methodological Foundations," in *The Handbook of Humanistic Psychology: Theory, Research and Practice*, 2nd ed., ed. Kirk J. Schneider, J. Fraser Pierson and James F. T. Bugental (Los Angeles: Sage Publications, 2015), 275–296.

49. Foucault, *History of Madness*, 241.

50. Foucault, *History of Madness*, 91. French: Foucault, *Histoire de la folie à l'âge classique* (Paris: Gallimard, 1972), 127.

51. Foucault, *History of Madness*, 463–511. The methods, for example, of the famous reformers Samuel Tuke and Philippe Pinel to manipulate guilt in their patients have in turn influenced practices used today.

52. For an excellent example of how to bring these perspectives together in relation to schizophrenia, see Louise Phillips, *Mental Illness and the Body: Beyond Diagnosis* (New York: Routledge, 2006).

53. While Merleau-Ponty's work on history was prematurely cut short, it still points to the necessity of including the historical element in our understanding of the human. His interest in history is seen in his *Adventures of the Dialectic*, trans. Joseph Bien (Evanston: Northwestern University Press, 1973) and other later works. If he had lived longer, many scholars argue that he would have continued to pursue the impact of history on human experience. Foucault, in his own way, carried on this project through his detailed philosophical explorations of history.

54. Merleau-Ponty, *Phenomenology of Perception*, 482–483.

Part II

Practical Phenomenological Applications of Merleau-Ponty's Theories of Normality, Abnormality, and Pathology

Chapter 6

Meandering Peripheries

A Ground without Figure for Relief

ADAM BLAIR

Introduction

In this chapter, I unground Merleau-Ponty's use of figure-ground structure. In the *Phenomenology of Perception*, Merleau-Ponty argues that a figure-ground structure is foundational to the sense-making of one's visual world.[1] Beginning from the most basic visual sensations, he builds upon the figure-ground of one's visual field as if from a cornerstone, translating it into isomorphic structures of attention,[2] decision making,[3] habit,[4] language,[5] desire (or, more broadly, affect),[6] and, in his later works, ontology[7] (where he also states that "to be conscious" is to "have a figure on a ground").[8] However, I want to revisit this very first moment when Merleau-Ponty establishes figure-ground as a basic fact of the visual field, taking for granted its necessity and ubiquity. Given Merleau-Ponty's methodological reliance on this initial claim regarding visual perception, undermining the necessary structuring of vision according to figure-ground would invite us to rethink the other existential modalities that build upon and make use of such a structure. This shattering of figure-ground as a necessary perceptual cornerstone would open new possibilities for all existential dimensions, revealing underexplored variations of bodily life and experience.⁹ By challenging the introduction of figure-ground, I hope to undermine Merleau-Ponty's overreaching claim to the ubiquity of one form of perceptual life.

I begin by performing a phenomenology of my own visual world. My right eye is "normal," while I characterize my left eye as opening upon a ground without figure. Through this critical phenomenological study, I think through what a visual field without a figure means, for vision and for perception itself. "Figure-ground" gives Merleau-Ponty the language to discuss a hinge between the determinate and the indeterminate—the real presence of ambiguity that tends toward clarity. By introducing an abnormal body into the discussion, I intend to show that the world does not always tend toward such determinacy. Furthermore, I argue that one need not always define indeterminacy in opposition to the determinate—thereby rendering it merely a negation—but that one can encounter indeterminacy on its own, generative terms. While Merleau-Ponty may have famously stated that we must "recognize the indeterminate as a positive phenomenon,"[10] I will show how his own treatment of indeterminacy implicitly undermines this commitment in favor of an indeterminacy that tends toward determinacy. I want to embrace Merleau-Ponty's promise of a positive indeterminacy without the crutch of an implicit optimality that never lets this indeterminacy run its course.

I am not turning my back on Merleau-Ponty to rethink perception from square one. Instead, I am exploring how a different relationship to figure-ground opens new and constructive horizons for our encounter with indeterminacy. I challenge here not the presence of figure-ground within ordinary perception and sense-making, but its ubiquity and necessity within all forms of perception and embodiment. Although Merleau-Ponty himself does describe perceptual forms that are not structured according to figure-ground, these cases are cited as pathological and debilitating in their deviation from the norm. For instance, when discussing language acquisition, Merleau-Ponty cites a case of paraphasia that is cast as a failure of the speaker to accomplish the "essential" task of differentiating figures from a ground.[11] Upon establishing figure-ground as necessary for visual perception, Merleau-Ponty presumes the structure to be an essential facet of all sense-making and thereby establishes a perceptual norm that enables him to diagnose pathological cases of perception as lacking in some important regard. By undermining the supposedly most elementary and ubiquitous instance of figure-ground perception, I call into question such overreaching claims. For Merleau-Ponty, the good type of ambiguity, or indeterminacy, is that which tends toward a determinate end—the pathological cases trapped in unending indeterminacy are, as we will see, a bad kind of ambiguity or indeterminacy. Rather than writing off such nonnormative bodies as exceptions that prove the rule, I will press upon Merleau-Ponty, refiguring and regrounding his tools and insights to uncover a path toward accounting for a greater variety of forms of perception and being-in-the-world. Let us look to an unresolvable, never-ending indeterminacy as a positive phenomenon, and see what happens to our world.

A Description of my "Dream Eye"

I begin with a scientifically objective account of my visual field: I was born with "normal" vision in my right eye and with what the doctors diagnosed as Morning Glory Syndrome in my left eye. This very rare birth "defect," as it is officially defined, is due to an underdeveloped optic nerve. A large cavity within my optic disc has led to an increased number of enlarged blood vessels around the optic nerve of my retina. The resulting knot of vessels and nerve fibers, spread too wide and containing a white center, resembles the Morning Glory flower. The optic nerve of my left eye still functions, but the result is a field of vision alien to my right eye.[12]

As a child, my family and friends would ask me about my left eye. My family knew of the abnormality, of course, but the strangeness would announce itself to others through my eye's tendency to wander on its own, never making eye contact with others or matching the direction of my right eye. I tried to explain how I saw the world through this strange opening, but words could never do the experience justice. One day I finally realized what the visual field felt like: "It's like when you're in a dream," I told my father. "Everything blurs, just out of reach. It isn't far away or dark, and you can't quite see it, but you still can. Almost. Like when it's hard to remember something." From then on, my family called it my "dream eye," and I am certain that my access to two different ways of seeing is what has brought me to phenomenology and questions of perception.

When I cover my right eye and look through my dream eye alone, I see a vague haze. I can make out fuzzy shapes, movement, and color but no definite lines, edges, or localizable qualities. At the heart of the strangeness of this vision is that it is only peripheral, with no ability to focus on a single point. There isn't a black hole or emptiness in the center of my visual field. It also isn't the case that everything is so blurry that the center is out of focus and blends with its surroundings. Instead, there is no focal center; the way that the visual field is structured is fundamentally different from that of my "normal" eye. The field as a whole strikes my eye all at once, with no condensed line of vision or direct gaze. The margins are defined spatially, perhaps, but not in terms of their focal relation to the center or my ability to grasp them. Instead, all areas of the visual field are equally accessible, all at once—and this access is slippery, distant, and restless. Due to my nerve fibers' wide spreading, my gaze is smeared across the whole field, never condensing, and thus never unified or unitary. It is not that I have multiple gazes incapable of finding a central focus; there is no condensing activity of vision at all. The field as a whole is homogeneously focused despite a heterogeneity of shape, color, and movement. I could equally observe that the field is homogenously unfocused—its homogeneity in relation to the grasp of its gaze defies our typical language about vision, for I precisely lack the contrast of "in focus" and "out of focus" that gives the act of focusing its meaning. The field is differentiated, yet I do not look at any one thing, as my look itself is all-at-once, spread and diffuse.

Several people have encouraged me to paint a picture of my dream eye's visual field to make its strangeness accessible to others, but this would not work. It isn't that I am not a good enough painter—the structural difference between my dream eye's gaze and any "normal" spectator's gaze is insurmountable based upon supposed perceptual content alone. If I painted the dreamy ambiguous haze, a normally sighted person would still be able to investigate it one point at a time. The visual field of my dream eye is alien not in *what* it is seeing, but in *how* it sees—precisely calling into question what "perceptual content" meaningfully refers to—given that perception is a living activity. My dream eye's power of vision is its unique grasp on the world, and therefore not located in the inert, empirical images that it encounters in some Cartesian theater.

When I cover my right eye, the habit of focusing with this "normal" eye forces me to orient my underused dream eye toward objects, trying to coax a gaze out of a gazeless field, edges and regions out of a distantly fluid atmosphere. I attempt to focus on one region of the distant blur. While I cannot visually focus, my attention can somewhat pick out familiar objects and shapes given cognitive mediation—especially if I have looked to the scene with my right eye already. But neither my gaze nor my attention can ever rest within the field of vision, as my attention is always swirling and meandering, always spread over the resistant fog. Seeing through my right eye in normal waking life has habituated me to attend directly to that which I visually focus upon. Therefore, when I attempt to focus upon something in the field of my dream eye, an irresolvable tension erupts as this singular attentive activity doesn't find a unified gaze to ride into the world or any things to focus upon. Any given region of the field inevitably escapes my attention and resists investigation; just like the feeling of a hazy dream or a distant memory, everything, even the "center" of the field, feels hollow and far off—always on the margin. I am grasping but cannot wrap my gaze around any object as it slips and slides away, melting into the all-at-once. My typical, thing-focused attention doesn't find a world that correlates to its activity—it finds only echoes and shadows, drifting away.

The best way to make this apparent is to ask you to perform a brief exercise. If you are sighted and able, cover or close one of your eyes to get the monocular vision that I see. Now, stare directly at a point somewhere near where you are—a corner of the room, a dark spot on a tree, or the pointed corner of this book. Don't let your eye leave this point. Next, shift your attention to something on the periphery of your visual field without redirecting your gaze. Try to investigate your surroundings, but never leave this point as your center of visual focus. Attempt to gather the colors in front of you, the pictures on the wall, your own hands moving around, the world out of the window beside you, the words on this page—but never let your gaze leave its focal anchor.

This exercise for a normal gaze remains radically different from my dream eye since normal sight experiences a focal center to its field in contrast to an unfocused periphery. However, having one's attention directed to the visual periphery begins to gesture toward the strangeness that I feel when I cover my right eye; there is an inherent tension in bringing one's focus to the visual field's margins, and, as I hope you noticed, it is difficult to do. The periphery is out of focus in a visual sense, but it is also attentively out of reach, outstripping it of a simple visual deficiency. The vision of my dream eye cannot *grasp* anything, for there is either no direct gaze or only direct gaze—I am precisely missing the contrast between a figure and a ground that mutually shape one another. Nothing settles into place, and everything remains hovering at a perpetual distance. An attentive drive habituated to a condensed gaze finds frustration or uneasiness in the vague haze of an unfocused field.

My visual field is not undifferentiated or homogenous, but it does feel shapeless. It is indistinct not only in the images it encounters but vague in its very hold on the world.

Merleau-Ponty on Figure-Ground in Vision

I will now show how Merleau-Ponty's development of figure-ground structure, from the very beginning, takes for granted the normal structuring of visual perception. It will then be clear how my abnormal visual field challenges some of his far-reaching conclusions, while also supporting some of his other central claims.

In the *Phenomenology of Perception*, figure-ground structure appears within the first few pages after the introduction—when Merleau-Ponty discusses the puzzle of sensation.[13] Others before him characterized visual perception as the sum of many "punctual jolts," claiming that one's body senses individual colors before they are arranged into something that "makes sense" for conscious awareness. However, Merleau-Ponty wants to criticize this notion of pure impressions by returning to perceptual experience: I never encounter a bare quality in the world, but sense is always already present within the perceptual field. In other words, there is never mere sensation, but there is always perception—an insight of Gestalt psychology.

Merleau-Ponty begins this argument with the most basic example: a "white patch against a homogenous background."[14] The borders of this patch are contiguous with its ground, and yet, the patch "stands out" from this ground, for the patch's "color is denser and somehow more resistant than the background's color."[15] Merleau-Ponty calls this patch a figure and notes that whether we look to this figure or its ground, each point of the image already speaks for more than itself, as each element is in a contextual relationship with the whole and the other parts. An individual point in this field is never merely this point alone—that is, it is not experienced as a mere sensation—but is experienced fundamentally in relationship to its participation as the "ground," the "figure," or the border in-between. Therefore, there are never pure impressions of mere sensation, but always perceptual sense.[16]

This example can be difficult to parse through, since Merleau-Ponty uses the terms "figure" and "ground" to refer to the elements of his example, as well as discrete conceptual tools used to describe structural aspects of the perceptual field which opens onto these same elements. To help with this distinction, keep in mind that he notes: "each point [of the visual field] in turn can only be perceived as a figure on a background."[17] Whether we look to a region of the white patch, to its ground, or to the border in-between, this visual focal point becomes our perceptual figure charged with the sense of its contrast with its periphery.

The important feature of the white patch on a ground of color is the presence of heterogeneity—such contrast is necessary for one to focus on a "point" to begin with, and thus for one to have a perceptual figure. This is precisely why Merleau-Ponty concludes from this discussion that "a truly homogeneous area, offering *nothing to perceive*, cannot be given to *any perception*."[18] Our most basic example must have at least two colors. Otherwise, one's gaze cannot grasp anything, for it lacks the contrast necessary to focus upon a point, which is, in other words, to bring forth a figure. As Merleau-Ponty asserts, the "very definition of the perceptual phenomenon" is "a figure against a background."[19]

Thus, Merleau-Ponty's critique of pure sensation gives rise to the figure-ground structure, since perception always finds the presence of immediate, contextual contrast within its heterogenous field. However, Merleau-Ponty's analysis of the patch example takes for granted that, for him, it is not only the differing of colors that provide the contrast necessary for perceptual sense but also a focal center that picks out a "point"—amidst a vague ground that then throws this point into relief. Merleau-Ponty assumes that the visual capacity of a given perceiver is capable of grasping the world through focusing. However, such an act of focusing may depend upon the contrast of a heterogenous field, and I argue that the heterogeneity necessary for there to be vision need not necessarily be in terms of clarity and indistinctness.

It is in taking for granted the structure of this figure and ground as one of focus and fog that Merleau-Ponty calls us to "recognize the indeterminate as a positive phenomenon," with the "region surrounding the visual field" described as "indeterminate."[20] Merleau-Ponty observes that in normal vision the indeterminate haze of my periphery is itself positive; its atmospheric vagueness throws the object of my gaze into sharp focus while being available as a possible future figure. To focus on something is precisely to have it emerge from an indeterminate background and become determinate by virtue of its contrast to this surrounding indeterminacy. In other words, the determinacy of a figure and the vagueness of its ground mutually constitute one another. According to Merleau-Ponty, if my visual world were not structured according to figure-ground, then sense-making in this dimension would be impossible.[21] The figure and the ground themselves are never absolutely determinable, but our field is always structured according to a tension between something that is in focus and its indistinct, unfocused background. Without the tension born of this contrast, there functionally would be no motivation or intentional mechanism to pull a figure into focus against its background, and therefore no way to look at any one thing. As Merleau-Ponty writes, "the perceptual 'something' is always in the middle of some other thing, it always belongs to a 'field.'"[22] As Merleau-Ponty demonstrates, to perceive by definition is to focus upon (visually or otherwise) one differentiated element against an indeterminate ground; to collapse an entire field into homogeneity is to remove the contrast necessary for focusing, and thus is to remove the very possibility of perceiving things to begin with. However, why must perception necessarily be tied to the activity of focusing upon things?

The description of my dream eye does not contradict the claim that we can never perceive a homogenous area. Likewise, the basic fact of sense always already being present within the perceptual field does not seem to be up for revision. My dream eye's visual field is not homogenous or void of sense, since it is differentiated. I can see a blue spot in a given direction that is likely a human body, or movement and light hovering in and around what seems to be a window, or some unreadable text on the page below. Each of these I can generally attend to, and each is broadly apprehended according to its contrast with its surroundings, yet I can never discretely attend to any one object or visually focus on one region of my field. Even in the case of my dream eye's visual field, Merleau-Ponty seems correct to argue that perceptual sense (and therefore any perception at all) needs the contrast of a heterogenous field. However, despite the heterogenous world of my dream eye, its grasp—the focus of its gaze—remains homogenous and constant throughout the whole of its field. This is something that Merleau-Ponty cannot account for in his leap to considering the focused-upon "points" of the field as its most elementary perceptual "figures." In other words, my dream eye attests that, while contrast is necessary for there to be perception, one's perceptual field need not be spatially organized as a figure upon a background nor according to a tension borne of a difference in clarity.

I can reliably attend to a region of the haze and apprehend its sense without absolutely grasping any one *thing*—and yet, the field is neither homogenous nor composed of mere impressions. It does not follow, as

Merleau-Ponty seems to imply, that if contrast is necessary for perception then a sharp figure of a thing against an indeterminate background is also necessary. Merleau-Ponty characterizes "things" as individuated perceptual stuff that we can dive into focusing upon ever narrower regions as new figures find relief in backgrounds.[23] Indeed, Merleau-Ponty defines visual objects as that which one can focus more and more finely (or broadly) upon within their perceptual field.[24] However, my dream eye cannot find the attentive attitude necessary to "gear"[25] in to any one thing. This inability accords with Merleau-Ponty: the world of my left eye finds no visual objects to begin with, since it lacks a controllable, unified gaze with which it can investigate its world. However, what Merleau-Ponty does not consider is that my left eye perceives nonetheless, despite its lack of focused, object-oriented exploration.

The deeper claim of Gestalt psychology—that sense is always already present—can still hold, but it need not arise from the contrast between the determinate and indeterminate. To be sensed, an experiential given need not be determinate nor tending toward determinacy nor even determinable. As the field of my dream eye attests, a heterogenous area can be explored generally and indeterminately while remaining perceptual and meaningful. I need not anchor myself in any one thing to perceive it, but I can coast over and around the whole ground all at once. It can be true that horizons give clarity to things, but all perception need not be of things (or their attendant horizons) to begin with. In the subsequent section, I will look more deeply into this notion of determinacy within Merleau-Ponty's theory of perception remaining true to Merleau-Ponty's overall philosophical enterprise while accounting for the possibility of an experience that lacks a normative figure-ground structure.

In/Determinacy

Through the aforementioned example of the colored patch, Merleau-Ponty's investigation of figure-ground structure begins from the "dense" and "resistant" color of the white patch and works backward.[26] Merleau-Ponty explains how the patch finds unity as a patch, before recognizing that this patch is placed upon its background.[27] The emphasis here reveals that the background is rendered secondary—it is that which gives definition to the figure. Though Merleau-Ponty himself might characterize the figure and the ground as mutually reciprocal, there seems to be a bias that places the determinate at the forefront; the indeterminacy of my peripheral vision is seen as a function of the perception of this determinate object. Indeed, the very use of the term "in-determinacy" shows that it is precisely that which is *not* determinate, a negation of what is under consideration. This emphasis on the determinate over the indeterminate orients Merleau-Ponty's phenomenology to privilege clearly defined objects, rendering a normativity to perceptual experience as he describes it.

Merleau-Ponty argues that objects themselves are unified within perception rather than unified after the fact through a principle of association. In an example that is worth quoting at length, Merleau-Ponty describes how he is walking on a beach toward a ship that has run aground. He notes that:

> [If] the funnel or the mast emerges with the forest that borders the dune, then there will be a moment in which these details suddenly reunite with the boat and become welded to it. As I approached . . . I merely felt that the appearance of the object was about to change, that something was imminent in this tension, as the storm is imminent in the clouds. The spectacle was suddenly reorganized, satisfying my vague expectation . . . The unity of the object is established upon the presentiment of an imminent order that will, suddenly, respond to questions that are merely latent in the landscape. It will resolve a problem only posed in the form of a vague uneasiness . . .[28]

He uses this example to argue that we do not encounter the world as either a sum of discrete impressions or an undifferentiated whole. He argues that if it is true that he felt this tension and then witnessed the ship correctly organize itself, then he could not have been the one to constitute the ship, nor could he have constructed a representation of it from given sense impressions. While I agree with Merleau-Ponty's conclusion that we do not encounter simple impressions and combine these into perceptual wholes, I want to pause and question how he arrives at this conclusion.

In this example of a ship that has run aground, Merleau-Ponty experiences a vague indeterminacy amongst the tangle of trees and the ship's wooden parts. In retrospect, after clarifying this tangle into its components, he notices that this indeterminacy was experienced as a felt tension. There is a "vague uneasiness" he feels when he confuses the mast of the ship with the trees on the beach. His perception is ambiguous, and this creates a felt tension as it strains toward determinacy. Following Husserl,[29] we can say that the perceptual field tends toward "optimality," wherein objects at the "proper" distance are perceived as they "ought" to be—as discrete, determinate, and unified. The indeterminacy, though a positive phenomenon, is nevertheless in service of this optimality. There is a normativity inherent to Merleau-Ponty's characterization of perception, wherein indeterminacy is present to be resolved. The ground is there to throw the figure into relief, or to become the next figure itself. Perception, therefore, becomes a perpetual process of pulling things out of an otherwise ambiguous atmosphere. Just as the conceptual work of the figure-ground structure ushers in a visual world of focal points and their defining margins, it assumes the body's world as one of thingly objects.

I, however, do not encounter discrete objects with my dream eye, for its strangeness is precisely that there is no thing thrown into relief. In this abnormal visual field, there is no individual, perceptual something but instead a field of qualities of varying degrees of determinacy. I have no figures, no objects, no self-contained wholes or felt tensions that solicit rearrangement—just the shock of open and smooth space, movement, and color.

This proposed and inherent normativity is further evidenced in the "Space" chapter of *Phenomenology of Perception*. Merleau-Ponty considers that illusions that present depth[30] are effective not due to their associational constructions but to the motivations inherent within my sense-giving.[31] He writes that "my gaze always attempts to see *something*," and that this "something" is established by a certain norm, such that we will inevitably tend to see a given organization as that which puts it into "perfect symmetry." He goes on to argue that "our visual field always tends toward the more determinate."[32] As we have seen, this is a reliance upon a visual field structured according to normal anatomy. It assumes not only that one can see objects determinately but also that one will prereflectively strive to see them in this clarifying light.

By employing the description of my left eye's visual experience, I challenge Merleau-Ponty's privileging of determinacy and seek to push on his theoretical agenda by thinking through a new starting point. Rather than assuming a perceptual field geared toward determination, I will start from the field of my dream eye. That is, I will begin with the pathological case rather than the norm to understand how this might change the reading of determinacy and perception as a whole. My dream eye experiences the aforementioned tension-toward-clarity, but perpetually and without any release or satisfaction. My consciousness strains in its desperate search for discrete objects, but it can never pin them down, as its world is one of margins, a field of confused peripheries-without-centers. The world of my dream eye is one in which the ship and trees never resolve into their "proper" and determinate unities and are only vague and atmospheric semblances to begin with, ceaselessly unsettled. The dreamy perceptual field can only ask general questions of my gaze, which it can never definitively answer. My gaze does not condense onto objects within its world, and therefore its world is not one of things in settled space—not the perfect perspectival equilibrium of Merleau-Ponty's harmonious horizons and thingly things. My gaze is a smearing, a suffusion, a spiraling dispersion—the field doesn't open onto a world, but it meanders just in front of the world, or perhaps just behind it. There is no descending of the gaze into objects, but airy light floating without respite. Merleau-Ponty argues against Descartes's claims that we cannot trust our sensations since we might be dreaming, for we already have a "sense of the real"[33] prior to any dream or experience of waking life. Despite this, my left eye's world is real *and* dreamy, and its dreaminess is its reality. Subsequently, it is necessary to rethink what the real is for perception to account for the experience of abnormal bodies.

As speculated in the chapter's first section, the felt tension in my dream eye may be due to my everyday reliance upon my right eye, which sees the world in a "normal" way (besides its monocular vision). When I look at a scene with my dream eye, it strains in vain to penetrate objects with a gaze, as my body seeks its familiar grasp on the world. This fuzzy, evaporating ground, just out of reach, foils my habit of attending to the visual world with a condensed gaze. My perceptual world's inherent normativity is born of my right eye's "normal" anatomy, thus creating a tension in my left eye that will never be satisfied.

I am in the unique epistemic position of being able to compare a field structured by figure-ground and one void of this structure. However, this also means I cannot entirely habituate myself to this strangeness, nor completely immerse myself in its unsettled world. It is conceivable that one might have a body that experiences its world entirely as my dream eye does—as an indeterminate flux without condensation. I very well might have been born with two dream eyes, and therefore not have been conditioned by the thingly world of my right eye's visual field. Such a case would not result in a senseless homogenous field or an absolute cacophony, for I still apprehend differentiations and can work over my dream eye's perceptual field. This form of indeterminacy would be on its own terms, rather than an indeterminacy defined by and against a normative determinacy. Such ambiguity would not be asking the same questions of its perceiver, just as such a perceiver would not feel an "uneasiness" in their world that needs resolution in clarity. This perceptual structure would take a shape entirely different from the call-and-response form that Merleau-Ponty experiences on the beach, and that my right eye feels in its comforting world of things.

The subject of determinacy is at the heart of Merleau-Ponty's project, and therefore the possibility of such a body has wide-ranging consequences. In fact, one can characterize the definitive activity of perception for Merleau-Ponty as making the indeterminate determinate, in varying degrees of existence. To perceive *this* piece of paper is to pick it out from the horizon of possible choices laid out before me. It requires me to focus on it over and against the indeterminate haze of the room that was in my periphery but a moment ago, and to activate my *general* power of expression by turning to *this* object and the word (along with its rich layers of inexhaustible sense) "paper." Perception perpetually makes figures out of grounds and grounds of figures, and, through this activity, it is able to always make sense of the perceptual field—one discrete and determined figure at a time.

But if determinacy did not figure in a perceptual world, it is conceivable that discrete objects as such would not present themselves—we find ourselves in the world first, but our world is dependent upon the powers of our body. If my body is incapable of grasping visual determinacy, then how would I find myself? What sort of finding might this be, and what sort of self? Considering such a radically different being-in-the-world requires us to rethink the body-schema, the division of the senses (and their synesthetic communication), and what reality is and means for perceptual life.

This line of questioning is counter to Merleau-Ponty's assumptions within the *Phenomenology of Perception*, as he assumes the necessary ubiquity of figure-ground structure within perception. My dream eye is therefore a perceptual experience that he never thematizes or entertains as a possibility. Merleau-Ponty goes on in the aforementioned passage on depth and illusion to describe how a clarifying, focusing gaze is inevitable for us because of the world we find ourselves in. Perception's activity of making-determinate is not a mere psychological curiosity—it has its roots in our very mode of being. He writes that the determinacy that my gaze tends toward is "recommended" by the way that phenomena present themselves to me:

> In a normal visual field the segregation of planes and contours is irresistible, and, for example, when I walk along the boulevard, I am unable to see the intervals between the trees as things and trees themselves as the background . . . I am aware in this experience of . . . gathering together a sense that is scattered throughout the phenomena, and of saying what they themselves want to say.[34]

In everyday perceptual experience, I encounter discrete and determinate objects through the "inspection of my gaze," a gaze that is "neither originary nor constituting, [but] solicited or motivated. Every focusing is always a focusing on something that presents itself as something to be focused upon."[35]

Merleau-Ponty here defines the gaze as "this perceptual genius underneath the thinking subject who knows how to give to things the correct response *they are waiting for* in order to exist in front of us."[36] He writes that to focus on something is, definitively, to "make it count as a figure."[37] This collection of claims throughout the *Phenomenology of Perception* point to Merleau-Ponty's reliance upon the determinacy of objects as normative both for visual experience and for the world itself, as it is the tree out there that solicits my vision to pick it out as one discrete thing. In being true to Merleau-Ponty's central project, rethinking the very structure of the gaze that is solicited by the world calls us to reconsider the world itself and the nature of its solicitation. If not a world of things, then a world of what?[38]

I understand Merleau-Ponty's project as an attempt to blur the boundary between the subject and the object, and as a gesturing toward an intentionality that uncovers what is already being offered to it by the world. Yet the picture becomes more complicated when we consider how a nonnormative body idiosyncratically encounters its world. While Merleau-Ponty delivers important insights regarding the interplay of body and world, we can no longer assume all of the structures that Merleau-Ponty offers as ubiquitous and necessary. Rather than simply writing off deviant perceptual lives as not "correct,"[39] we ought to allow their fruits to enrich our phenomenological frameworks. Rather than explaining away abnormal perceptual forms to maintain the world of the anatomically average, classical phenomenologist, we ought to allow our notion of the world itself to be expanded by the experiential possibilities offered by different bodies. What would it mean for the world itself to be "waiting for" my dream eye to see it in an inherent, irresolvable ambiguity?

The gaze of my dream eye has no correct response for the world within the terms set by Merleau-Ponty (and by my right eye), as it is unable to shift its focus or to settle upon any one thing. Therefore, if it were habituated to its own world, this world would not be "waiting" for its indeterminacy to be resolved, nor would it be asking visual questions of my body through confused fields or obscured perspectives, for my body would not be situated as one that could be called upon in such a way to begin with. Merleau-Ponty is correct to argue that my gaze does not constitute its world, nor is it merely passive in the face of a wholly active world—but the reciprocal play of perception between my dream eye and its world is not one of figure-ground. As Merleau-Ponty notes, in ordinary vision my gaze is solicited to see things according to a determinate arrangement of optimally unified and discrete objects. This tendency is not wholly constituted by my gaze nor imposed upon by the world, but it is in their union that my visual field is able to find things "where they are" as they present themselves to me. I am both active and passive before a world that is also both active and passive.

In the case of my dream eye, it is simultaneously true that the field washes over me, pressing up against me out of my control while also remaining static and at a distance in its indistinctness. The holistic sense and style of my world is radically different through my dream eye, as I lack a distinct handle on things. I am less a participant in a felt location holding the world at a distance, and more of an openness that is spread out, smeared between here and there, hovering—evaporated and dissolved more than condensed. The important facts underlying figure-ground remain: the field is differentiated in a very basic way, I have a perspective, I am neither wholly constituted nor constituting, and I am free to shift my attention or have it solicited by the world, but by losing the traditional structure of figure-ground, each of these perceptual facts gains new meanings and possibilities. The body is still my transcendental possibility for perceiving the world, but by rethinking what is necessary regarding the structure of these powers, it is possible to more deeply appreciate the many varied ways a human can live their world. And since this world itself is what calls upon a given body to act, the world itself will shift its contours for the different powers open to different bodies.

Some may wonder how a body that lacks a traditional hold on things will achieve any kind of practical action in the world. How could one eat a meal, talk with friends, or ride a bike in a perceptual world wholly structured like the field of my dream eye? I cannot say what leading this life would be, for I have not lived it. However, I think we ought to consider Merleau-Ponty's insight that our bodies develop in conjunction with their worlds. Therefore, we should not consider the complement of an indeterminate milieu as a disadvantage in our world (except for, of course, in the environments and social worlds already crafted for normal bodies). Instead, I hope this exploration has opened the door to considering what one's entire being-in-the-world might be from an indeterminate perceptual field to begin with. We should not presume a perceptual apparatus incapable of clarity as a lack. Consider a body habituated to indeterminacy, a mind that flows rather than anchors, a field that spreads instead of condenses, an eye that encounters its field as you see your periphery. While we cannot live a life other than our own, I hope that the intellectual play can help to open the perceptual possibilities of our worlds—and also help us better reflect upon our theoretical suppositions.

Conclusion

In conclusion, I will gesture toward some future regions of exploration that the possibility of my dream eye has opened up, and that I could not expand upon here. The first avenue of inquiry that this study opens up is to consider how indeterminacy might become a constructive force, rather than something only to resolve. Merleau-Ponty in his discussion of habit embraces the tension between the determinate and indeterminate—pinpointing this shared, in-between space as the place where we can build and revise our habits.[40] As we concretize indeterminate possibilities, we have a degree of freedom in determining them, and by selecting repeated possibilities, we can incorporate this horizonal possibility deeper and deeper into our bodily powers. However, by devalorizing determinacy, we can ask: what would it mean to look to the other side of this in-between space? Rather than using the in-between space where determinacy and indeterminacy are both present to increasingly shape our world's possibilities through habituation, what if we unraveled our own habits and expectations by tipping the scale toward the indeterminate?

We could introduce more novelty into our worlds by pushing ever closer to the horizon rather than using the horizon to more finely shape the figure of our present through habit.

Further, this shift of emphasis within Merleau-Ponty's thought calls upon us to reconsider his ontological foundation. The "flesh" embraces—and perhaps is—the process of making the indeterminate determinate, particularizing the general possibilities of a body and its world as a metaphysical principle.[41] But this focus on determination leads us back, in my view, to an object-oriented view of the world. I want to complicate this picture by pressing on the hard line Merleau-Ponty seems to draw between the determinate and indeterminate, which is traceable to his ocularcentrism. This ocularcentrism reveals itself, I believe, through a normative drive for control and clarity in the face of an ambiguous world. Indeed, in "Child's Relations with Others," Merleau-Ponty highlights that "it is by the means of vision that one can sufficiently dominate and control objects,"[42] and vision is the paradigmatic perceptual experience in both "Eye and Mind" and *The Visible and the Invisible*.[43]

But what would it look like (or sound like, or feel like) to think of the world not as a vague horizon becoming particularized through the activity of perception, but as a constant mixing and mingling together of different degrees of indeterminacy as various horizons interact and resonate?[44] If we started from my dream eye, the resonance in the music of a non-melodic composition[45] would be closer to a paradigm of Being than a Cézanne painting. As soon as the listener's attention tries to settle on a melodic line, it is pulled in another direction, spread thin, and then pushed in all directions—never able to find clear direction, where one's attention fails to settle on a single thing and attends only to a vague constellation of shifting, multiplicitous impressions.[46] If this were taken as our (figureless) ground of Being, what possibilities might open? We can also revisit where Merleau-Ponty isomorphically institutes the figure-ground structure from desire and attention to intersubjectivity and freedom, in order to rethink how these different perceptual dimensions could be understood in terms of a generative indeterminacy. How do we consider the structure of a desire that does not take a discrete object as its end, or a decision that is not made based upon determinate choices but an open and irresolvable field, or a self that never reflects upon itself as an individual?

Finally, I believe that this current investigation calls upon us to reconsider Merleau-Ponty's use of pathology. Rather than considering Schneider's strangeness as an exception that proves the rule,[47] what would it mean to consider his perceptual world on its own terms, and attempt to account for it in our theory of perception? As we have seen, we need not contradict Merleau-Ponty entirely. However, we can instead press upon his claims of ubiquity and necessity, thereby allowing for a wider range of possible bodies and experiences to be accounted for.

Rather than constructing a thoroughgoing argument or exegesis, I have sought in this chapter to critique and complicate the role of the figure-ground structure within Merleau-Ponty's project. By considering a nonnormative body—specifically the visual field of my dream eye—I have explored the nature of determinacy within perception. I hope that this conversation has left us with more questions than answers, and with a deeper appreciation for the possibilities of human experience. We should try to see the world through our peripheries and see what it might mean to be in a world of airy light and dancing shapes rather than fixed objects. Our worlds become stale as soon as we let our bodies become too familiar. Let's reawaken the drive of phenomenology to begin in "wonder."[48] See your world anew, and never forget that the world is not fixed but is always open, grasped (or not grasped) through any number of different bodies.

Notes

1. Maurice Merleau-Ponty, *Phenomenology of Perception*, trans. Donald A. Landes (Routledge, 2012), 7.

2. Merleau-Ponty, *Phenomenology of Perception*, 32–33. For instance, to give my attention to one thing is precisely to let other matters fall into the periphery of my current awareness.

3. Merleau-Ponty, *Phenomenology of Perception*, 451. For instance, deciding upon a matter today is to take this choice itself as a figure against the grounds of my past personal life and my impending future possibilities.

4. Merleau-Ponty, *Phenomenology of Perception*, 86–87. Merleau-Ponty's model of the sedimentation of habit finds one's current activity as a *focused* participation in a larger *background* of past organic and motor activity.

5. Merleau-Ponty, *Phenomenology of Perception*, 201. Merleau-Ponty here describes the "sense" of a spoken word as drawing from an inexhaustible background of personal and cultural life, citing a pathological case of motor aphasia as "due to a lack of the ability to differentiate 'figure' and 'background.'"

6. Merleau-Ponty, *Phenomenology of Perception*, 172. Merleau-Ponty explains sexuality as an ambiguous atmosphere that privileges certain relations—such an atmosphere motivates explicit perceptual figures as their affective background.

7. In addition to Merleau-Ponty's own ontological writings, other contemporary thinkers have teased out important through-lines in his thinking, revealing how the structures in the early moments of *The Phenomenology of Perception* are carried through his later works; see David Morris, "The Enigma of Reversibility and the Genesis of Sense in Merleau-Ponty," *Continental Philosophy Review* 43, no. 2 (May 2010): 141–165. https://doi.org/10.1007/s11007-010-9144-7; and Don Beith, *The Birth of Sense: Generative Passivity in Merleau-Ponty's Philosophy* (Athens: Ohio University Press, 2018).

8. Maurice Merleau-Ponty, *The Visible and the Invisible: Followed by Working Notes*, trans. Alphonso Lingis (Evanston, IL: Northwestern University, 1968), 197. Though drawing the connection more explicitly would call for a larger argument, let it suffice to say that in equating the "element of Being," flesh, with "generality," Merleau-Ponty motivates the ontological process by which particular things as figures emerge from this processual background of generality (114).

9. Other contemporary thinkers have also found counterexamples relevant for rethinking Merleau-Ponty's core commitments. An important contribution relevant here, which also touches upon figure-ground relationships, is found in Susan M. Bredlau, "A Respectful World: Merleau-Ponty and the Experience of Depth." *Human Studies* 33, no. 4 (December 1, 2010): 411–423. https://doi.org/10.1007/s10746-011-9173-1

10. Merleau-Ponty, *Phenomenology of Perception*, 6–7.

11. Merleau-Ponty, *Phenomenology of Perception*, 201.

12. MD, Mitchell B Strominger. "Morning Glory Syndrome." *American Academy of Ophthalmology*, November 9, 2017. www.aao.org/disease-review/neuro-ophthalmology-morning-glory-syndrome

13. Merleau-Ponty, *Phenomenology of Perception*, 4.

14. Merleau-Ponty, *Phenomenology of Perception*, 4.

15. Merleau-Ponty, *Phenomenology of Perception*, 4.

16. Merleau-Ponty, *Phenomenology of Perception*, 4.

17. Merleau-Ponty, *Phenomenology of Perception*, 4.

18. Merleau-Ponty, *Phenomenology of Perception*, 4, his emphasis.

19. Merleau-Ponty, *Phenomenology of Perception*, 4.

20. Merleau-Ponty, *Phenomenology of Perception*, 6–7.

21. Merleau-Ponty, *Phenomenology of Perception*, 4.

22. Merleau-Ponty, *Phenomenology of Perception*, 4.

23. Merleau-Ponty, *Phenomenology of Perception*, 313–314.

24. Merleau-Ponty, *Phenomenology of Perception*, 332.

25. Merleau-Ponty, *Phenomenology of Perception*, 291.

26. Merleau-Ponty, *Phenomenology of Perception*, 4.

27. Merleau-Ponty, *Phenomenology of Perception*, 4.

28. Merleau-Ponty, *Phenomenology of Perception*, 17–18.

29. Husserl, Edmund, *Analyses Concerning Passive and Active Synthesis*, trans. Anthony J. Steinbock (Dordrecht: Kluwer Academic Publishers, 2001), 61.

30. Not to confuse the central claim I make here, but it is also worth noting that such illusions assume a binocular viewer—these illusions do not work for my monocular vision.

31. For a further discussion of normativity in Merleau-Ponty as it relates to spatiality, see Maria Talero, "Perception, Normativity, and Selfhood in Merleau-Ponty: The Spatial 'Level' and Existential Space." *The Southern Journal of Philosophy* 43, no. 3 (2005): 443–461. https://doi.org/10.1111/j.2041-6962.2005.tb01962.x; and David Morris, *The Sense of Space*. (Albany, NY: SUNY Press, 2013).

32. Merleau-Ponty, *Phenomenology of Perception*, 274.

33. Merleau-Ponty, *Phenomenology of Perception*, lxxx.

34. Merleau-Ponty, *Phenomenology of Perception*, 275.

35. Merleau-Ponty, *Phenomenology of Perception*, 275.

36. Merleau-Ponty, *Phenomenology of Perception*, 276; my emphasis.

37. Indeed, Merleau-Ponty does characterize a perceptual field void of things, further in the "Space" chapter. This is the "spatiality of the night," which Merleau-Ponty seems to posit in order to argue that a thingly world of figures upon grounds is at the very foundation of "normal" selfhood. However, carrying our current conversation into selfhood is larger than the scope of this chapter, though it is worthy of consideration. See Merleau-Ponty, *Phenomenology of Perception*, 275.

38. Merleau-Ponty, *Phenomenology of Perception*, 296; my emphasis.

39. Merleau-Ponty, *Phenomenology of Perception*, 276.

40. Merleau-Ponty, *Phenomenology of Perception*, 143.

41. Merleau-Ponty, *The Visible and the Invisible*, 139.

42. Maurice Merleau-Ponty, *The Primacy of Perception and Other Essays on Phenomenological Psychology, the Philosophy of Art, History, and Politics*, trans. James M. Edie (Evanston, IL: Northwestern University Press, 1964), 138.

43. Many cite chapter 4 of *The Visible and the Invisible* as highlighting tactility for Merleau-Ponty, given his oft-quoted treatment of the reversibility of two hands touching (134). However, careful readers will note that Merleau-Ponty uses this tactile reversibility to ultimately make a point about the reversibility of the visible dimension.

44. Several phenomenological investigations into aesthetic experience help to illuminate the possible horizons for new experience that emerge if we move past our typical, taken-for-granted figure-ground structuring of perceptual life; see Michael Schreyach, "Pre-objective Depth in Merleau-Ponty and Jackson Pollock," *Research in Phenomenology* 43, no. 1 (2013): 49–70, doi-org.proxy.library.stonybrook.edu/10.1163/15691640-12341243; and Galen A. Johnson, "The Invisible and the Unrepresentable: Barnett Newman's Abstract Expressionism and the Aesthetics of Merleau-Ponty," *Analecta Husserliana* 75 (2002): 179–189.

45. For a musical example of what I "see" in my left eye, listen to Julia Wolfe (2008). *Stronghold*. The Hartt School. https://juliawolfemusic.com/music/stronghold

46. Such an ontological program finds resonances with Jean-Luc Nancy's anti-ocularcentric program in Jean-Luc Nancy (2007), *Listening*, trans. Charlotte Mandell (New York: Fordham University Press).

47. Merleau-Ponty, *Phenomenology of Perception*, 115.

48. Plato, *Theatetus*, 155d, in *The Dialogues of Plato*, 4th ed., vol. 3, trans. B. Jowett (Oxford: Clarendon Press, 1953), 251.

Chapter 7

The Insight of Dispossession

Examining the Phenomenological and Political Significance of Merleau-Ponty's Account of the Spatial Level

WHITNEY HOWELL

Introduction

In the opening pages of the chapter on "Space" in part two of the *Phenomenology of Perception*, Merleau-Ponty acknowledges a fundamental difficulty in accounting for the basic lived experience of "up" and "down." He writes: "We cannot grasp this experience in the everyday course of life, for it is already concealed beneath its own acquisitions. We must look to some exceptional case in which it breaks down and rebuilds itself before our eyes [. . .]."[1] Specifically, Merleau-Ponty looks to an experimental study of a subject whose vision has been modified by means of goggles to prevent the retinal inversion necessary for normal sight. Upon donning the goggles, "the whole landscape at first appears unreal and inverted."[2] Merleau-Ponty examines the stages through which the subject's experience of the landscape is eventually restored as "real" and "upright." His intent is to discern by means of their absence in abnormal experience the "acquisitions" upon which normal experience depends and which it conceals. In this chapter, I consider why this turn toward abnormal experience is especially instructive for understanding our experience of space in both phenomenological and political terms. I begin by considering Merleau-Ponty's claim that "up" and "down" are meaningful designations according to the prior establishment of a "spatial level." I focus on his characterization of the spatial level as a matter of "possession" between inhabitant and environment.[3] Specifically, I consider how we possess space and how space possesses us. Next, I show that our possession of and by space always involves a consequent failure to recognize other nascent possibilities. I then consider the role of others in our possession of space and their implication in this failure. I focus on ways in which abnormal moments of "dispossession" of space reveal the more fundamental contingency that Merleau-Ponty describes as underlying the established spatial level and, in turn, potentially open our experience to others' perspectives. In the third and final section, I examine the political ramifications of the experience of spatial dispossession. Specifically, I propose an important continuity between experiences of spatial and political dispossession.

Possession

In the course of everyday experience, questions regarding spatial orientation often arise en route to a particular destination, and they are most often answered with reference to fixed landmarks. For example, in response to a man who has just stopped me on the street to ask where the library is, I may tell him to continue walking on the same street until he crosses the large parkway, and to look for the Beaux-Arts building on his right. It is likely I will also turn my body toward the direction I suggest he take, adding further emphasis by pointing and gesturing. This example reveals that spatial orientation is not abstract; rather, it always expresses a concrete relation between my body and an environment that also involves the things that populate and distinguish that environment. In other words, spatial orientation—that is, knowing which way to go and how to get there—draws on determinate features of particular places and my bodily relation to them. These spatial orientations serve as what Merleau-Ponty refers to as "anchorage points," establishing a concrete sense of "here" and "there."[4]

However, Merleau-Ponty further argues we cannot turn to the body or to concrete features of particular places given in our sensory experience as furnishing absolute "anchorage points" that determine our sense of spatial orientation. This is because, as the experiment with the subject in the goggles demonstrates, the same contents given in sensory experience can at different times indicate different directions, conflicting orientations.[5] More specifically in the case of the experiment, prior to donning the goggles, the subject experiences his body as upright within a correspondingly upright world. The goggles, which prevent the retinal inversion that produces upright images in normal vision, upend his perception of the landscape.[6] Though his normal perception gradually returns after wearing the goggles for a couple of days, the subject still experiences his own body as "inverted."[7] After about eight days, however, "the body is progressively brought upright."[8] In this experiment, neither the subject's visual perception of the world around him nor his tactile perception of his own body maintains a constant sense of orientation even though the contents of his perception remain the same.[9]

Merleau-Ponty's analysis suggests that in order to understand spatial orientation, we must attend to its concrete specificity—that is, to its implication within the body and its rootedness in a particular place—while at the same time recognizing that it is not fixed absolutely in either the body or the particular place in which one is situated. Indeed, under normal circumstances my sense of spatial orientation seems to precede and inform my experience of my body and place in an already-established relation between them such that each is implicated in the other.[10] In the case of my giving directions, for example, it is this already-established relation that organizes the streets and buildings around me. This is expressed in the bodily gestures that attempt to convey this organization to the man with whom I am speaking. Merleau-Ponty's notion of the "spatial level" captures the coordination between bodily capacity and environmental opportunity experienced in normal spatial orientation. In keeping with Merleau-Ponty's earlier analysis, this level is not fixed absolutely in the landscape, things, or the body, but rather sets the terms according to which each is in meaningful relation to the other. For example, ordinary movements—in the tilt of my head or the quickening of my pace or the flow of traffic—do not disrupt my spatial orientation. Thus, the spatial level functions as an established precedent that orients us toward potential interaction with the world.

Merleau-Ponty describes more specific consequences of the coherence between body and world in the spatial level:

> My body is geared into the world when my perception provides me with the most varied and the most clearly articulated spectacle possible, and when my motor intentions, as they unfold, receive the responses they anticipate from the world. This maximum of clarity in perception and action specifies a perceptual *ground*, a background for my life, a general milieu for the coexistence of my body and the world.[11]

In this passage, Merleau-Ponty argues that a sense of orientation informs meaningful perception and, more specifically, is the necessary ground for vivid and nuanced perception. For example, his point here is evident in the contrasting experience of being overwhelmed by your first impressions of an unfamiliar city: it is precisely because you are not oriented there that you do not know what you are looking at and you may fail to actually see much of what is around you. Indeed, the notion of a first "impression" is especially instructive here, since it suggests one's passivity in relation to the novel environment, such that the distinctions characteristic of more meaningful perceptual experience are absent. The unfamiliar city affects you—it impresses itself upon you—but you are not yet prepared to make sense of it. Merleau-Ponty gives his own example of his first impression of Paris: "And when I arrived there for the first time, the first streets that I saw upon leaving the train station were—like the first words of a stranger—only manifestations of a still ambiguous, though already incomparable essence."[12] Merleau-Ponty describes his first impression of Paris as having a distinctive appearance and feel—an "incomparable essence" available even to the newcomer—but nevertheless "ambiguous": the streets lack the coherence of meaningful details that constitute and define this essence. In contrast, the more established city inhabitant recognizes these details as individual "confirmations" of "a certain style or a certain sense of Paris."[13] In understanding its language, so to speak, she is capable of noticing modulations in how the city speaks through these details. Unlike the newcomer, who may be overwhelmed and intimidated by the uninterpretable patterns of this particular mode of urban life, she will discover in them solicitations for her involvement: the cafés, shops, and sidewalks, along with the flow and clusters of pedestrians, accommodate her interests and movements, which "receive the responses they anticipate from the world."[14]

This example of the city inhabitant further illustrates how the establishment of a spatial level is reflected in bodily capacity. Not only is the inhabitant's perception of the world more vivid than that of the first time visitor, but, correspondingly, her capability within the world is more refined as well. Merleau-Ponty describes this sense of bodily capacity in relation to the environment in the spatial level as a form of "possession." On this point, he writes:

> The spatial level is [. . .] a certain possession [*possession*] of the world by my body, a certain *hold* my body has on the world. [. . .] It sets itself up when, between my body as the power of certain gestures and as the demand for certain privileged planes, and the perceived spectacle as the invitation to these very gestures and as the theater of these very actions, a pact is established that gives me possession [*jouissance*] of space and gives to the things a direct power upon my body.[15]

In this passage, Merleau-Ponty describes how the spatial level effects a sense of continuity and reciprocity between bodily capacity and world. As a result of the "pact" I have established with the world, I belong there, but also, correspondingly, I am freed to act within it.[16] This passage conveys the intimate relation between possession as a claim, a "hold" [*possession*], and possession as a sense of disposal, of leeway to enjoy [*jouissance*]. In securing the anchorage points that constitute the spatial level, I achieve a platform for action; I am no longer passive in relation to the environment, subject to being impressed upon by it, but rather am attuned to and integrated within what animates it. Nevertheless, as this passage also suggests, there is a sense in which my possession of the world in the spatial level opens up a degree of nonoptional responsiveness. Just as my literacy makes it impossible for me not to read the words on a sign or billboard in front of me, so does my inherence in the spatial level make it impossible for me not to follow the cues of the world. In a certain sense, the spatial level imposes intelligibility on my experience of the environment, which has the dual effects of securing my hold on it as interpretable [*possession*] and also unlocking the opportunities for action it makes available [*jouissance*]. Insofar as these interpretations and opportunities are rooted in that space and specific to the capacities of my body opened up by the spatial level, I am also "held" to the standards set in the spatial level and, in effect, committed to the "pact" I have made with it as a "privileged" plane.[17]

To examine what this possession—of the body by space, and of space by the body—is like in lived experience, let us turn to a couple of examples. Consider first the conscientious college student who attends class regularly. A few weeks into the semester, he has already established "his" seat in the classroom, which determines his orientation within the room. Upon walking through the door, he moves directly to his seat; he settles into it, and the room settles around him. The spatial level that characterizes his orientation here includes organization of its sensory contents: he has become accustomed to the "feel" of the wall to his right, which offers a sense of protective security. Rows of students intervene between him and the professor at the front of room, providing the suggestion of privacy under her gaze, and, perpendicular to those, rows of other students occupy the appreciable distance between him and the far wall of windows to his left, of which he takes almost no notice. When he first arrived in class at the beginning of the semester, the new faces, the lighting, the decoration and decay of the walls and floors, and the arrangement of desks in the room all imposed upon him, but now his familiar place has established them as the ground against which more relevant and more nuanced perceptual details emerge. Taking his seat "frees" his attention to focus on the lecture and discussion. Moreover, whenever he is in the room he feels the "pull" of his established place, such that to be displaced from it is uncomfortable (indeed, students can be quite territorial about "their" seats, and are often resistant to the suggestion of changing or rearranging seats). However, this discomfort is not simply a matter of arbitrary preference, but rather a testament to the necessary conditions for meeting the normal demands of this environment. A student has a claim to his seat, but his seat also claims him insofar as it unlocks capacities for settling into his body, listening, thinking, and learning, which are accommodated by the room.

The talented tennis player in the midst of a match provides a further example of how the spatial level organizes one's experience of space. Unlike the student, the tennis player is not rooted in a specific spot on the court; instead, the game requires that she move around freely and resist committing to a particular corner or line. The dimensions of the court and the shots of the opposing player are felt as demands answered in the pace of her movements, the reach of her racket, and the speed of her strokes.[18] In this example, the spatial level is dynamic: it is not anchored in stationary points, but rather in the system of relations that govern the possible plays. Becoming a skilled tennis player requires possession of the space of the court—an intimacy with its possibilities—that, as this example illustrates, further involves a ready responsiveness to the claims it makes on her movements. Thus, the space of the game—both the dimensions of the court and the array of possible plays within it—also possesses her and animates her bodily capacities.

Both of these examples further demonstrate that the spatial level achieved in relation to a specific environment may also provide a point of entry into other, similar environments.[19] While these other spaces may require modulations in comportment, they nevertheless evoke the body's established sense of continuity with the world as a ground for action. Thus, the tennis player may find an analogous facility at the ping-pong table. The conscientious university student settles into other classrooms with a similar sense of focus and dedication reflected in his orientation toward this kind of environment. In these examples, we can see that the spatial level is not rigidly fixed, but rather serves as the dynamic ground for further interactions.[20] Moreover, this sense of orientation according to the established spatial level brings both the body and the world into definition. Indeed, this is Merleau-Ponty's point in the above passage about the refinement of perception in an environment in which one is oriented: body and world are more articulate and more defined. Beyond (though related to) perceptual experience, one's sense of oneself and one's place is also defined in the spatial level. I am a tennis player because of the relation I have to the court; I am a student because of the relation I have to the classroom. Thus, in coming into possession of space in the establishment of the spatial level, we define ourselves in terms of the capacities activated by that space.

Merleau-Ponty's analysis of the spatial level as a matter of possession reveals the established sense of continuity between body and world in normal lived experience. We have considered how this sense of continuity is reflected in bodily capacities developed in relation to a specific environment that may in turn provide a more general ground for further action. While our bodily capacities give us possession of space, they also give space possession of us insofar as it evokes our responsiveness to it. For this reason, Merleau-Ponty writes in the passage cited above that the spatial level "gives [. . .] things a direct power upon my body."[21] In the next section, I will consider how we experience this power not only in our successful responsiveness to the demands of a particular environment but also in our failure to recognize features of it.

Dispossession

At the end of the chapter on "Space," Merleau-Ponty cites his experience of Paris to demonstrate that "lived space" is characterized by a sense of its distinctive "style," rather than by a collection of discrete perceptions.

I discussed this example in the first section of this chapter in order to consider how this style develops in conjunction with the establishment of the spatial level, which informs our meaningful perception of and our sense of bodily capacity within that space. Merleau-Ponty's reference to urban experience is especially instructive on this point: because of their density and diversity, urban environments require highly developed coordination between individual and environment. As we saw above, the city inhabitant will see more of the city—its sensory details and its solicitations for her involvement—and will consequently navigate it more capably than the tourist visiting for the first time. Arguably, however, there is also much the seasoned city inhabitant will fail to see. Her familiar routes of engagement will direct her focus toward "invitations" for action, anticipating and answering her developed capacities but also excluding other forms of involvement. In this section, I consider how the establishment of the spatial level and the sense of possession it develops further entail a degree of obliviousness in one's relation to their familiar environment. More specifically, I show how the development of certain capacities necessarily forecloses others. I further consider how our relations with others are implicated in our relations with space. I argue that breaks in contiguity between body and environment that disrupt the developed sense of possession—what I refer to as dispossession—open the possibility of recognizing others' perspectives.

The example of the city inhabitant who both sees and fails to see aspects of her familiar urban environment is creatively portrayed in a recent novel by China Miéville, *The City & the City*, in a way that reflects and deepens Merleau-Ponty's phenomenological analysis of the experience of space. As the title suggests, the novel is set in two fictional cities—Besźel and Ul Qoma—that occupy the same geographical area as different political and cultural entities, each with its own distinctive architecture, language, food, and style of dress. However, the cities are not merely contiguous with one another; that is, they do not merely share a single border. Rather, they are interwoven through each other such that borders are internal and frequent, and are, for the most part, maintained by the distinctive cultural styles and bodily comportment of the inhabitants of each place. In addition, while each city has its own police force, the borders are strictly monitored by a mysterious independent entity known as "Breach," which is responsible for addressing transgressions, whether by "disappearing" an inhabitant of one city who has crossed over into the other (whether intentionally or unintentionally), or by cleaning up a car accident that affects the streets of both cities. The narrator of the novel describes how childhood development takes place in the context of these distinctive cultures that are further policed by "Breach." He writes:

> The early years of a Besź (and presumably an Ul Qoman) child are intense learnings of cues. We pick up styles of clothing, permissible colours, ways of walking and holding oneself, very fast. Before we were eight or so most of us could be trusted not to breach embarrassingly and illegally, though licence of course is granted children every moment they are in the street.[22]

Because each city is geographically continuous with the other, the young inhabitants become habituated not only to the cues of their own culture but also to cues that distinguish their city's culture from the other. They learn to read cultural commitments in aesthetic style, and they learn to demonstrate these commitments—to give the relevant cues—in their own appearance and comportment. These aesthetic distinctions are further enforced by stories:

> How could one not think of the stories we all grew up on, that surely the Ul Qomans grew up on too? Ul Qoman man and Besź maid, meeting in the middle of Copula Hall [a municipal building that serves both cities], returning to their homes to realise that they live, grosstopically, next door to each other, spending their lives faithful and alone, rising at the same time, walking crosshatched streets close like a couple, each in their own city, never breaching, never quite touching, never speaking a word across the border.[23]

Such a story explores possible romantic dimensions of the cities' lived realities that are explicitly forbidden, namely, the mingling of inhabitants across borders. The narrator's neologism describing the inhabitants as "grosstopically" near each other refers to their literal physical proximity. Nevertheless, cultural and political boundaries are ultimately more powerful and dictate what the residents of each city perceive and how they comport themselves. By means of these cultural cues, residents from each city navigate around an other, different form of urban life in their midst.[24]

This fictional setting highlights a number of important points about the nature of our possession of space. Most prominently, it suggests that physical, geographical designations are neither the only nor even the primary means of delineating spatial boundaries. That is, even though the citizens of Besźel and Ul Qoma physically occupy the same space, their different relations to that space organize it as separately (and distinctively) inhabited places that further determine what they can do and also what they perceive. Indeed, there are frequent examples throughout the novel of "unsensing" perceptual details that indicate the existence of the other city.[25] While some of the descriptions of "unsensing" seem extreme—such as "unsmelling" the scents of foreign food or "unhearing" the bark of a dog[26]—they put on explicit display the extent to which our possession of space always entails exclusions, even as it activates our capacities in a particular environment. More specifically, once we have established our familiar modes of interaction within the spatial level, other possibilities retreat below our awareness, such that they are not even part of the implicit ground against which we undertake our more explicit projects.

The fictional worlds of Besźel and Ul Qoma demonstrate how individuals' coordinated ways of inhabiting their respective cities maintain and reinforce separate collective grounds of action. However, it also often happens that others with whom we share a collective ground of action challenge our sense of enjoying exclusive claims within it. In a well-known passage in *Being and Nothingness*, for example, Jean-Paul Sartre describes how the presence of another person crossing a city park causes "a pure *disintegration* of the relations which [he] apprehend[s] between the objects of [his] universe," such that his own orientation there "flees" from him.[27] Sartre's example emphasizes how the presence of others illuminates nascent—and competing—spatial relations within a shared environment. Nevertheless, moments like this leave the spatial level intact, though they rearrange, as it were, the coordinates of possibility within it. In other words, while Sartre's presumed claim to a particular place is challenged, his actions remain viable: he could still sit on that bench and enjoy the park, though it is now currently "occupied by" someone else whose interests and attention have charged and reorganized the environment.

In both the contrasting fictional worlds of Besźel and Ul Qoma in *The City & the City* and in Sartre's encounter with a rival other in the public park, we can see how one's possession of space—made possible in the establishment of the spatial level—obscures other forms of spatial relations. In an important sense, we replace the potential to recognize these other forms with our specific capacities, which, as we have seen, both open up a particular world to us and orient us toward established routes of engagement within that world. Consequently, our normal experience of space is characterized by familiarity and unreflective facility. Merleau-Ponty claims that, by contrast, encountering the potential of our relation to space *as* potential is unsettling and nausea-inducing:

> At the core of the subject, space and perception in general mark the fact of his birth, the perpetual contribution of his corporeality, and a communication with the world more ancient than thought. And this is why they saturate consciousness and are opaque to reflection. The lability of levels gives not merely the intellectual experience of disorder, but also the living experience of vertigo and nausea, which is the consciousness of, and the horror caused by, our contingency. The positing of a level is the forgetting of this contingency, and space is established upon our facticity.[28]

Merleau-Ponty emphasizes the metaphysical significance of the spatial level in anchoring our experience as coherent and our being as stable. We are integrated meaningfully and capably into the world by "forgetting" the contingency of our relation to it. Indeed, this contingency is covered over by its resolution in a seemingly "ancient" past that precedes our decisions and is reflected in our "blind adhesion to the world, [. . . our] prejudice in favor of being."[29] While we implicitly rely on this contingency and the flexibility it affords us in our adaptations—such as in the case of the college student who carries his studious comportment into different classrooms—we nonetheless maintain a sense of the stability of our being in our inherence in the spatial level.

Though we typically exist within an atmosphere of spatial stability, it can be disrupted with important implications for our relations with others. In order to examine more closely the relation between moments of spatial instability and our relations with others, let us consider a further experiment that Merleau-Ponty cites in his discussion of the spatial level. Merleau-Ponty describes the situation of a man viewing a room through a mirror tilted at a 45-degree angle.[30] While initially the man sees the room and everything in it as correspondingly tilted, the "oblique" orientation soon establishes itself as a new vertical. Describing this shift in spatial level, Merleau-Ponty writes:

> Everything happens as if certain objects (the walls, the doors, and the body of the man in the room), determined as oblique in relation to the given level, aspired by themselves to provide the privileged directions, played the role of "anchorage points," and caused the previously established level to tilt.[31]

While it took up to a week for the subject wearing the goggles to perceive a normal landscape and body position—the latter achieved "above all when the subject [was] active"[32]—in this experiment "there is an instantaneous redistribution of up and down without any motor exploration."[33] In accounting for this shift in spatial level, Merleau-Ponty reiterates his earlier claim that the orientation of the body "as a mass of tactile, labyrinthine, and kinesthetic givens" does not determine the experienced spatial level.[34] Rather, it is the "body as an agent [. . . that] plays an essential role in establishing a level."[35] Thus, the man looking through the mirror that reflects the room at a tilt finds the *virtual* powers of his body activated in his perception of an inhabitable scene, such that the room calls for and answers his own proposals of what he could do. His own possibilities for movement inform a new spatial level.

Arguably, we experience something similar in viewing a modern dance performance when we are, in Maxine Sheets-Johnstone's words, "*kinetically attuned* to the qualitative dynamics of movement that we are visually experiencing and that constitute the dance."[36] In watching a scene from Pina Bausch's "Vollmond," for example, I marvel at the fluidity of the dancers' bodies, which appear to be swimming backward through the air while simultaneously moving forward in tandem.[37] Their movements manifest an imaginative exploration of bodily possibilities that defies the familiar spatial level of normal experience. An exhilarating feature of watching the performance is that I virtually inhabit the alternative spatial level enacted in their movements through my own bodily possibilities; I even feel the dancers' joy in opening up the space around them.[38]

While both the subject looking through the mirror at the tilted room and the audience of the dance performance can *virtually* inhabit an alternative spatial level through the activation of their bodily possibilities, the experience of *actually* adjusting to a new spatial level arguably takes a somewhat different form. Projects such as washing the outside of windows on the top floors of a tall building, rock climbing, and even knot-tying or knitting require that one abandon the established spatial level of normal upright experience in order to achieve and inhabit a new level that enables the current task.[39] For the sake of its contrast with our examination of watching the performance piece discussed above, consider further the experience of learning to dance as the performers do, which requires moving the body through space in an unaccustomed way. For the beginner, it is contingency—specifically, the openness of space and the malleability of bodily movement—that makes this project especially difficult. Indeed, she must loosen her commitment to the vertical of the established spatial level, as it is not the predominant "pole" of orientation within the piece, and her habituated attempts to appeal to it as such undermine her capacity to inhabit the spatial world of the dance. She does not yet have a "hold" on this world and thus, in her first attempts, she is dispossessed—enacting a break in the contiguity she normally experiences between her body and the environment. Notice, however, that the sensory facts of both her body and the environment remain the same. It is her orientation that must change: she aspires to accomplish a new spatial level that will open up new possibilities. While these possibilities are "hers," the space is not—at least, not *yet*. She recognizes others' possession of it in the facility of their movements, which suggest its openness, in principle, to her, if she can adjust to its spatial level and learn to respond to the cues of the perceptual world it grounds.

This experience is abnormal insofar as it involves acknowledgment of one's own incapacity as foregoing possession of space. Indeed, the beginner who wants to learn to dance must relate to her environment as offering solicitations—cues—to which she is not yet prepared to respond. This further involves attention to and patience with her failures to pick up on those solicitations within a world that is not "hers." In order to explain more fully the point I am making here, and to elucidate what I see as the relevant features of this example, I will turn briefly to an essay by Simone Weil. In "Reflections on the Right Use of School Studies with a View to the Love of God," Weil claims that our failures develop capacities unrelated to the task at which we are failing.[40] On this point she writes: "If we concentrate our attention on trying to solve a problem of geometry, and if at the end of an hour we are no nearer to doing so than at the beginning, we have nevertheless been making progress each minute of that hour in another more mysterious dimension."[41] More specifically, Weil argues that the student is developing a mode of attention suited to helping others in need.[42] The mode of attention required by "school exercises" is different from that required in the course of normal experience because, according to Weil's account, it involves "waiting upon truth, setting our hearts upon it, yet not allowing ourselves to go out in search of it."[43]

We can consider Weil's analysis in terms of Merleau-Ponty's account of the spatial level. The "waiting" she describes differs markedly from the anticipation and nonoptional responsiveness we have in relation to familiar environments grounded in an established spatial level. Specifically, in attempting to learn something new, we inhabit a different form of temporality in relation to our own development that we would otherwise fail to notice as part of what Merleau-Ponty describes as our "ancient" past. These experiences require patience with ourselves as beginners, but, Weil suggests, they also transform our relations to others. I propose that this transformation happens through the experience of dispossession. In the course of normal experience, the presence of others may either reinforce or challenge our possession of space, but almost always according to the terms of the established spatial level. Recall the conscientious university student: other students may secure his possession of the space by populating a familiar constellation around him, or they may challenge it by taking his seat. In either case, however, the spatial level remains intact, even when the student's capacity for familiar engagement is thwarted; the basic terms of his spatial involvements remain meaningfully in place. By contrast, the beginner learning to dance contends with the absence of an established spatial level. Specifically, she contends with this absence *as* potential—as the nascent possibility of forms of engagement that while not yet available *to her* are nevertheless available. She sees her own incapacity in relation to the contingency of its development. While our normal experience of facility within an environment—grounded in the spatial level—inevitably implicates others who support or challenge the projects we pursue there, it does so according to unreflectively familiar terms: the space and its possibilities *belong* to us. However, when, like the beginner learning to dance, we are dispossessed, we cannot maintain the illusion of furnishing these terms ourselves, or of their belonging to us absolutely as a result of their foundation in an "ancient" past. As a result, we are able to recognize what we are otherwise normally oblivious to—namely, the potential of space to accommodate unfamiliar forms of engagement and the corresponding potential within ourselves to adapt to these forms.[44]

Politics of Belonging

Many of the examples we have considered to understand the role and import of the spatial level have revealed its interpersonal and cultural dimensions. Indeed, as our phenomenological analysis of urban experience makes clear—in the fictional cities of Besźel and Ul Qoma, but also in Merleau-Ponty's encounter with Paris—the spatial level is not merely a bodily dimension of our comportment but also further entails significant political ramifications. These political ramifications are often brought to the fore in abnormal experiences of dispossession that demonstrate the more fundamental contingency of our relation to space and raise questions that otherwise go unexamined in normal experience, namely: To whom does this space belong? What or whom does our possession of space exclude? What are the relevant terms that make possible our sense of belonging to and capability within a particular space? These are political questions that we are always implicitly answering in our relations with individual others, but also in our implication in and relations toward more general social groups that unavoidably constitute and shape our experience of space. What we see and fail to see—in objects, in routes of involvement, and even in others—reflects a specific perceptual and social world opened up by our inherence in an established spatial level.[45] However, notice that the examples drawn from urban experience juxtaposed with the example of the novice dancer suggest an important distinction between forms of dispossession that we touched on briefly in the previous section: we may be dispossessed due to what I have referred to as an absence of coordinates of possibility, in which the more fundamental spatial level remains intact, or we may be dispossessed because the spatial level itself has been disrupted or upended. Let us examine the cases more closely to consider their political implications and whether there is a relation between them.

An unfamiliar place—such as a neighborhood in the city where one lives but never has occasion or reason to visit—may be disorienting because it requires that one contend with an absence of coordinates and, consequently, an absence of cues and capabilities. Nonetheless, in situations such as this, the established spatial level remains intact. That is, one is dispossessed of one's familiar world, but not of the more fundamental ground out of which that world is articulated. Thus, it is possible that a person may visit a different neighborhood or travel to a foreign country *without* experiencing the contingency of the spatial level, and without, in turn, recognizing the contingency of her own and others' possession of space. In her book *Queer Phenomenology*, Sara Ahmed describes a possible reaction one can have to experiences such as this, as well as its further political implications:

> Bodies that experience disorientation can be defensive, as they reach out for support or as they search for a place to reground and reorientate their relation to the world. So, too, the forms of politics that proceed from disorientation can be conservative, depending on the "aims" of their gestures, depending on how they seek to (re)ground themselves.[46]

As Ahmed notes here, disorientation may motivate our defense of those worlds that support our developed capacities. However, such defense may amount to criticizing or even living in denial of the worlds in which we find ourselves dispossessed of such capacities.[47] In the chapter on "Race, Space, and Place" in *Revealing Whiteness*, Shannon Sullivan provides an example of what this defensiveness may look like. Sullivan recalls a white relative feeling discriminated against in a Latinx grocery store in south Dallas, and then "somewhat angrily complaining" about his treatment.[48] In her analysis of this experience, Sullivan notes her relative's presumption of having a "right" to that space—and, more specifically, to feeling comfortable and legitimate within it—as evidence of white privilege, the denial of which motivates his criticism of the store.[49] Sullivan's discussion of the ways in which space lacks racial neutrality in white racist society presents contemporary lived correlates of the forms of spatial exclusion imagined in *The City & the City*. The exclusive co-existence of Besźel and Ul Qoma creatively portrays the political and often racial divisions that are more explicitly enacted in social and economic policies, redlining, gerrymandering practices, and even literal wall-building that emphatically separate communities that nevertheless share a common ground—reinforcing the development of different worldviews and capacities. As Sullivan's example suggests, while one may be disoriented and dispossessed in their encounter with an unfamiliar world, it does not follow that they will reflect critically on the ground of their own capacities or consider the situation of others who are more at home there, especially if they typically experience space as supportive.

I have suggested, however, that the experience of the more fundamental dispossession of the loss of the spatial level does not admit of a similar strategy of defense. Indeed, as the novice dancer demonstrates, such experiences force us to confront the contingency of our capabilities in our attempts to establish a ground. Ahmed's choice of the term "regrounding" in the above passage explicitly evokes Merleau-Ponty's notion of the spatial level and thus seems to conflate the disorientation that results from entering an unfamiliar world with the more fundamental dispossession of the loss of the spatial level. However, Ahmed goes on to offer an observation that suggests an important continuity between these two phenomena:

> Disorientation is unevenly distributed: some bodies more than others have their involvement in the world called into crisis. This shows us how the world itself is more "involved" in some bodies than in others, as it takes such bodies as the contours of ordinary experience. It is not just that some bodies are directed in specific ways, but that the world is shaped by the directions taken by some bodies more than others. It is thus possible to talk about the white world, the straight world, as a world that takes the shape of the motility of certain skins.[50]

As Ahmed points out in this passage, the experience of entering an unfamiliar world is not for many people an optional consequence of, for example, travel, but is rather the very condition of their experience.[51] More specifically, it is a political condition. As we have seen, the established spatial level may lend itself to the simultaneous articulation of different and conflicting worlds. The subjects of disorientation Ahmed describes consistently find themselves in a world that does not reflect and support their capacities, even as it reflects and supports the capacities of others. Though the spatial level remains intact, it may not provide them with a hold on the world and its possible routes for involvement. In this sense, their experience of dispossession is similar to that of the subject who seeks a new vertical, not merely because the one lacks a metaphorical ground of support for their projects but because the other lacks the ground of the spatial level. Rather, both situations motivate recognition of the fundamentally contingent ground of one's own and others' capacities.[52]

Conclusion

Merleau-Ponty's account of the spatial level demonstrates the implicit coordination between body and world necessary for meaningful perception and action. His account further demonstrates that while this coordination is metaphysically significant for the stability of our being, it is not anchored in either the body or the world. Though we normally operate with a sense of "up" and "down" that informs our capabilities, our spatial orientation is not fixed absolutely. Merleau-Ponty turns to abnormal experiences, such as the subject wearing the retinal inversion goggles and the subject looking through the tilted mirror, that reveal a more fundamental "lability of levels" and, in turn, our capacity to make adjustments and establish new grounds for meaningful perception and action.[53] Merleau-Ponty argues that such experiences make apparent the contingency of our relation to space, which can take forms other than those that are most familiar to us. Though "the positing of a level is the forgetting of this contingency,"[54] moments of dispossession, I have argued, can serve as reminders. More specifically, in experiences such as learning to dance, when we suspend or lose altogether our normal relation to "up" and "down," we reckon with the contingent development of our capacities and, in turn, with the openness of space to forms of engagement unfamiliar to us. Meaning and movement become obscure. In situations such as these, we are vulnerable because we lack the ground upon which we normally and unreflectively depend. Consequently, it may be impossible for us to gauge whether or not we are making progress. This situation is akin to that of the student Simone Weil mentions who fails to solve the geometry problems but continues to work through their difficulty. Weil claims that the student makes progress "in another more mysterious dimension" in which they become more attuned to others.[55] This experience of struggle and attunement that Weil describes is perhaps more common among children, whose capacities are still in the process of developing. Those with more developed capacities, and with well-established routes of involvement in the world that support and facilitate them, may rarely encounter—let alone seek out—experiences that render them vulnerable by disrupting their reliable correspondence with the world. In turn, their perspective on themselves and others is limited by their familiar involvements. By contrast, the vulnerable situation of learning to dance, for example, transforms that established perspective, potentially opening it to new insights into one's own and others' capacities.

This attunement to others and, more specifically, to the ground of their and our own capacities, may be exhilarating in the context of dance. However, as Ahmed's emphasis on the "uneven distribution" of disorientation makes clear, the insight of dispossession often comes at a higher and more damaging personal cost for those who are more consistently denied unproblematic involvement in the world. Such experiences of dispossession demonstrate the political dimensions of coordination between subject, world, and others that further defines the spatial level. As we have seen, this coordination is neither fixed nor neutral. While it enables and empowers the movements of some, it restricts those of others. Thus, recognizing the contingency of the spatial level entails also recognizing the contingency of the uneven political ground of our involvements in the world. This is perhaps especially important for those who for the most part experience this ground as stable and supportive, and thus as securing their possession of and leeway within space. Becoming aware of the unjust inequities between their own and others' capacities opens the possibility of more actively working against those inequities.[56]

Notes

1. Maurice Merleau-Ponty, *Phenomenology of Perception*, trans. Donald A. Landes (New York: Routledge, 2012), 254–255 [291]. Page numbers in brackets, in this and subsequent citations, refer to the French original, *Phénoménologie de la perception* (Paris: Gallimard, 1945).

2. Merleau-Ponty, *Phenomenology of Perception*, 255 [291].

3. Merleau-Ponty, *Phenomenology of Perception*, 261 [298].

4. Merleau-Ponty, *Phenomenology of Perception*, 259 [296]. This insight challenges what Merleau-Ponty refers to as "intellectualist" accounts of orientation, which emphasize the role of the mind in constituting space. He argues that such analyses overlook this necessary specificity for orientation and, in doing so, "[lack] an actual starting point or an absolute here that could gradually give a direction [*sens*] to all the determinations of space" (258 [295]).

5. Merleau-Ponty, *Phenomenology of Perception*, 257 [294].

6. Merleau-Ponty, *Phenomenology of Perception*, 255 [291].

7. Merleau-Ponty, *Phenomenology of Perception*, 255 [292].

8. Merleau-Ponty, *Phenomenology of Perception*, 255 [292].

9. Merleau-Ponty, *Phenomenology of Perception*, 257 [294]. For an excellent discussion of how Merleau-Ponty's analysis of this experiment attends to the existential significance of vision, see Susan M. Bredlau, "Monstrous Faces and a World Transformed: Merleau-Ponty, Dolezal, and the Enactive Approach on Vision without Inversion of the Retinal Image," *Phenomenology and the Cognitive Sciences* 10 (2011): 481–498.

10. Merleau-Ponty sets up his analysis of the spatial level by writing that "It remains to be shown precisely what this level is that always precedes itself,

every constitution of a level presupposing another preestablished level [. . .]" (259 [296–297]).

11. Merleau-Ponty, *Phenomenology of Perception*, 261 [298].

12. Merleau-Ponty, *Phenomenology of Perception*, 294 [333].

13. Merleau-Ponty, *Phenomenology of Perception*, 294 [333].

14. Merleau-Ponty, *Phenomenology of Perception*, 261 [298].

15. Merleau-Ponty, *Phenomenology of Perception*, 261 [298], original emphasis.

16. See Maria Talero, "Perception, Normativity, and Selfhood in Merleau-Ponty: The Spatial 'Level' and Existential Space," *The Southern Journal of Philosophy* 43 (2005): 443–461," for an excellent discussion of the spatial level as a "fundamental normativity" that not only establishes preferential conditions for motor action within a particular world but also functions as an existential ground on which "my agential actions and decisions can take hold" (448–451).

17. In the following section, I will consider more specifically how one's possession of and by space in effect limits what one can see and do within it.

18. For a discussion of a similar example in terms of Merleau-Ponty's analysis of habituation, see Whitney Howell, "Learning and the Development of Meaning: Husserl and Merleau-Ponty on the Temporality of Perception and Habit," *The Southern Journal of Philosophy* 53, no. 3 (September 2015): 311–337.

19. See Kirsten Jacobson, "A Developed Nature," A Phenomenological Account of the Experience of Home," *Continental Philosophy Review* 42 (2009): 355–373, especially 367–372, for a detailed analysis of the way in which the childhood home functions as a "level" that makes possible navigation of environments beyond the childhood home. Jacobson emphasizes the passive character of the developed spatial level, which, in its tendency to remain in the background, provides the stability for our more active projects.

20. Merleau-Ponty makes a similar point earlier in *Phenomenology of Perception* in his discussion of habit in the chapter "The Spatiality of One's Own Body and Motricity." There he describes the organist who, though he has developed skills in relation to a particular instrument, is nevertheless "capable of playing an organ with which he is unfamiliar and that has additional or fewer keyboards, and whose stops are differently arranged than the stops on his customary instrument" (146 [180–181]).

21. Merleau-Ponty, *Phenomenology of Perception*, 261 [298].

22. China Miéville, *The City & the City* (New York: Random House, 2010), 66.

23. Miéville, *The City & the City*, 133–134.

24. Most city inhabitants would readily identify with the narrator's description of how the deployment and reading of "cues" constitute a form of urban choreography in public spaces in which diverse groups of people converge. Moreover, these cues not only influence comportment and movement but also

determine whether and to what extent people feel comfortable around each other. In *The Cosmopolitan Canopy*, sociologist Elijah Anderson discusses how race informs visual cues in contemporary urban environments and affects city inhabitants' sense of comfort or discomfort in public spaces: "A hierarchy of comfort can be discerned: white women, black women, white men, and then black men. In public, ethnicity is not always visible and discernible, but color and gender are. When people look for and read visual cues, these characteristics become significant, and even operative, in determining who means what to whom in the public space. White women and their male counterparts may tense up around lone black males, moving away or clutching their pocketbooks. Through such actions, all are taught about what to expect in public" (226). See Elijah Anderson, *The Cosmopolitan Canopy: Race and Civility in Everyday Life* (New York: W.W. Norton & Co., 2011), especially 225–238. I discuss the role of race in organizing space and movement in the final section of this chapter.

25. Miéville, *The City & the City*, 65.

26. Miéville, *The City & the City*, 54, 264.

27. Jean-Paul Sartre, *Being and Nothingness*, trans. Hazel E. Barnes (New York: Washington Square Press, 1992), 343.

28. Merleau-Ponty, *Phenomenology of Perception*, 265 [302–303].

29. Merleau-Ponty, *Phenomenology of Perception*, 265 [302].

30. Merleau-Ponty, *Phenomenology of Perception*, 259 [296].

31. Merleau-Ponty, *Phenomenology of Perception*, 259 [296].

32. Merleau-Ponty, *Phenomenology of Perception*, 255 [292].

33. Merleau-Ponty, *Phenomenology of Perception*, 259 [296].

34. Merleau-Ponty, *Phenomenology of Perception*, 260 [297].

35. Merleau-Ponty, *Phenomenology of Perception*, 260 [297].

36. Maxine Sheets-Johnstone, "Moving in Concert," *Choros International Dance Journal* 6 (Spring 2017): 1–19, at 14, original emphasis.

37. Pina Bausch, "Vollmond," Dance Performance, online video accessed July 18, 2019, Daily Motion. https://dai.ly/x11kljy

38. In her article "Emotion and Movement," Sheets-Johnstone provides a compelling analysis of the kinetic foundation of emotion, arguing that "movement *creates* the qualities it embodies and that we experience" (268). Following her analysis, I am suggesting here that in watching the performance, the viewer identifies not only with the bodily possibilities realized in the dancers' movements but also, as a result, with the emotions they embody. See Maxine Sheets-Johnstone, "Emotion and Movement: A Beginning Empirical-Phenomenological Analysis of Their Relationship," *Journal of Consciousness Studies* 6.11–12 (1999): 259–277.

39. I thank Kirsten Jacobson for her suggestions of these examples, particularly knot-tying and knitting, which require one's adjustment to micro-spatial levels that necessarily obscure, if not wholly exclude, the established spatial level

we normally inhabit. Indeed, as she points out, observe what happens when an intricate knitting or knotting project is interrupted by something outside its spatial level: the urgencies guiding and orienting the project may be lost entirely.

40. I thank Patricia Locke for suggesting that I look at this essay for a phenomenological analysis of the role of failure in developing the capacity to recognize others' perspectives.

41. Simone Weil, "Reflections on the Right Use of School Studies with a View to the Love of God," in *Waiting for God*, 57–65, trans. Emma Craufurd (New York: Harper Perennial Modern Classics, 2009), 58.

42. Weil, "Reflections on the Right Use," 64–65.

43. Weil, "Reflections on the Right Use," 63.

44. Sheets-Johnstone arrives at a similar conclusion in her analyses of different examples of "moving in concert." She argues that when we attempt to coordinate our movements with others, we become aware of our common humanity and its expression in the "mother tongue" of movement (8). Moreover, she points to the experience of improvising with others in dance performance as especially illuminating because it awakens a feeling of "aliveness" and motivates recognition of our shared capacities and the creative possibilities they give rise to (10–12). See Sheets-Johnstone, "Moving in Concert," 1–19.

45. See Helen Ngo, "Racist Habits: A Phenomenological Analysis of Racism and the Habitual Body," *Philosophy and Social Criticism* 42, no. 9 (2016): 847–872, especially 855–860, for an excellent discussion of the ways in which "modes of racialized perception" determine what we see and fail to see in others. In accounting for this selectivity, Ngo provides a compelling analysis of the "orientating power of habit [to] entail an orientation away from certain people and possibilities" (859). Unsurprisingly, and consistent with Ngo's phenomenological account of the role of habituation in shaping our vision, what is seen in one perceptual and social world may be overlooked in another. In his analysis of contemporary urban workspaces, Anderson notes that "as they go their separate ways, black professionals I've gotten to know complain that in chance encounters on the streets, in local cafés, and on public transportation their white co-workers, eyes glazing over, sometimes act as though they didn't know their black colleagues, as though they had never met them before" (164). While Anderson observes that the general impersonality of urban environments may in part account for this phenomenon, this example nevertheless illustrates the extent to which the particularity of one's perceptual and social world—and, more specifically in this case, its attitude toward race—determines what one acknowledges as significant within it. See Anderson, *The Cosmopolitan Canopy*, especially the chapter "The Color Line and The Canopy," 152–188.

46. Sara Ahmed, *Queer Phenomenology: Orientations, Objects, Others* (Durham, NC: Duke University Press, 2006), 158.

47. Jacobson's analysis of "spatial neglect" in people who fail to acknowledge the "side" of the world that corresponds to the paralyzed side of their body provides a helpful example of the latter phenomenon. See Kirsten Jacobson, "Neglecting Space: Making Sense of a Partial Loss of One's World through a Phenomenological Account of the Spatiality of Embodiment," in *Perception and Its Development in Merleau-Ponty's Phenomenology*, 101–122, ed. Kirsten Jacobson and John Russon (Toronto: University of Toronto Press, 2017), especially 104–111.

48. Shannon Sullivan, *Revealing Whiteness: The Unconscious Habits of Racial Privilege* (Bloomington: Indiana University Press, 2006), 164–165.

49. Sullivan, *Revealing Whiteness*, 165. Sullivan further notes the "fittingness of psychological discomfort" that white people may experience in nonwhite spaces (164). Arguably, such spaces serve an important function for communities of color in a white racist society. Anderson points to this function in his account of the Gallery Mall in Center City Philadelphia as "a black community under a canopy [. . .] where diverse elements of one racial community may mingle peacefully and express themselves more fully" (93). In terms of Anderson's analysis, the discrimination Sullivan's relative experienced in the grocery story was perhaps a response to the threat he represented to the non-white "canopy" within which the Latinx community enjoyed comparative freedom of association and expression.

50. Ahmed, *Queer Phenomenology*, 159–160.

51. Compare Lugones's account of "world"-traveling: "Most of us who are outside the mainstream of, for example, the United States' dominant construction or organization of life are 'world' travelers as a matter of necessity and of survival. It seems to me that inhabiting more than one 'world' at the same time and traveling between worlds is part and parcel of our experience and our situation" (88–89). See María Lugones, "Playfulness, "World"-Traveling, and Loving Perception," in *Pilgrimages/Peregrinajes: Theorizing Coalition against Multiple Oppressions*, 77–100 (New York: Rowman & Littlefield, 2003).

52. By contrast, as I suggest in my discussion of the established spatial level as a form of "possession," the ground of our capacities often goes unnoticed. Ruth Frankenberg's work in *White Women, Race Matters* on "the social geography of race" provides an interesting illustration of this point. Drawing on a number of in-depth interviews with white women, Frankenberg examines their impressions of race and racism in childhood and early adolescence. She notes that while one of the women she interviewed was aware of the social and economic oppression faced by black Americans in her segregated southern town in the late 1960s and early 1970s, she failed to notice the relative privilege she enjoyed (49). For example, while she criticized as racist the behavior of neighbors who attempted to prevent a black family from moving into their all-white neighborhood, she does not, as Frankenberg notes, observe that "the very existence of a neighborhood whose residents are all white itself bespeaks a history of racist structuring of

that community" (47). In effect, the stability of her social situation enabled her to overlook the contingency of its political grounding, even as she recognized the latter in the situation of her black neighbors. See Ruth Frankenberg, *White Women, Race Matters: The Social Construction of Whiteness* (Minneapolis: University of Minnesota Press, 1993), 43–70. I thank Gail Weiss for sharing this text with me.

53. Merleau-Ponty, *Phenomenology of Perception*, 265 [302].

54. Merleau-Ponty, *Phenomenology of Perception*, 265 [303].

55. Weil, "Reflections on the Right Use," 58.

56. My conclusion follows Sullivan's argument that the assumed "neutrality" of space risks perpetuating racism. On this point, she writes that "The conception of space and habits of lived spatiality as race-free constitutes a false neutrality that makes invisible the inequalities of raced space, rendering one powerless in the fact of, and often complicit with, racism. We can more fully combat racial oppression when we are better aware of how racialized space and habits of lived spatiality impact human existence. As long as racial inequalities exist, striving to make the racialization of space visible will be crucial to the fight against racism" (158).

Chapter 8

Moving without Movement

Merleau-Ponty's "I can" and
Memoirs of Bodily Immobility

JAMES RAKOCZI

Introduction

The past thirty years have seen a proliferation of life-writing concentrated around a condition known as locked-in syndrome. Locked-in syndrome, or LIS, was first coined by American neurologists Fred Plum and Jerome B. Posner in the 1960s to describe a state in which a patient experiences near-total motor paralysis but retains full cognitive capacity.[1] Its most common causes are stroke, brain injury, and late-stage amyotrophic lateral sclerosis (ALS). The condition is usually considered permanent, though some definitions do acknowledge temporary forms of LIS such as sleep paralysis and the effects of incorrectly administered anesthetic or certain forms of spider and snakebite venom. The challenge of communication from a subject-position of bodily immobility is immense, both due to the centrality of movement and gesture to language, but also because of the ways in which people fail to recognize the subjecthood of those who cannot move. In clinical settings this can manifest in misdiagnosis and mistreatment when immobile people are presumed to also have nonfunctioning minds. Furthermore, immobility is frequently figured in sociocultural contexts as a form of death. For example, two nineteenth-century French novels are often cited in LIS research to demonstrate literature's credentials for having "highlighted the locked-in condition before the medical community did."[2] But what is rarely attended to is how these novels pursue a representation of immobility as deathlike: Alexandre Dumas describes Monsieur Noirtier de Villefort as "a corpse with living eyes,"[3] whilst Émile Zola depicts a paralyzed woman as "alive but buried deep within a dead body."[4]

This chapter attends to the ways in which Maurice Merleau-Ponty's account of bodily movement in his most influential work, *Phenomenology of Perception*, is helpful in illuminating how clinicians, neurologists, medical humanists, cognitive scientists, and phenomenological philosophers understand the life-writing and communicative capacities of people who live with total or near-total bodily immobility. However, I also wish to show how we should be cautious of the grounds of this helpfulness. Turning to LIS life-writing, I will demonstrate how such texts are not simply descriptions of immobile experience—furnishing theories of movement with example or counterexample—but rather act as sites which themselves interrogate philosophical-phenomenological imaginaries of bodily movement. I argue that Merleau-Ponty's project, commendable in its commitment to the body-subject, nevertheless helped instantiate a conceptualization of bodily integrity that both aids a harmful occlusion of the immobile body and makes certain kinds of theoretical thinking about bodies that cannot move heuristically impossible.

This chapter is, therefore, structured around a pair of questions: what does a Merleau-Pontian toolset allow us to notice about memoirs of bodily immobility, and what does it conceal from us? In section one, I offer a brief survey of current discussions that surround immobility memoirs. Noting that the problem of continuity has emerged as a central point of philosophical anxiety around LIS, I show that in order for debates to converge around this topic the role of movement and nonmovement is precluded. In section two, I turn toward Jean-Dominique Bauby's *The Diving-Bell and the Butterfly* to outline how Merleau-Ponty's phenomenological explanation of a condition known as anosognosia allows us to engage with movement in LIS memoirs and consequently resolve a number of conceptual difficulties of these texts. Yet it is precisely the success of this reading, the utilization of Merleau-Ponty's bodily "substitutive equilibrium" to help explain (or rather, *explain away*) the exegetic difficulties in LIS memoirs, that I wish to interrogate in section three. There, I use the immobility memoirs themselves to critique Merleau-Ponty's philosophy. Merleau-Ponty's *Phenomenology of Perception* ambitiously builds on his earlier account, in *The Structure of Behavior*, of consciousness and the nervous system as a shared system of self-organization to reach a conception of the lived body via phenomenology that is free of any trace of body–mind dualism. In doing so, however, it produces a conception of bodily movement that is bound to self-organization. I aim to show how this philosophical move, grounded in what I will term a therapeutics of the "I can," throws up existentially significant challenges to the interpretation of LIS description and experience.

Continuity and LIS

As Fernando Vidal notes, there has yet to be a "systematic" phenomenology of global bodily immobility,[5] and this neglect parallels the social and ontological exclusion of people who cannot move. Nevertheless, in the past ten years LIS has emerged as a troublesome site for phenomenologically inflected accounts of personhood. This scholarship can be divided by two motivations. First, there is research seeking to describe what the experience of being locked-in is like. This work tends to align toward a bioethical desire to ascertain the quality of life of LIS patients and to call for consequent legal, technological, or health care–based interventions. Second, there is research that investigates LIS not on its own descriptive terms but rather as a limit-case that can be used to guide philosophical, neurological, or theoretical intuitions about so-called normal human experience and consciousness. Marie-Christine Nizzi, for example, has constructed a survey questionnaire for LIS patients that is explicitly for the use of philosophers to think about "*real* patients" as opposed to thought experiments or "fictional cases."[6] Both strands of research often revolve around the question of the continuity of personal identity in locked-in syndrome. Two possibilities tend to be considered when defining the extent of continuity: the direct loss of bodily movement or, more commonly, the breakdown of interpersonal relations.

In the first case, the claim is as follows: given theories that posit bodily movement or sensorimotor apparatuses as integral to embodiment, social identity, or self-experience,[7] global bodily immobility would therefore necessarily make coherent self-experience impossible. However, recent secondary literature on this topic rarely takes this threat too seriously. Miriam Kyselo and Ezequiel Di Paolo, for example, formulate LIS as a "radical" but ultimately "crude challenge" for theories of embodied cognition. They note that the objection circulates informally amongst cognitive scientists but is rarely committed to publication.[8] That said, many texts written by people with LIS do not share this sense of the problem's disposability. Robert Murphy's memoir of a spinal tumor, for example, insinuates an interplay between the progression of his body's immobility and his thoughts: "the slow process of paralysis of my limbs was paralleled by a progressive atrophy of the need and impulse for physical activity. I was losing the will to move."[9] Murphy suggests here that the loss of movement correlates with his mind's capacity to desire movement. I will address the extent and consequence of Murphy's rendering of the impact of not-moving upon his mind in section two.

Yet a large number of locked-in memoirs *prima facie* do insist on the irrelevance of the issue and are in fact preconditioned precisely by an operative textual or narrative strategy that the mind is intact whilst the body cannot move by employing a first-person, stable narrative voice. Vidal points out that LIS is distinguished in clinical and bioethical practice "as precisely *not* being" a disorder of consciousness.[10] Correspondingly, a stable continuity of voice enables what a reader of a memoir about locked-in syndrome might anticipate: the horror of being trapped in one's own body or the triumph of the will over extreme material and bodily circumstances. Kate Allatt's memoir of a rare recovery from LIS is almost fervent in its affirmation of a mind that continues to function quite well despite her inability to move. The text frames its body–mind dualism as therapeutically integral: a "fit Kate inside my head," alongside a "bloody-mindedness" and a "concentration to 'will' my limbs to move by staring at them and thinking 'move, damn you'" was pivotal to Allatt's getting better.[11] In addition, her continuity of self (the "old Kate" who regularly ran seventy kilometers per week on the Yorkshire fells) is repeatedly described as a moving self within her present interiority. When outlining her approach to physiotherapy, the memoir describes a "running psyche" based on "the importance of setting objectives beyond my ability."[12] In Allatt's account of her unusual case, this internalized metaphorical movement translated back into literal movement. For her, it was clear that the temporalities of her past memories and a clinical logic of motricity, where the faintest "flickers of movement" (the slight twitching of Allatt's right thumb) in the ICU ward are taken as signs of rehabilitative possibility,[13] intertwined to achieve a therapeutically successful outcome.

A similar tension plays out in the title of actor Christopher Reeve's memoir, *Still Me*. The title suggests a double meaning, oscillating between a me that has been stilled, and a me that is the same as it ever was, which in Reeve's infamous case was a hypermobile, ultra-ablebodied "Superman." In contrast to Allatt's success, however, Reeve outlines how his body's lack of recovering signs of movement foreclose therapeutic possibility. A high-profile campaigner for further research into spinal cord injury, Reeve argued that the "search for a cure for paralysis" has "never captured the public interest" because "it had always been considered impossible."[14] Allatt's and Reeve's advocacy work has been criticized by disability activists who note the ableism at work in their refusal to accept a shift in bodily circumstances.[15] That said, both also allow us to glimpse an important mapping of immobility and not-moving as being beyond therapeutic recognition, which occurs through the binding together of bodily movement with mind or cognitive capacity.

The more commonly discussed measure of continuity in LIS is the breakdown of interpersonal relations, although it is primarily LIS life-writing that provides explicit accounts of how lack of bodily movement institutes interpersonal exclusion. Andrea Ostrum outlines how her loss of bodily movement following a brain injury altered her relational sense of self in perception: "Voices actually become louder and people seem taller than they really are," and "home health aides who do not occupy a powerful socioeconomic position are perceived as very powerful."[16] In addition, though Ostrum insists on being her "old self" on the "inside," she writes that "because I was trapped in a badly injured body and because the medical books said it was not possible, I no longer existed."[17] Julia Tavalaro's memoir *Look Up for Yes*, alongside Martin Pistorius's *Ghost Boy*, similarly describe instances of the sustained failure of medical and health care staff to notice that the writers were conscious. Tavalaro lived on a ward for six years, known dismissively to staff as "the vegetable," before she was diagnosed with LIS.

Out of health care settings, Albert Robillard's autoethnographic work *Meaning of a Disability* details via ethnomethodological analysis how his bodily immobility excludes him ontologically from social interaction. Analyzing an incident in which it proved impossible for him to hold a seat for his wife in a restaurant, Robillard outlines how ALS led him to discover how bodily movement is "the foundation of mutually understood, coordinated integration" that "compose[s] our everyday existence with others."[18] Simon Fitzmaurice likewise interprets the averted gaze of others when he is in a public space as the social refiguring of his immobile body as "a totem of fear. Sickness, madness, death . . . a touchstone to be avoided." The exception is children, who "do not look away" because they are still "looking for the definition" of humanity.[19]

Within academic debates that surround LIS, life-writing's textured articulation of the role of nonmovement in social exclusion is displaced in favor of a focus on the interpersonal threat to continuity itself. For example, where Nizzi, Veronique Blandin, and Athena Demertzi insist on the imperative of "recognition" by describing how "personhood in LIS is progressively regained as the widening circle of others recognizes them as persons,"[20] Dan Zahavi counterargues that such an account conflates "two quite different normative conceptions" of personhood.[21] Zahavi's concept of "minimal self" prevents him from being able to accept a notion of social death. He argues that it cannot be the case that "personal identity is dependent upon social interaction to such an extent that I will cease being a person if the latter is interrupted."[22] He also rejects Kyselo's insistence that to be a self—even a minimal self—is to be self-organizational and social, instead arguing that "to distinguish oneself from others" occurs on the basis of "ontological or physiological" and not "processual and organizational" boundaries.[23] Bracketing this debate, I wish to observe how both Kyselo and Zahavi's analyses conceal the mechanisms by which the marginalization or exclusion of immobilized body-subjects occurs and instead prefigures the self-evidentness of experiential continuity in LIS. There is strikingly little mention of the role of nonmovement in their analyses. For Zahavi, LIS is simply a bad example to discuss the (dis)continuity of selfhood: "If there is something in particular (the study of) LIS can teach us," he concludes, it is to "appreciate the resilience of human beings," and to not "operate with too narrow a conception" of a meaningful life.[24] For Kyselo, who does consider LIS a threat to experiential continuity, the challenge of LIS is figuring out how to extend and reestablish the possibilities of sensorimotor capacities for the patient and across the patient's intersubjective network.[25] Each views LIS as exemplary of the body's potential to reorientate itself to new life projects. Similarly, Marie-Aurélie Bruno, Nizzi, Steven Laureys, and Olivia Gosseries appeal to the capacitation of "homeostatic resources" in their interpretation of a "'happy' subgroup of LIS survivors" reported by Nizzi's 2012 survey:

these are individuals "capable of high flexibility and plasticity who have fully succeeded in recalibrating, reprioritizing, and reorienting" their needs, values, and judgments.[26]

Whether arguing for the continuity or discontinuity of the experience of immobility, both sides emphasize the recapacitating potential of living with an extreme disability such as LIS. This entails the foregrounding of therapeutic movements—what Merleau-Ponty would refer to as substitutive equilibrium—in a condition that is precisely about the challenge of bodily nonmovement. In the following section, I will use Merleau-Ponty to uncover the processes of therapeutic movement at work in a single LIS memoir. Through this reading, however, I aim to also map how this secondary literature's emphasis on resilience, or intersubjective recapacitation, rests on a potentially misleading or harmful inattention to the phenomenological characteristics of bodily immobility itself.

Butterflies

[I] am beginning to forge glorious substitute destinies for myself.[27]

The most well-known and cited memoir of LIS is editor of French *Elle* magazine Jean-Dominique Bauby's *Le scaphandre et le papillon*, translated into English as *The Diving-Bell and the Butterfly* just a few months after Bauby's death in 1997. In 1995, at the age of forty-three, Bauby suffered a severe stroke that rendered him almost completely immobile for the rest of his life. In this time, Bauby wrote his memoir and founded ALIS, which continues to sponsor and collaborate with researchers of LIS to this day. The memoir's translated title gestures temptingly toward a reading of Bauby's memoir as a dualistic tale in which the body exists as a prison from which the mind can occasionally escape. A 1997 *New York Times* review declares: "The diving bell of Bauby's title is his corporeal trap, the butterfly his imagination."[28] However, rather than embracing the dualism that Bauby's deteriorating mobility seemed to instantiate, a number of critical readings instead explore how Bauby's account of LIS might square with an ontology or phenomenology that seeks to privilege the body, or even bodily movement, as constitutive activity.

Richard Zaner, for example, argues that the memoir's "powerful attraction" is its ability to represent "the sheer density of embodiment *in extremis*," and suggests that the text's staging of its own means of production (encounters with speech therapists, descriptions of the laborious writing process) demonstrates its concern with embodied forms of consciousness and interaction.[29] However, Zaner also views Bauby's "unbidden flights of fancy" as an increasing inability "to stay in touch with the surrounding milieu of people, things, environing spaces and places," a sentiment that tacitly endorses the dualism of "the butterfly."[30] Lisa Diedrich attempts to resolve the dualism by noting how Bauby's memoir insists that the diving-bell holds "his *body*, not his *mind* prisoner." She argues that "the diving bell does not signify a mind/body split" but, following Merleau-Ponty, a "phenomenal/objective body split: his phenomenal body is contained within an objective body (the diving bell) that then mediates his being-in-the-world."[31] Conversely, she suggests that Bauby's "condition of utter passivity—his extreme suffering, his solitude, and his nearness to death" precipitates a crucial qualitative difference to the form of consciousness he now experiences compared to that of his previous life. Lacking "*active intentionality*," Bauby's consciousness has become like a phenomenological reduction, not "directed outward in a taken-for-granted manner," but instead "directed inward and back upon itself."[32]

Yet in *Phenomenology of Perception*, Merleau-Ponty insists that the principal lesson of the phenomenological reduction is the "impossibility" of a "complete reduction."[33] Thus, under Diedrich's formulation, the impossibility of active intentionality in cases such as Bauby's LIS is itself impossible. This impossibility of an impossibility is evidenced by the ways in which the memoir represents Bauby's imagination:

> My mind takes flight like a butterfly. There is so much to do. You can wander off in space or in time, set out for Tierra del Fuego or for King Midas's court.
>
> You can visit the woman you love, slide down beside her and stroke her still-sleeping face. You can build castles in Spain, steal the Golden Fleece, discover Atlantis, realize your childhood dreams and adult ambitions.[34]

The text takes care in its use of verbs to assert the bodily capacity required for each of the escapist adventures evoked. Bauby does not just appear where he wants in time and space but has to take "flight," "wander off" or "set out." The butterfly simile is not merely a disembodied witness, but instead a rendering of the mind as an embodied presence that constantly metamorphoses, so that it can attend to and interact with its environment ("slide down beside her . . . build castles . . . steal the Golden Fleece"). From its subject-position of bodily immobility, then, the text might be said to uncover a similar insight to that of Merleau-Ponty's philosophy: a bodily "I can" exists as integral to our imagination as well as our perception. Just as perception requires a "tacit understanding of what our corporeal possibilities are at any given point in time,"[35] so too does imagination. This is not because imagination defers to perception, but because both perception and imagination are phenomenally imbricated in a world that "at every moment . . . demands a complete response."[36] Such a complete response is fulfilled by the privilege of having a body and *being able to move that body*. Merleau-Ponty writes:

> A "corporeal or postural schema" gives us at every moment a global, practical, and implicit notion of the relation between our body and things, of our hold on them. A system of possible movements, or "motor projects," radiates from us to our environment . . . Even our most secret affective movements . . . help to shape our perception of things.[37]

According to Merleau-Ponty, when there is a loss of bodily possibility, this "global, practical" notion does not go away. The body instead develops alternate strategies to articulate its complete response to the world. In Bauby's case, his descriptions of imaginative scenes can themselves be understood as such an articulation. The text can be read as the trace of this substitution, a tool that *incorporates itself* as Bauby's mobile body.

This conceptualization can be further illuminated by turning to Merleau-Ponty's account of cases of anosognosia in paralysis. Anosognosia is a condition in which a patient denies the existence of their ailment; its etiology remains contested. In Weinstein and Kahn's 1955 psychodynamic interpretation, the condition is considered to be "a psychological defensive mechanism," a repression or "reaction aimed to protect the self from the potential distress deriving from suffering."[38] More recent correlative theories posit that anosognosia accompanies the brain lesion directly. K.M. Heilman's "feed-forward" account, for example, suggests that the ability to intend to make movements is lost directly with the body's inability to make those movements.[39] Yet correlative theories fail to account for how anosognosic patients can be highly inventive in explaining away their inability to move.[40] Patients might insist they have made movements when they have not or claim they are not moving for another reason such as laziness, nervousness, or propriety.

Because of this lack of scientific clarity, Merleau-Ponty's phenomenological explanation of anosognosic perception remains a plausible defense of prereflective motor-intentionality. Merleau-Ponty characterizes actions that deny the existence of a "defect" as a "phenomenon of substitution." Through this phenomenon, we "discover the movement of being in and toward the world." Merleau-Ponty considers the case of an insect that has its leg tied as analogous, because the creature instinctively attempts to continue using its leg: "the impulse of activity that goes toward the world still passes through that limb."[41] This reveals a prereflective "movement" toward the world also visible in humans experiencing anosognosia of paralysis:

> What refuses the mutilation or the deficiency in us is [. . .] an *I* that continues to tend toward its world despite deficiencies or amputations and that to this extent does not *de jure* recognize them. The refusal of the deficiency is but the reverse side of our inherence in the world, the implicit negation of what runs counter to the natural movement that throws us into our [. . .] familiar horizons.[42]

Robert Murphy's memoir, *The Body Silent*, cites Colin Smith's translation of this passage—providing an opportunity to consider the impact of Merleau-Ponty's account within a self-description of immobility. Murphy considers the way in which "paralytics say that they no longer feel attached to their bodies" as a way of "expressing the shattering of Merleau-Ponty's body–mind system."[43] Murphy reads into Merleau-Ponty's description of a disabled body's "adherence" to its world (in cases of phantom limb or anosognosia) a violent mode of being. Because of the failure of "adherence," anosognosic phenomenality entails a ceaselessly felt sense of loss. The "amputee is missing more than a limb: He is also missing one of his conceptual links to the world, an anchor of his very existence."[44] Furthermore, Murphy notes an even more pernicious lack for the immobilized body-subject: the "delicate feedback loops between thought and movement" have themselves "been broken." Bodily movement is the actualization as well as the articulation of thought, and this means that "writing has become almost an addiction"—which is conceptualized by Murphy as the accomplishment of Merleau-Ponty's lived body's "refusal of disablement." The ambiguity of Murphy's account resides in how paralysis threatens thought by destroying the will but also by unmooring it from the possibility of its actualizing into motion. As in Zaner and Allatt's reading of Bauby, this "leaves one adrift in a lonely monologue, an inner soliloquy without rest or surcease."[45]

It is only once Merleau-Ponty has argued that anosognosia demonstrates the existence of "natural movements" that he introduces the distinction between the habitual and actual body (underpinning Diedrich's phenomenal/objective reading of Bauby). For Merleau-Ponty, the habitual body's natural movements act, in the case of people who cannot move, as a kind of guarantor for an immobilized actual body. When the body stops being able to move or to interact with its world in some way, it retains the residual and habitual shadows of those "natural movements" developed when it could move. It is for this reason that people with anosognosic paralysis are able to retain the belief that they can move.

Merleau-Ponty's analysis, I suggest, is immensely helpful in attending to the ways Bauby's text operates in both discreet and explicit ways as a form of persistent movement. In what ways could a genre of memoir distinguished by its depiction of the spatial, material, and corporeal labor of its own making be described as anosognosic? In *The Diving-Bell*, Bauby describes blinking his left eyelid to indicate what next letter should be transcribed by a bedside listener. The listener read off an alphabet board "until with a blink" of his eye, Bauby stopped them at "at the letter to be noted [46] He writes:

> My main task now is to compose the first of these bedridden travel notes so that I shall be ready when my publisher's emissary arrives to take my dictation, letter by letter. In my head I churn over every sentence ten times, delete a word, add an adjective, and learn my text by heart, paragraph by paragraph.[47]

Immediately after learning this, however, we are told how a duty nurse "interrupts the flow" of Bauby's thoughts. The text describes her "well-established ritual": "she draws the curtain, checks tracheostomy and drip-feed, and turns on the TV so I can watch the news."[48] The description of Bauby's writing-labor is thus instantly subverted by the description of a nurse's labor around his body. In the description of this interruption, the bodily writing-labor has been immediately transformed and redescribed as a flow of thoughts experiencing a situation. The text conceals its methods of production the moment it has revealed them. In two paragraphs, what little bodily movement Bauby has is transformed into a flow of thoughts, and what we have just been told is a carefully crafted text, learned by rote, disappears into this flow.

The memoir's final chapter, "Season of Renewal," exemplifies this theme of textual production exceeding itself. It is a scene of someone "reading out these pages we have patiently extracted from the void every afternoon for the past two months."[49] Yet the text is telling us about this scene of its own recounting. It creates the sense of existing outside of its own textual production. Using Merleau-Ponty, we can resolve this ambiguity as an anosognosic impulse, and the text's movements become understandable neither as anachronistic nor solipsistic. The text imitates the "natural movements" of perception. It allows what little movement Bauby has to flourish into transcendental movement, into language—springing forth an able, moving self: an "I can." By reading the memoir through Merleau-Ponty, we are able to see the text as a therapeutic strategy in which the act of describing the diving-bell produces the movements of a butterfly.

This has a crucial consequence for the reading of immobility memoirs. When they have been taken up in the secondary literature, they are often thought of as a means to understand the experience of being unable to move. Bauby's text, for example, has been described as an "exemplar" resource for medical students looking to learn about, or sensitize themselves to, the bodily realities of LIS.[50] A reader of *The Diving-Bell* learns "how it is to be locked-in" and is "forced to look at this situation through the eyes of a sufferer."[51]

Phenomenological readings have tended to describe illness life-writing in two ways. First, as Diedrich notes, they have understood them as "case studies that seek to describe . . . the disabled body in the world,"[52] attempts to capture rather than alter the texture of experience. Second, in order to adhere to a medical humanist imperative, they often enact a dualistic tendency to regard the phenomenal body of the text as in some way distinct from the objectified and immobilized body of medical treatment. What Merleau-Ponty helps us recognize is that to view the text as merely a representation of LIS (a what-it-is-like-ness) is to misunderstand the text as a static rendering of events rather than a movement in and of itself. Immobility narratives are not a *representation of sick bodies* (an "I think") but a *therapeutics of sick bodies* (an "I can"). In this light, we can see the work that such texts do in producing the continuities of experience and the subject.

Merleau-Ponty and Bodily Movement

Merleau-Ponty has allowed us to resolve the body–mind contradictions of immobility life-writing by identifying them as anosognosic texts. In phenomenological terms, through their construction of a perceptual-narrative flow (a motor-sensory seamlessness), these texts reveal a capacitating orientation to the world on a prereflective level. My task now, however, is to unpack an uneasiness I have about these capacitating therapeutics and to examine the subjectivities that become unthinkable through this Merleau-Pontian heuristic. I wish to consider here what is shared with the sublimation of nonmovement into questions of continuity within the philosophical and bioethical debates that surround LIS. Turning the critical gears the other way, I will now apply LIS life-writing to Merleau-Ponty's account of movement in the *Phenomenology*. My concern is with the supposed illegibility of not-moving, and how the experiences of people who are unable to move are subsumed into phenomenological logics of therapy—the "I can," the intentional arc, substitutive equilibrium—that are grounded in ceaseless and adaptive movement. Merleau-Ponty's account affords a cultural primacy to movement so total that not-moving is always already writing itself out of existence and, in the case of LIS memoirs, quite literally. With this observation, I hope to tease out how various orthodoxies of movement have become commonplace and unnoticed.

In her reading of Julian Schnabel's film adaptation of Bauby's memoir, Megan Craig notes some of the exclusionary consequences of Merleau-Ponty's theory of embodiment. For her, the significance of LIS is in how it "forces us to reevaluate the attribution of consciousness or degrees of consciousness via visible clues (i.e., he *looks* conscious) or linguistic ability (i.e., he *tells* us he is conscious)."[53] As a consequence of Merleau-Ponty's account of bodily movement as not only the signifier of consciousness but the actualization of consciousness, Craig worries that his philosophy of the body is, in fact, a narrowing humanism. Her analysis concentrates on a section of *Eye and Mind* that becomes "disturbing . . . in relation to Bauby." Merleau-Ponty writes that a body with no ability to cross-blend its visual field—a body, as Craig reads it, with only one working eye—would "be an almost adamantine body, not really flesh, not really the body of a human being. There would be no humanity."[54] Sharing her concern with bodily exclusion, I would add that Craig does not recognize the role that bodily movement is doing in her own account of bodily organization. By focusing her reading on "the flickering, darting organ" of Bauby's eye, she views this movement as an instantiation of transcendental forms of being: "an acrobat—a butterfly."[55] But what if this interpretation, which we have seen Bauby's text is frequently interpreted as drawing us toward, is itself implicative of a normative—or rather *pseudo-normative*—therapeutic imaginary of movement? In other words, although Craig incisively draws attention to the ways Merleau-Ponty's account excludes certain forms of disabled embodiment from the category of the human,[56] her principal response is to foreground the bodily movements of which Bauby remains capable. This strategy thus participates in Merleau-Ponty's own presumptions about movement and its therapeutic grounds of belonging in the world. What remains unattended is the immobility and disintegration that also accompanies Bauby's human life. This elision typifies a phenomenon that Katherine Morris notes: authors who use Merleau-Ponty to analyze illness seem to only emphasize "healthy" responses to illness.[57]

I contend that Merleau-Ponty's "I can" gestures toward a self-organizing network of movements that precedes the tactile kinesthesis of the body. It is a therapeutic, as much as it is a bodily, philosophical intercession. To demonstrate this, I would like to consider the way in which the *Phenomenology of Perception* introduces the "I can" and how the "I can" relates to Merleau-Ponty's use of pathology. We find the "I can" introduced into the text only after another concept—the intentional arc—is presented. The intentional arc extends the concept of intentionality into the body, motor-intentionality, and further expands the concept into an all-encompassing account of the complexity of what it is like to live in that body. By extending and expanding intentionality into an all-encompassing arc, Merleau-Ponty draws attention toward the intertwined vulnerabilities of thinking, moving, speaking, perceiving, and living. The arc is a philosophical concept that accounts not for how consciousness works, as intentionality itself does, but rather how "consciousness can be ill."[58] Talia Welsh characterizes pathologies as a disruption of the intentional arc,[59] but it is worth empathizing here that Merleau-Ponty rarely characterizes such disruption as a rupture or breakage. Instead, disorders alter the topography of the arc: it "goes limp."[60] Sickness remains a "complete form of existence," for Merleau-Ponty, to the extent that we can never "fully be sick."[61]

Unpacking this idea further, we can notice how Bauby's representation is hypothesized as itself a movement, and how—as Merleau-Ponty puts it—representation is always "simultaneously a de-presentation."[62] Such an emphasis on movement that then allows for representational mutability is precisely what the bodily "I can" substitutes for the Cartesian "I think." "I think therefore I am" becomes "I am therefore I think," only this "I am" is explicitly couched by Merleau-Ponty *as* movement: the "movement of transcendence of the 'I am.'"[63] It is in this way that movement becomes the condition of possibility of existence. The "I can" is mediated and sustained by movement, and this movement is always a movement-away-from decapacitation, an "I cannot." As an example, Merleau-Ponty describes a blind person's cane as "an instrument *with* which" they come to perceive: "an extension of the bodily synthesis."[64] Unable to see, the blind person incorporates the cane within their bodily schema. Merleau-Ponty describes this as "a new knot of significations" in which "previous movements are integrated into a new motor entity." What makes the emergence of this new knot possible is how it is "anticipated in our experience through a certain lack." The blind person moves toward an "equilibrium" by moving away from the "lack" of their sightlessness.[65] The intentional arc explains how canes, alternate body parts, memories, and ultimately texts can all be substituted for one another in the development of this equilibrium of self. The continuity of personal identity, under this account, relies on the capacitation of a body's movements toward the completion of its body.

Not only is this rendering of movement integral to the intentional arc but it is also critical in interpreting Merleau-Ponty's difficult relationship to the role of dualism in the experience of pathology. In the *Phenomenology of Perception*'s final chapter, "Freedom," Merleau-Ponty seemingly oscillates between critiquing Sartre's account of free will in *Being and Nothingness* and also endorsing it. He begins by discussing how even in cases of "sick-consciousness" a wholeness of perception is maintained:

> We are often amazed that . . . the person suffering from a disease can bear the situation. But in their own eyes they are not disabled or dying . . . Consciousness can never objectify itself as sick-consciousness or as disabled-consciousness . . . In returning to the core of his consciousness, everyone feels himself to be beyond his particular characteristics and so resigns himself to them. They are the price we pay, without even thinking about it, for being in the world, a formality we take for granted.[66]

This somewhat Sartrean claim, that there is always a first-personal consciousness at work viewing the sickness (that is therefore not really sick), appears to conflict with the explanatory framework of the intentional arc. Yet a similar idea can also be found in *The Structure of Behavior*, as Merleau-Ponty discusses how there is "always a duality which reappears at one level or another" in instances of bodily limitation.[67] Though this might accord with the perpetuation of interiority in self-descriptions of LIS, it has the odd consequence of Merleau-Ponty seeming to be unable or unwilling to unpack the full implications of his body-subject precisely in cases when bodies make their most radical interventions.

This exegetic difficulty is resolved once we consider how Merleau-Ponty's notion of duality in these instances is in fact predicated on the phenomenality of this "consciousness of" that perceives one's own disabled body. This phenomenality is—as Merleau-Ponty unpacks throughout parts one and two of *Phenomenology of Perception*—constituted by the perceptions and movements of "worldliness." We cannot, as he writes in part one, "relate certain movements to the bodily mechanism and certain other ones to consciousness," and therefore we must recognize that "there are *several ways for the body to be a body, and several ways for consciousness to be consciousness.*"[68] All these "*ways*" are movements that reside, and must be thought, at a level of phenomenality that allows for the body's myriad and parallel processes to be understood together. In his account of the phenomenon of movement itself, in part two, Merleau-Ponty writes that if "we can ever speak of a movement without a moving object, then it is surely in the case of one's own body. The movement of my eye toward what it will focus upon is not the shifting of one object in relation to another object; it is a march toward the real."[69] What enables Merleau-Ponty's pairing of movement and therapeutics is precisely this concern with the mutual imbrication of higher psychical processes and motor innervation. Bodily movement must always be thought of as the completion of an organizing system.

This is illuminated by considering the *Phenomenology of Perception*'s brief engagement with neurologist Hugo Liepmann, whose pioneering work on apraxia Merleau-Ponty considered instructive because apraxia can be accounted for neither as a nervous problem nor a psychological problem. Merleau-Ponty constellates his engagement with Liepmann around the following question: if bodily movements themselves produce the representative function, how can we conceptualize the anticipation of individual movements as non-representational? Merleau-Ponty notes how difficult it is "to bring pure motor intentionality to light," because it "hides behind the objective world that it contributes to constituting."[70] Liepmann's diagnostic of apraxia both encounters this difficulty and indicates its solution through how it discloses that our relationships to objects must be as much practical as they are theoretical. The distinction "between the body as mechanism in itself and consciousness as a being for itself" collapses: consciousness is the actualization of the body, and the body is the actualization of consciousness.[71]

Under Merleau-Ponty's formulation, then, two quite dramatic shifts are occurring in the understanding of bodies. First, we see the privileging of a therapeutic self—a self always already seeking to move beyond itself, to "get better," a self entirely consonant with a number of theoretical ideas that have emerged from Merleau-Ponty's thinking: for example, Francisco Varela's autopoiesis, Catherine Malabou's plasticity, Frantz Fanon and Sylvia Wynter's sociogenesis, as well as biomedical notions of ecological prosthesis. Second, we see how this therapeutic self is not so much a notion of therapeutics but a motion. Consequently, people who cannot move—who are unable to partake in these processual, organizational movements—are excluded from recognition. Or, at the very least, their not-moving is incorporated into schemas of movement's legibility. Otherwise they are coded, as witnessed in contemporary LIS scholarship's quick allusions to Dumas and Zola, toward death, and their immobility remains an existential and experiential ground-zero of death in life. The "I can" is a *therapeutic originary* precisely to the extent by which movement remains possible.

Through the bidirectional configuring of LIS life-writing outlined in this chapter, I have aimed to catch hold of the subtle and multitudinous ways in which not-moving has been made unthinkable: a horizon of death beyond therapeutic possibility. It is into the midst of these grounds of unthinkability that I argue life-writing of bodily immobility must make its intervention. Immobility life-writings are readable not only as emblematic of the movement therapeutics they inherit, as I suggested in section two, but also through their imbrication within such dilemmas of movement. They subversively—even radically—attend to qualitative features of bodily immobility which Merleau-Pontian thought neglects. LIS memoirs should be taken neither straightforwardly as a transmission of experience (description, exemplars, cases), nor as adaptations of a corporeal schema (resilience, continuity, plasticity), but rather as what Bauby styles as "*samizdat* bulletins."[72] Immobility writing functions, in other words, to expand clandestinely upon an aspect of lived experience which—in phenomenological, neurological, bioethical, and indeed ontological imaginaries—is excluded from both language and life.

Notes

1. Jerome B. Posner, Clifford B. Saper, Nicholas D. Schiff, and Fred Plum, *Plum and Posner's Diagnosis of Stupor and Coma*, 4th ed. (Oxford & New York: Oxford University Press, 2007), 7.

2. Marie-Aurélie Bruno, Marie-Christine Nizzi, Steven Laureys, and Olivia Gosseries, "Consciousness in the Locked-in Syndrome," *The Neurology of Consciousness*, 2nd ed., eds. Steven Laureys, Olivia Gosseries, and Giulio Tononi (San Diego & London & Waltham: Academic Press, 2016), 189.

3. Alexandre Dumas, *The Count of Monte Cristo* (London: Wordsworth Editions, 1997), 474.

4. Émile Zola, *Thérèse Raquin*, trans. Andrew Rothwell (Oxford: Oxford University Press, 1992), 158.

5. Fernando Vidal, "Phenomenology of the Locked-in Syndrome: An Overview and Some Suggestions," *Neuroethics* (2018): 1. https://doi.org/10.1007/s12152-018-9388-1

6. Marie-Christine Nizzi, Athena Demertzi, Olivia Gosseries, Marie-Aurélie Bruno, François Jouen, and Steven Laureys, "From Armchair to Wheelchair: How Patients with a Locked-In Syndrome Integrate Bodily Changes in Experienced Identity," *Consciousness and Cognition* 21 (2012), 432.

7. Merleau-Ponty presents a philosophical account that accords bodily movement this constitutive role. Also instructive in this regard are a few sociological subdisciplines and aesthetic projects that Merleau-Ponty influenced from the 1960s, such as Harold Garfinkel's ethnomethodological program or Maxine Sheets-Johnstone's phenomenology of dance. See Harold Garfinkel, *Studies in Ethnomethodology* (Englewood Cliffs: Prentice-Hall, Inc., 1967) and Maxine Sheets-Johnstone, *Phenomenology of Dance*, 50th anniversary ed. (Philadelphia: Temple University Press, 2015).

8. Miriam Kyselo and Ezequiel Di Paolo, "Locked-In Syndrome: A Challenge for Embodied Cognitive Science," *Phenomenology and Cognitive Science* 14 (2015): 519.

9. Robert F. Murphy, *The Body Silent* (New York & London: W. W. Norton, 1990), 88.

10. Vidal, "Phenomenology," 13.

11. Kate Allatt and Alison Stokes, *Running Free* (Bedlinog, Wales: Accent Press, 2011), 96, 209.

12. Allatt and Stokes, *Running*, 132.

13. Allatt and Stokes, *Running*, 192.

14. Christopher Reeve, *Still Me* (London: Century, 1998), 132.

15. Eli Clare, *Brilliant Imperfection: Grappling with Cure* (Durham, NC & London: Duke University Press, 2017), 12.

16. Andrea E. Ostrum, "Brain Injury: A Personal View," *Journal of Clinical and Experimental Neuropsychology* 15, no. 4 (1993): 632.

17. Andrea E. Ostrum, "The 'Locked-In' Syndrome—Comments from a Survivor," *Brain Injury* 8, no. 1 (1994): 97.

18. Albert Robillard, *Meaning of a Disability: The Lived Experience of Paralysis* (Philadelphia: Temple University Press, 1999), 105.

19. Simon Fitzmaurice, *It's Not Yet Dark* (Boston & New York: Houghton Mifflin Harcourt, 2017), 2.

20. Marie-Christine Nizzi, Veronique Blandin, and Athena Demertzi, "Attitudes towards Personhood in the Locked-in Syndrome: From Third- to First-Person Perspective and to Interpersonal Significance," *Neuroethics* (2018): 8. https://doi.org/10.1007/s12152-018-9375-6

21. Dan Zahavi, "Locked-In Syndrome: A Challenge to Standard Accounts of Selfhood and Personhood?" *Neuroethics* (2019): 4. https://doi.org/10.1007/s12152-019-09405-8

22. Zahavi, "Locked-In," 5.

23. Zahavi, "Locked-In," 6.

24. Zahavi, "Locked-In," 7.

25. Miriam Kyselo, "More than Our Body: Minimal and Enactive Selfhood in Global Paralysis," *Neuroethics* (2019): 16. https://doi.org/10.1007/s12152-019-09404-9

26. Bruno, Nizzi, Laureys, and Gosseries, "Consciousness," 197.

27. Jean-Dominique Bauby, *The Diving-Bell and the Butterfly*, trans. Jeremy Leggatt (London: Harper Perennial, 2004), 124.

28. Thomas Mallon, "In the Blink of an Eye," *New York Times*, June 15, 1997. www.nytimes.com/1997/06/15/books/in-the-blink-of-an-eye.html?mtrref=www.google.com&gwh=544F2E74E44F33E3C3AD24E37873F4C3&gwt=pay

29. Richard M. Zaner, "Sisyphus without Knees: Exploring Self-Other Relationships Through Illness and Disability," *Literature and Medicine* 22, no. 2 (2003): 194, 191.

30. Zaner, "Sisyphus," 196. Zaner is paralleling Allatt's dismissal of Bauby's memoir: "Unlike Bauby I could not, and would not, allow my imagination to run away with me. In my mind imagination was an indulgence, and . . . only distracted me from the road ahead—getting better" (Allatt and Stokes, *Running*, 148–149).

31. Lisa Diedrich, "Breaking Down: A Phenomenology of Disability," *Literature and Medicine* 20, no. 2 (2001): 220.

32. Diedrich, "Breaking," 221.

33. Maurice Merleau-Ponty, *Phenomenology of Perception*, trans. Donald A. Landes (Abingdon: Routledge, 2012), lxxvii.

34. Bauby, *Diving-Bell*, 13.

35. Gail Weiss, *Body Images: Embodiment as Intercorporeality* (New York & London: Routledge, 1999), 17.

36. Jessica Wiskus, *The Rhythm of Thought: Art, Literature, and Music After Merleau-Ponty* (Chicago: University of Chicago Press, 2013), 56.

37. Maurice Merleau-Ponty, *The Primacy of Perception*, trans. James M. Edie (Evanston, IL: Northwestern University Press, 1964), 5.

38. Gabriella Bottini, Eraldo Paulesu, Martina Gandola, Lorenzo Pia, Paola Invernizzi, and Anna Berti, "Anosognosia for Hemiplegia and Models of Motor Control: Insights from Lesional Data," in *The Study of Anosognosia*, ed. George P. Prigatano (New York: Oxford University Press, 2010), 18.

39. K.M. Heilman, "Anosognosia: Possible neuropsychological mechanisms," in *Awareness of Deficit after Brain Injury: Clinical and Theoretic Issues*, eds. George P. Prigatano and Daniel L. Schacter (New York: Oxford University Press, 1991), 53.

40. C.D. Frith, S.J. Blakemore, and D.M. Wolpert, "Abnormalities in the Awareness and Control of Action," *Philosophical Transactions of the Royal Society of London; B Biological Sciences* 355, no. 1404 (2000): 1771.

41. Merleau-Ponty, *Phenomenology*, 80.

42. Merleau-Ponty, *Phenomenology*, 83–84.

43. Murphy, *Body Silent*, 102.

44. Murphy, *Body Silent*, 99.

45. Murphy, *Body Silent*, 102.

46. Bauby, *Diving-Bell*, 28.

47. Bauby, *Diving-Bell*, 13.

48. Bauby, *Diving-Bell*, 14.

49. Bauby, *Diving-Bell*, 138.

50. P.J. Kearney, "Autopathography and Humane Medicine: *The Diving Bell and the Butterfly*—An Interpretation," *Medical Humanities* 32 (2006): 113.

51. Joost Haan, "Locked-in: The Syndrome as Depicted in Literature," in *Literature, Neurology and Neuroscience: Neurological and Psychiatric Disorders*, eds. Stanley Finger, François Boller, and Anne Stiles (Amsterdam: Elsevier, 2013), 28.

52. Diedrich, "Breaking," 209.

53. Megan Craig, "Locked In," *Journal of Speculative Philosophy* 22, no. 3 (2008): 146.

54. Maurice Merleau-Ponty, "Eye and Mind," in *The Merleau-Ponty Aesthetics Reader: Philosophy and Painting*, ed. Galen A. Johnson (Evanston, IL: Northwestern University Press, 1993), 125.

55. Craig, "Locked-In," 149.

56. Disability theorist Tobin Siebers describes such cultural exclusions as exemplifying what he terms an aesthetics of human disqualification. See Tobin Siebers, *Disability Aesthetics* (Ann Arbor: University of Michigan Press, 2010), 23.

57. Katherine J. Morris, *Starting with Merleau-Ponty* (London & New York: Continuum Books, 2012), 129.

58. Merleau-Ponty, *Phenomenology*, 139.
59. Talia Welsh, "Many Healths: Nietzsche and Phenomenologies of Illness," *Frontiers of Philosophy in China* 11, no. 3 (2016): 340.
60. Merleau-Ponty, *Phenomenology*, 138.
61. Merleau-Ponty, *Phenomenology*, 110.
62. Merleau-Ponty, *Phenomenology*, 381.
63. Merleau-Ponty, *Phenomenology*, 403.
64. Merleau-Ponty, *Phenomenology*, 154.
65. Merleau-Ponty, *Phenomenology*, 155.
66. Merleau-Ponty, *Phenomenology*, 458–459.
67. Maurice Merleau-Ponty, *The Structure of Behavior*, trans. Alden L. Fisher (Pittsburgh: Duquesne University Press, 2015), 210.
68. Merleau-Ponty, *Phenomenology*, 125.
69. Merleau-Ponty, *Phenomenology*, 291.
70. Merleau-Ponty, *Phenomenology*, 523.
71. Merleau-Ponty, *Phenomenology*, 525.
72. Bauby, *Diving-Bell*, 89.

Chapter 9

A Whole New World

Reimagining Divergent Sensory and
Perceptual Experience in Autism through
Merleau-Ponty's *Phenomenology of Perception*

JENNIFER E. BRADLEY

Introduction

Autism is a complex social and clinical phenomenon that has been subjected to extensive inquiry across various disciplines. It has challenged researchers in the social sciences to reconsider long-sedimented theories regarding core aspects of human experiences such as sociality, emotionality, and, more recently, sense and perceptual experience.[1] A key feature of autism is divergent sensory and perceptual experience.[2] More than 80 percent of individuals diagnosed with autism have reported some degree of sensory difficulties.[3] Meryl Alper referenced four sensory processing difficulties that can "emerge in environments that are not configured for an individual's differences: high threshold and passive response (low sensory registration), high threshold and active response (sensory seeking), low threshold and passive response (sensory sensitive), and low threshold and active response (sensory avoiding)."[4] These sensory sensitivities have been consistently reported throughout the literature and reviews.[5] Research further suggests these divergent sensory experiences may be implicated in the social and communication deficits, as well as in the repetitive behaviors, that are key features of autism.[6]

In her review *Autism and the Senses*, Olga Solomon outlines two polarizing lenses through which autism is conceptualized. The first is the biomedical and clinical lens, which understands autism as a neurodevelopmental disorder. Within this biomedical model, research is aimed at uncovering the etiology of autism, clarifying its symptomatic presentation, and testing and assessing clinical and medical interventions.[7] The second approach that Solomon identifies is an ethnographically informed research model that conceptualizes autism as "a personal, family and community/ social group experience."[8] Researchers in the social sciences and humanities who adopt this approach attempt to generate knowledge about autism through exploring the lived experiences of individuals with autism and their families, and examining how normative social and cultural discourses inform how autism is conceived.[9] In recent years, ethnographic studies have explored the social, cultural and phenomenological dimensions of sensory experience.[10] In Meryl Alper's article, "Inclusive Sensory Ethnography: Studying New Media and Neurodiversity in Everyday Life," she illustrates her ethnographical approach to studying the sensory experience in relation to interactive media use.[11] According to Alper, "inclusive sensory ethnography allows for more nuanced observation of the social, the sensory, and their co-configuration, particularly among the autistic population . . ."[12] An inclusive sensory approach further attends to the embodied and emplaced dimensions of sensory experience.

In this chapter, I hope to contribute to this burgeoning field of work by exploring divergent sensory and perceptual experiences evident in autism within a phenomenological framework. My interest in working clinically and academically in the area of autism and neurodivergence stems from my experiences working with and advocating for children and adults with autism and their families in Canada and the United States. An ongoing challenge for individuals that I worked with, who predominately identified as boys and men, was an extreme sensitivity to the sensory elements of their everyday environments. Where they encountered the most difficulty were public spaces such as the classroom, grocery stores, malls, and outdoor parks not designed or structured with neurodivergence in mind. Listening to their painful reports of trying to survive in a world designed exclusively for neurotypical people, as well as observing their participation in these public spaces and with others, drew my attention toward the spatial dimension of sensory and perceptual experience. Throughout this chapter, I will share insights and experiences from my previous work as an inclusive support worker and training psychotherapist in multiple clinical and educational settings. All identifiable information, including names, of the individuals mentioned in this chapter have been altered to preserve their anonymity and confidentiality. By drawing on Merleau-Ponty's discussion of sense, space, and things in the *Phenomenology of Perception*, as well as my own personal accounts from working with children and adults with autism, I aim to present a more nuanced understanding of how exceptional sensory experiences shape the individual with autism's relationship to the world and others.

Autism: A Brief Overview

Autism is generally understood as a neurological developmental condition characterized by limited social interaction or interest, communication and language delays or challenges, restricted interests, and/ or repetitive behaviors.[13] Dominant etiological theories espouse autism as a disorder marked by neurocognitive dysfunction.[14] Cognitive deficit theories such as weak central coherence theory and theory of mind deficit continue to inform clinical conceptions of autism and shape the clinical interventions implemented to address the behaviors that emerge as a consequence of these so-called deficits.[15] In "Autism and the Pathology Paradigm," Nick Walker problematizes the characterization of autism as a disorder or condition marked by deficiency. He argues that:

> the pathology paradigm's medicalized framing of autism and various other constellations of neurological, cognitive, and behavioral characteristics as "disorders" or "conditions" can be seen for what it is: a social construction rooted in cultural norms and social power inequalities, rather than a 'scientifically objective' description of reality.[16]

In response to this negative characterization, Walker instead proposes that we embrace a neurodiversity paradigm, which recognizes autism as a form of neurodivergence. According to Walker, "neurodivergence can be largely or entirely genetic and innate, or it can be largely or entirely produced by brain-altering experience, or some combination of the two."[17] Within this paradigm, autism is no longer regarded as a pathology but rather as a style or approach to neurocognitive functioning that "diverges from societal norms."[18] Throughout this chapter, it is my hope that, through Merleau-Ponty's insights, we can begin to appreciate how the sensory and perceptual features of autism also constitute one's approach or style of being in the world.

Autism and the Senses

In Temple Grandin's autobiography, *Thinking in Pictures: My Life with Autism*, she evocatively describes her experience of the sensory world. When discussing auditory problems in autism she describes her auditory experiences as often feeling like "a dentist's drill hitting a nerve."[19] She further explains: "[sounds] actually caused pain. I was scared to death of balloons popping, because the sound was like an explosion in my ear . . . when I was in college, my roommate's hair dryer sounded like a jet plane taking off."[20] Alex, a man with autism whom I worked with for several months in a community mental health clinic, often described his sensory experience as an attack. Similar to Grandin, he was pained by loud sounds and expressed feeling as though sound cut into his body. Another boy, Andrew, whom I worked closely with in an early childhood classroom, was often found spinning his body around while covering his ears when the classroom became too busy and noisy. His gestures and frequent repetition of the phrase: "no, no, no" revealed an intense distress. As mentioned earlier, sensory sensitivity and reactivity is common among individuals with autism; they will often develop behaviors or adaptive strategies to cope with an overwhelming or underwhelming sensory environment.

Repetitive behaviors or "stimming," for example, is an adaptive strategy used to calm and reorient the body or to evoke sensory stimulation.[21] Danny, a school-aged boy, would frequently rub his knee when the room was loud with chattering, moving children. The pressure and familiar motion helped to calm him when the noise and motion of the other children became too overwhelming. For Andrew, spinning his whole body around and around was a kinesthetic movement that helped him stay calm when the classroom became too loud and rowdy.

How we sense the world is intimately tied with our perception of it. One shared perceptual phenomenon reported by individuals with autism is the tendency to "perceive everything as it is."[22] Where a neurotypical person might see the "whole" of an image or situation before noticing or attending to its discrete parts, an individual with autism may first attend to the parts of a situation before integrating it into a whole. Thus what is foregrounded and significant for the person with autism might be minute, seemingly irrelevant details of a much larger and more complex situation. They might get lost in the details, losing sight of the overall meaning or purpose of the activity or other activities around them. For example, Andrew, a five-year-old boy in one of the early childhood classrooms where I worked as an educational assistant, frequently engaged in a serious project of organizing dinky cars according to their color and shape. He would spend a great deal of time visually inspecting each discrete element of the dinky car. This activity consumed his attention so much that he did not hear when the fire alarm rang for a fire drill. Furthermore, experiencing such acute attention to all aspects of a situation can also interfere with completion of tasks and larger projects, which has implications for education and learning. For example, when I encounter a situation such as working in a coffee shop, my attention yields to my computer and my coffee mug. In order to engage effectively in the tasks of writing and drinking, all other elements of my experience, such as the background music, people chattering, and glasses clinking, must recede into the background so that I can exclusively attend to the meaningful task of writing this chapter. Many individuals with autism are unable to establish an efficient figure-ground relationship with the world because "what is background to others may be equally foreground to them; they perceive everything without filtration or selection."[23] In other words, for a person with autism, all of the discrete components of a phenomena become meaningful—making it difficult to determine what needs to be foregrounded from what can be left to recede into the background. What this perceptual style does afford, however, is a greater capacity to perceive vast amounts of information with clarity and accuracy, which can be considered an asset in some situations or professions.

Within a pathological paradigm, these deviations from what are considered to be typical modes of sensing and perceiving the world imply a dysfunction at the level of sensory processing and integration (i.e., a disruption occurring somewhere in the brain). In order to understand how the process is disordered, it is helpful to briefly discuss how "normal" sensory processing is conceptualized. Contemporary theories of sensation and perception maintain that sensory and perceptual processing are physiological processes.[24] Sensation refers to the immediate stimulation experienced from an external stimulus, which causes a reaction from a sensory system. Our sensory systems are olfaction (the sense of smell), gustation (the sense of taste), vision, hearing, vestibular sense (sense of balance and gravity), proprioception (kinesthetic sense) and finally, tactility (the sense of touch). Our sensory receptors respond to external stimuli such as lights and sounds by transforming the external stimuli into nerve signals. The nerve signals are then organized and interpreted in specialized areas of our brains. [25] Thus, perception is understood as the process of integrating and making meaning from our sensory inputs.

By reducing the meaning and significance of our sensory engagement with the world to a process in the brain, we inadvertently turn a blind eye to the role that the environment has in shaping our sensory experiences. Behaviors evoked as a response to the sensory world, particularly those that appear to deviate from socially and culturally prescribed norms like stimming, become interpreted by others (e.g., medical professionals, educators, parents, and peers) as a symptom or consequence of a dysfunctional brain system and are not recognized or appreciated as a response to an environment that is not conducive to one's style or way of being in the world. The contemporary model for conceptualizing sensory processing and integration thus characterizes autism as a disorder or pathology. Danny's rubbing and Andrew's investment in organizing cars are problematized because they are missing out on opportunities to connect with their peers. Jacob's spinning becomes concerning because he could get dizzy and hurt himself. Such consequences of the stimming behaviors are possible. However, so too is the fact that these behaviors, which are shaped by the individual's relationship with the world and others, afford experiences of pleasure, regulation, control, and agency. In addition, as I will argue in the next few sections, these behaviors afford a sense of *orientation*. In order to even begin understanding and appreciating the nature of these affordances, we must move beyond the pathological lens to attend to how experiences and behaviors related to autism are functional rather than dysfunctional. Since contemporary theories of sensation and perception rely on an assumption that there is a "normal" way of sensing and perceiving the world, we must also reimagine how these processes work outside the bias of normality.

Phenomenology of Sensation and Perception

In the *Phenomenology of Perception*, Maurice Merleau-Ponty begins with a critique of intellectualist and empiricist approaches to understanding human experience. He argues that the reduction of human experience to the objective qualities of the physical world and physiological body cannot not account for our actual, lived experience of the world. Drawing from phenomenology, Gestalt psychology, and psychoanalysis, Merleau-Ponty reenvisions perception as an act of meaning-making that emerges through our lived, embodied relation to the world.[26] This approach to perception has implications for addressing the sensory and perceptual challenges faced by individuals with autism. In the sections to follow, I will draw on Merleau-Ponty's *Phenomenology of Perception*, namely his discussions on sense, space, and things to formulate a phenomenological understanding of the common sensory and perceptual experiences reported by individuals with autism.

The understanding of sensory processing described earlier is rooted within reductionistic and physiological models of sensation and perception. To regard sensory integration as merely a physiological *process* (i.e., stimulation-response) that the body undergoes reduces the significance of the body to its biological or physiological capacities. The body, through this reductionistic lens, is understood as a passive recipient of the sensory field. For Merleau-Ponty, the body's significance is its capacity to structure and orient one's experience of the world. It is through the lived body that one encounters and is shaped by the sensuous world. He asserts that the relationship between the body and the sensory field is not one of passivity: rather, our relationship with the sensory field exists as a dialectic. The body presses upon and gestures toward the sensory world with its own curious attunement. The sensory world, in turn, calls forth particular gestures and responses from the body. He claims that "the subject of sensation is neither a thinker who notices a quality, nor an inert milieu that would be affected or modified by it; the subject of sensation is a power that is born together with a certain existential milieu or that is synchronized with it."[27] The sensory world extends various invitations that one can choose to accept and participate in or decline. When an invitation is accepted, and body and milieu are engaged in a reciprocal dialogue with one another, meaning emerges. This is what is meant when it is said that the body, as it is *lived* in relation to the world, is central to perception. However, this is not because the body is where the transformation of sensations into perceptions takes place, but because it is the point at which what is sensed and what is perceived are simultaneously realized—a realization made possible only by space. For Merleau-Ponty, "space is not the milieu in which things are laid out, but rather the means by which the position of things becomes possible."[28] In other words, space is not some geographical area that our physical body and material objects occupy; rather, space is what allows our encounters with sensations, things, and others to become possible. Space is thus understood as the moment where the sentient being and the sensible make contact and existence unfolds.

This coexistence with our sensory field anchors us in our perceptual experience(s). For a neurotypical person, the sensory field forms a gestalt with a figure and a ground, which allows her to foreground certain experiences and allows others to recede into the background. For instance, as I am writing this chapter in a local café, my computer and the project of writing capture my attention and direct my activity. In order to successfully engage in this activity, however, I must allow other experiences to fall out of my awareness such as the conversations at the cash register and the music playing over the speakers. As mentioned before, the sensory field for someone with autism is reportedly not experienced as a gestalt with a clear figure against a background. It seems that for many individuals with autism, the whole sensory field can be experienced as fragmented, without a clear center, and it invites meaningful engagement with many discrete details of experience. For the neurotypical person, many situations have an obvious orientation—I'm at the café to work, so I ignore the chatter of others—but for the person with autism, lived situations are lived in with an immediacy that makes backgrounding disturbances difficult to ignore. According to Merleau-Ponty, "things, in the most general sense of the word, only figure within the confused mass of impressions if they are put into perspective and coordinated by space."[29] Space for the body is action space, a space where potential change, habits, or deeds become enacted. It is the body's action within this sensory field that allows for orientation and situatedness. The body in and of itself is, however, not responsible for orientation, but rather it is the body—situated within a milieu and its affordances—that does the orienting. This is clear when

Merleau-Ponty writes that "what counts for the orientation of the spectacle is not my body, such as it in fact exists, as a thing in objective space, but rather my body as a system of possible actions, a virtual body whose phenomenal 'place' is defined by its task and by its situation."[30] For individuals with autism, their everyday tasks and situations may call forth their immediate attention to all of the discrete things and relationships made possible in a given situation.

Thus, what is referred to as "stimming" or, in the case of Andrew and his toy cars, intense focus on a singular activity, may be an intentional and perhaps aggressive gesture toward specific phenomena—usually those that evoke stimulation of the one of the five senses in order to establish a figure-ground relationship that puts the world into perspective and provides orientation. Based on my observations of individuals with autism, it seems as though they have often preferred one sense over others, and would attempt to elicit certain sensations over and over again in order to feel calm and grounded in times where sensory activity is heightened. To illustrate this point, I will share my experience with Jacob, a young child with whom I worked as his assistant for several months in the United States. Jacob received a dual diagnosis of pica and autism. Pica is a psychiatric condition marked by persistently eating nonedible things.[31] Jacob was often found chewing or holding nonedible items such as crayons, rocks, tacks, and toilet paper in his mouth. His specialist and I struggled to understand why he was constantly putting these things in his mouth. We ruled out hunger early on because Jacob loved to eat different kinds of food. We also ruled out texture because Jacob showed no preference for one textured thing over another. After several months of working closely with Jacob, I began to notice a pattern: Jacob put nonedibles in his mouth only when he transitioned to a different area in the classroom or outside. For example, if Jacob sat down at the drawing table, he would instantly put a crayon in his mouth. Sometimes he did not even chew it—he would just hold it in his mouth. When we would go outside on the playground, Jacob would find rocks to hold in his mouth while he was outside. It was as if, when Jacob encountered a new field of phenomena, he needed to experience holding something in his mouth in order to orient himself to his immediate milieu.

When the body is in action, it is constantly encountering a field of phenomena with varying invitations or possibilities. For a neurotypical person, the possibilities that become foregrounded or warrant attention are shaped by intentions, mood, past experience, or other elements. As a child, I loved going on the swings at the park. As I would walk toward the park, my attention and focus would be directed toward the swings, and as such, the swings would become figures in my experience and direct my activity. However, for an individual with autism, a multitude of possibilities may become foregrounded when transitioning to a space, even when it is familiar. For example, Andy, an adult whom I worked with for several months, would often dread going to the mall. Even though he went to the same mall and the same stores at the same time each week, he feared the potential unknowns of the sensory field. "Would there be a fire drill when he was there? Would there be more people because of a sale? Would they be playing the music louder than usual?" These were all questions that he mulled over each time he needed to go to the mall. In order to control and modify his sensory experience so that it became more tolerable, Andy often took ear plugs with him everywhere he went. The ear plugs served to ground Andy, helping him to orient to the intensely stimulating sensory world. With ear plugs, he could drown out some of the noise, allowing it to recede to the background so that he could focus and engage in his task of shopping. I believe for Jacob the sensation of holding something in his mouth served a similar function. Unlike Andy, Jacob could not speak, and thus could not express why he was putting things in his mouth and what feeling was experienced when doing so. However, given that he engaged in this behavior only during times of transition suggests that engaging the holding sensation was his way of finding orientation in a mass of sensory impressions competing for his attention.

Various behavioral interventions were implemented to address Jacob's pica. Most times, the intervention was to remove the object from his mouth, place his hands on his lap, and say firmly "No." It was presumed that by stopping him before he put the object in his mouth, he would eventually learn that crayons, rocks, and toilet paper were not for *eating*. While interventions were necessary because there was a risk of choking, and Jacob did put some things in his mouth that would cause a great deal of harm if swallowed, the assumption and interpretation that he wanted to *eat* the things simply because he put them in his mouth warrants further consideration.

Things and Orientation

In the chapter "Thing and the Natural World" in *Phenomenology of Perception* Merleau-Ponty posits that "things" are understood as phenomena that structure our existence and corporeality, rather than mental representations. Merleau-Ponty claims that:

> The thing can never be separated from someone who perceives it; nor can it ever actually be itself because its articulations are the very ones of our existence, and because it is posited at the end of a gaze or at the conclusion of a sensory exploration that invests it with humanity . . . After all, we only grasp the unity of our body in the unity of the thing, and only by beginning with things, do our hands, our eyes, and all of our sense organs appear to us as interchangeable instruments.[32]

Things are connected to each other and articulate certain spatial fields. They also evoke possibilities (e.g., imaginative, emotional or behavioral) as well as memories. Merleau-Ponty emphasized that the possibilities of things are neither circumscribed nor determined. This is perhaps most clear when we think of young children and imaginary play. A cardboard box for the young child can be experienced as a house or a car just as it can be the thing that the television came in. In his description of the opacity of things, Merleau-Ponty claims that the "thing and the world only exist as lived by me, or as lived by subjects like me, since they are the interlocking of our perspectives; but they also transcend all perspectives because this interlocking is temporal and incomplete."[33] Here, Merleau-Ponty opens up a new way of thinking about our relationship with the world of things, as well as our observations and interpretations of how *others* relate to their world and things.

The everyday physical spaces that we inhabit are imbued with things prescribed with neurotypical meanings and functions. Further, we ascribe neurotypical meanings to certain behaviors and activities. For example, a neurotypical interpretation of Jacob's pica would be: if he puts a crayon in his mouth and chews it, his intention must be to eat it. These interpretations consequently inform the type of intervention used to alter or eliminate the behavior. As mentioned earlier, the interventions developed to address Jacob's pica required me to either prohibit Jacob from putting something in his mouth (e.g., grabbing the object out of his hand) or removing the object from his mouth. In both situations, Jacob became quite distressed, often crying and grabbing frantically at my hand that held the desired object. Witnessing such distress forced me to stop and shift my attention away from trying to understand why he was trying to eat nonedible things and toward his body in space. What was he *doing?* I asked myself. It was then that I really began to notice that he put things in his mouth only when he transitioned to different areas of the classroom. I also discovered that he rarely, if ever, ingested the things he was putting in his mouth. I was so quick to interpret the "putting things in his mouth" behavior as a desire to eat that I missed some very obvious clues that the *things* for the mouth held a completely different meaning for Jacob. While I will never fully know what the things being held in the mouth meant for him, it did seem as though holding onto some*thing* when arriving in a new and perhaps overwhelming sensory milieu connected and anchored Jacob to the space in some way.

Through these close observations of what I would describe as his "holding behavior," its meaning for me shifted. I saw how calm he became when he did manage to escape my efforts. When he had something in his mouth, he was at ease. I began to hold a tension between wanting Jacob to be able to hold things in his mouth while feeling terrified of that possibility. There was a legitimate safety concern here that could not be ignored. These observations did, however, lead me to think more creatively and expansively about how to "intervene" in such a way that actually facilitated orientation for Jacob. Some of the nonedible things that Jacob really liked to put in his mouth were the rocks outside on the playground. Because I could not always be with Jacob outside, there was concern he might put rocks in his mouth and they would go unnoticed. One day I took a small tin lunchbox out to the backyard. Each time Jacob put a rock in his mouth, I opened up the tin box and gestured to him to put the rock(s) inside. I showed him how to lock it and then handed it to him. He quickly realized that he could take the box with him wherever he went. Being able to carry the rocks around in the tin can while he was outside seemed to be grounding enough, and soon he stopped putting the rocks in his mouth. I will never know if the tin can served as a true substitute for the holding sensation provided by the mouth, and I can never be sure that my interpretation of his behavior was correct or appropriate. I am, however, confident that by suspending my neurotypical assumptions about Jacob's behavior and its function, and engaging in a close, curious observation of how he engaged and participated in our shared milieu, I was able to recognize his style or way of orienting to the world and things.

It is important to reiterate here Merleau-Ponty's assertion that "we only grasp the unity of our body in the unity of the thing, and only by beginning with things, do our hands, our eyes, and all of our sense organs appear to us as interchangeable instruments."³⁴ The experience of capturing and being captured by the things of the world are what afford our meaningful engagement and participation in it. Our relationship with things, both the sensible qualities and the concrete objects in our milieus, further remind us of our capacity for agency and action. They gesture to us, and we respond. If we think of this in relation to Jacob's experience, the experience of discovering and holding things from his immediate milieu may have been his way of finding his body situated in the world and among others. This leads me to wonder what he was experiencing when I intervened in his attempts to put something in his mouth. When people's relationships with the sensuous world and things are severed, or when they are denied access to certain affordances of a thing (e.g., no longer being able to experience holding a rock in one's mouth), what happens to their capacity to respond and act upon the world? What if they are denied access to affordances that situate them in the world and give shape and meaning to their interactions? I would argue that when one's tie to the world is severed, one becomes disoriented, lost, and confused. I do not raise these questions to evoke guilt or to discourage the use of behavioral interventions. In fact, I think that behavioral assessment tools and plans can be useful as a template or approach to closely observing lived experience. For example, Functional Behavioral Assessments (FBAs) are commonly used in educational settings to assess behaviors considered "problematic" because they are interfering with the child's capacity to learn, or are harmful to the child or others. The goal of these assessments is to understand fully the function of the behavior by observing and recording the antecedents (what preceded the behavior), and the consequence (s) (i.e., how was the behavior managed/negotiated) in order to make sense of how the behavior is functioning or serving the child. These assessments (i.e., interpretations of behavior) then become translated into a concrete plan to address the behavior by trying to modify or eliminate it completely.³⁵ What I do not find to be helpful with these tools is that they are situated within a pathological paradigm of autism. The whole notion of behavior modification rests on the assumption that there is a functional or healthy way to engage in the world and with others. The underlying intention for implementing interventions such as behavioral modification is thus to normalize the behaviors of those with autism and to force them to adapt and survive in built environments designed and intended for neurotypicality and not neurodiversity. These tools, namely, functional behavioral assessments, could be used as a guide to observing behaviors, insofar as they aim to aid in our understanding of how the individual with autism is participating, engaging, and relating to their world. The end goal here would be to use these findings to develop individualized supports so that the individual with autism can feel comfortable in their everyday environments. In some cases, this may involve behavior modification, but it could also include redesigning public spaces to be more inclusive of neurodivergent experiences or reorganizing social practices and expectations.

As I conclude this chapter, I am reminded of Andy and his frequent laments about how dreadfully painful it was to live in a world designed for neurotypical people. Merleau-Ponty's insights, particularly those presented in this chapter from his *Phenomenology of Perception*, afford a way of attending to lived, sensory, and perceptual experience that honors the distinctive ways that each of us, including those with autism, engage with the sensuous world. By appreciating perception as an active and dynamic engagement between body and world, and not merely mental or physiological activity, he invites us to look beyond the body (i.e., the individual) when understanding behavior and action. He further calls us to look at the world of sensations, things, and others, and at how our relationship with these things orients and structures our very being in the world. Responding to this call in my own clinical and academic work has meant orienting my attention more intentionally to the physical milieu, that is, the shared public spaces whose affordances only often serve neurotypical people, and to reimagine these shared spaces—the classroom, the grocery stores, and the public parks—with neurodivergence in mind. It is through Merleau-Ponty's approach to sense and perception that new possibilities and deeper modes of understanding lived experience emerge in a way that can inspire new and creative ways to connect with and support individuals with autism.

Notes

1. Meryl Alper, "Inclusive Sensory Ethnography: Studying New Media and Neurodiversity in Everyday Life," *New Media and Society* 20, no. 10 (2018): 3561; Chloe Silverman, "Fieldwork on Another Planet: Social Science Perspectives on the Autism Spectrum," *BioSocieties* no. 3 (2008): 325; Olga Solomon,

"Sense and the Senses: Anthropology and the Study of Autism," *Annual Review of Anthropology* 39 (2010): 242.

2. Alper, "Inclusive Sensory Ethnography," 325; Olga Bogdashina, *Sensory Perceptual Issues in Autism and Asperger Syndrome: Different Sensory Experiences— Different Perceptual Worlds*. (London: Jessica Kingsley Publishers, 2003); Temple Grandin, *Thinking in Pictures: And Other Reports from My Life with Autism* (New York: Vintage, 1997); Solomon, "Sense and the Senses."

3. Jane Case Smith, Lindy L., Weaver, and Mary A. Fristad, "A Systematic Review of Sensory Processing Interventions for Children with Autism Spectrum Disorders," *Autism: The International Journal of Research and Practice* 19, no. 2 (2015): 133.

4. Alper, "Inclusive Sensory Ethnography," 3563.

5. Case Smith, Weaver, and Fristad, "Systematic Review of Sensory Processing Interventions," 133–134; Bogdashina, *Sensory Perceptual Issues in Autism*, 44–51.

6. Bogdashina, *Sensory Perceptual Issues in Autism*, 25.

7. Solomon, "Sense and the Senses."

8. Solomon, "Sense and the Senses," 241.

9. Ariel Cascio, "Cross-Cultural Autism Studies, Neurodiversity, and Conceptualizations of Autism," *Culture, Medicine, and Psychiatry: An International Journal of Cross-Cultural Health Research* 39, no. 2 (2015): 207–212; Elinor Ochs, Tamar Kremer-Sadlik, Karen Gainer Sirota, and Olga Solomon, "Autism and the Social World: An Anthropological Perspective," *Discourse Studies* 6, no. 2 (2004): 147–183; Elizabeth Fein, "Making Meaningful Worlds: Role-Playing Subcultures and the Autism Spectrum," *Culture, Medicine, and Psychiatry: An International Journal of Cross-Cultural Health Research* 39, no. 2 (2015): 299–321; Jennifer C. Sarrett, "Custodial Homes, Therapeutic Homes, and Parental Acceptance: Parental Experiences of Autism in Kerala, India and Atlanta, GA USA," *Culture, Medicine and Psychiatry* 39, no. 2 (2015): 254–276.

10. Alper, "Inclusive Sensory Ethnography"; Ann Donnellan., David Hill, and Martha Leary, "Rethinking Autism: Implications of Sensory and Movement Differences for Understanding and Support," *Frontiers in Integrative Neuroscience*, no. 28 (2013).

11. Alper, "Inclusive Sensory Ethnography."

12. Alper, "Inclusive Sensory Ethnography," 3562.

13. *Diagnostic and Statistical Manual of Mental Disorders: DSM-5*. Arlington, VA: American Psychiatric Association, 2013.

14. Elisabeth L. Hill and Uta Frith, "Understanding Autism: Insights from Mind and Brain," *Philosophical Transactions: Biological Sciences* 358, no. 1430 (2003): 281–289.

15. Hill and Frith, "Understanding Autism."

16. Nick Walker, June 23, 2016. "Autism and the Pathology Paradigm" Neurocosmopolitanism (blog). https://neurocosmopolitanism.com/autism-and-the-pathology-paradigm

17. Nick Walker, September 27, 2014, "Neurodiversity: Some Basic Terms & Definitions," Neurocosmopolitanism (blog). http://neurocosmopolitanism.com/neurodiversity-some-basic-terms-definitions

18. Walker, *Neurodiversity*

19. Grandin, *Thinking in Pictures*, 63.

20. Grandin, *Thinking in Pictures*, 63.

21. Bogdashina, *Sensory Perceptual Issues in Autism:* Stimming refers to the elicitation of a behavior that can intensify a sensation. Stimming is understood as a helpful and adaptive strategy that is experienced as grounding when feeling either over- or understimulated.

22. Bogdashina, *Sensory Perceptual Issues in Autism*, 45.

23. Bogdashina, *Sensory Perceptual Issues in Autism*, 29.

24. Bogdashina, *Sensory Perceptual Issues in Autism*, 30–43.

25. Bogdashina, *Sensory Perceptual Issues in Autism*, 29.

26. Maurice Merleau-Ponty, *Phenomenology of Perception*, trans. Donald Landes (London: Routledge, 2012).

27. Merleau-Ponty, *Phenomenology of Perception*, 219.

28. Merleau-Ponty, *Phenomenology of Perception*, 254.

29. Merleau-Ponty, *Phenomenology of Perception*, 225.

30. Merleau-Ponty, *Phenomenology of Perception*, 260.

31. American Psychological Association, *Diagnostic and Statistical Manual of Mental Disorders*

32. Merleau-Ponty, *Phenomenology of Perception*, 334.

33. Merleau-Ponty, *Phenomenology of Perception*, 334.

34. Merleau-Ponty, *Phenomenology of Perception*, 334.

35. Nathan Call, Mindy C. Scheithauer, and Joanna Lomas Mevers, "Functional Behavioral Assessments," in *Applied Behavior Analysis Advanced Guidebook: A Manual for Professional Practice.*, ed. James K. Luiselli (San Diego: Elsevier Academic Press, 2017), 41–71.

Chapter 10

Health and Other Reveries
Homo Curare, Homo Faber, and the Realization of Care

JOEL MICHAEL REYNOLDS

To endeavor to shape people and populations to conform to an "imagined future" in which the present ascendant values, understandings, and intentions are manifest . . . is not only eugenic but also an untenable enterprise.

—Rosemarie Garland-Thomson[1]

"It would be naïve to seek solidity in a heaven of ideas or in a *ground (fond)* of meaning—[. . .] the very idea of objective knowledge and . . . the idea of an object that informs itself and knows itself are, as much as any other ideas, and more than any other, supported by our reveries."

—Maurice Merleau-Ponty[2]

Introduction

Modern scientific methods have allowed humans to significantly extend their average lifespan, create life under circumstances previously thought impossible, and maintain life after both environmental and genetic events that in centuries past would have meant immediate or inevitable death.[3] Whether one looks to the policies of the NIH, UN, or Gates Foundation, this wealth of scientific knowledge about the human body has transformed how we think about individual humans as well as the fundamental framework and goals of their sociopolitical existence. Governments govern, communities coalesce, and individuals choose by and in parameters set by the value of health and the many private and public entities that produce its power, knowledge, and guidance. Yet, modern scientific methods and their manifold effects have also put within reach the total annihilation of our species and set into motion global processes that will powerfully curtail, if not hasten the end of, human life on Earth. Initially, this potential extinction will likely come through the widescale death and suffering of historically marginalized groups and the economically disadvantaged.[4] Both at the level of knowing and of praxis, the methods and modes that underwrite the rise of the biopolitical—and, increasingly, the infopolitical—are the very methods and modes that have underwritten processes of global injustice the scale of which are unparalleled across recorded history.[5] Where, precisely, does *health* fit in this history?

Socially and politically, modern conceptions of health function as a stratagem or gambit. They assume a certain naiveté regarding the mortal necessity and curious transitions of aging, the social construction of normality, and the biological ambiguity of typicality—of the *typos*, the kind. This naiveté is profoundly productive. The fear of death and the changes it occasions are best tamed by never rising to the level of a fear: *I'm not afraid of dying; I just want to live life to the fullest*. The desire to be normal, to not be a *misfit*, is best tamed by being framed as a desire for flourishing: *I'm not against being different; I just want things to go more easily as I pursue my goals*.[6] The instinct to categorize things absolutely is best tamed by an impassioned fidelity to scientific method, the density of fact, and the gravity of the mean: *I'm not saying there aren't variations; I just want you to know how evolution has structured things*. Each of these strategies contribute in fundamental ways to the positive production of health, a production that garners and leverages untold amounts of capital and, far too often, functions to cover over a litany of historic and contemporary injustices baked into the fabric of each society it touches. The truism that "everyone wants to be healthy" is superseded in rank only by the assumption that there is such a thing as health—that health is an objective fact of the world by which we can produce objective knowledge about morbidity and mortality, functioning and flourishing, and forms of life. Is health, then, a *reverie*?

In the epigraph above from *The Visible and the Invisible*, Merleau-Ponty claims that "the very idea of objective knowledge [is] supported by our reveries."[7] My aim in this chapter is to interrogate this claim with respect to the phenomenon of health. In section one and as a case study for the analysis to follow, I look at a contemporary, highly specific site of health screening: return of results of incidental variants or variants of unknown significance with respect to the use of genetic and genomic screening technologies (GSTs) in newborn and pediatric contexts. These screenings, undergirded by decades of basic, applied, and transitional work in genomic medical sciences as a whole, produce situations wherein parents might face knowing, or face potentially knowing, the health fate of their own children—a fate that could include early and inevitable death. Drawing on a range of Merleau-Ponty's texts, but with a special focus on his Collège de France lectures on the concept of nature, I show how this scene of care reveals a tension between the macro and the micro, between medical research and practice as a science of the general and the patient's interest in medical care as an art of treating the individual.

In section two, I further develop this concern by arguing that genomic medical sciences reveal an even more fundamental tension between two distinct ways of conceiving of the human: *homo faber*, the human understood as controller of fate through the creation and use of tools, versus what I term *homo curare*, the human understood as conspiring with fate through the guidance and practice of care. Each of these conceptions lead to distinct interpretations of the proper role and balance between the macro and the micro. I argue that by looking to Merleau-Ponty's concept of the flesh it becomes clear that homo faber and homo curare are but two modalities of the relationship between fleshly beings like us and the concept of health.

In the final section, I examine the aforementioned arguments in the context of larger issues of social justice. With respect to the studies that I examine and given the demographics of those with access to technologies like GSTs, I suggest that under the aegis of homo faber, health functions as a reverie that creates and upholds white, cishet, able-bodied, settler colonialist, upper-middle-class privilege. This, then, is "health" not as a harmless reverie, but a dangerous reverie particularly apt to contribute to and maintain injustice in both theory and practice. It is only by better balancing homo faber and homo curare, the human as *maker* and the human as *carer*, that the idea of health will transform from a dangerous reverie into a more just reality.

An initial caveat is in order concerning how this piece fits in relation to the large body of scholarship on Merleau-Ponty. Research engaging central figures in Continental/European philosophy typically takes two forms today. There is figure scholarship, which works out philosophical problems directly through or within the oeuvre of the thinker or thinkers in question. There is also problem-based scholarship, which uses the insights of a thinker or thinkers to address and gain understanding concerning a problem. This chapter is an instance of the latter. Both approaches strike me as valuable, for different though at times overlapping purposes. Still, it is worth noting that a problem-based use of continental figures is arguably more common in the social sciences than it is in the humanities (just consider the wide range of use of figures like Michel Foucault, one of the more cited figures in the twentieth century as a whole). One reason for this is that the social sciences are, at least typically, oriented toward building knowledge about various sorts of social phenomena as opposed to learning more about a particular thinker. I adopt a problem-first method here because while working upon ethical, legal, and social issues related to genomics, I found myself turning again and again to Merleau-Ponty for insights concerning the debates at play—whether with respect to return of results of secondary findings or the psychosocial impact of genomic knowledge upon people more generally. In short, it was by turning to Merleau-Ponty for discernment and understanding of pressing concrete problems that this project came to fruition, and this chapter engages Merleau-Ponty in that admittedly applied spirit.

Would You Like to Know When Your Child Will Die?

Your young child is exhibiting unusual physiological or behavioral symptoms. You have anguished over their meaning, maybe for months or even years—anguished over what may or may not be the case. At the suggestion of your medical provider, you agree to whole genome sequencing. You do so because you think it is the best way, and perhaps also the last way, to figure out what is going on in order for you to know how to care for your child. Not another's child or children in general, but your *child. Genomic information will help one do this.*

The assumption concerning the helpfulness of genomic information in this vignette in fact runs counter to the methodological milieu of modern medical science as well as modern medical care. The ultimate focus of the primary institutions of modern medicine turns not on the person as unique microcosm—one laden with a singular history, personal, biological, genomic, and the like, and with unique cares, traumas, fears, desires, and plans—but on the person as macrocosm, as a particular instance of homo sapiens or of some specific population of homo sapiens.[8] In *Nicomachean Ethics*, Aristotle writes, "for what the doctor appears to consider is not even health, but human health, and presumably the health of this human being even more, since he treats one particular patient at a time."[9] In this terse formulation, Aristotle lays out the complex relationship between the practice of individualized care, of *singular, micro-level treatment*, and the reflective, knowledge-building processes concerning human health, of *general, macro-level* considerations. Although there is a singular patient before a clinician, the knowledge brought to bear on that patient is knowledge ultimately developed in and derived from the vast body of modern scientific knowledge about humans and about patients—knowledge that has grown exponentially in recent decades. Yet, as Aristotle contends, the end of medical care is nevertheless presumed to be the care of the specific patient a clinician is treating. As calls for the import of narrative medicine as well as values-based practice makes clear, focus on the patient as an individual is not today the norm.[10] At the heart of modern medicine, at least, lies a tension between the micro and the macro.

Merleau-Ponty, in the context of a larger critique of a statistical approach to evolution, puts a finer point on the issue, writing "in all the sciences, there is a distinction of the micro and the macro, beyond the principle of causality . . . the schema are everywhere the same, absorbing the 'historical given.' The macroscopic facts of evolution do not bring out more of this analysis than does the aerial photo of the electronic microscope."[11] A few lines later, he argues, "geneticists study evolution from the point of view of *Homo faber*."[12] Within Merleau-Ponty's view, genetics (and what would later be called genomics) is a macro-level study of the structures of natural development carried out under the auspices of being able to change human fates; genomics plays out on one side of the medical tension Aristotle describes.

Laying the groundwork for later historians and critics of genetic and genomic sciences such as Lily E. Kay, Troy Duster, Nathaniel Comfort, and Colin Koopman, Merleau-Ponty understands contemporary genomics as an instance of third-person, modern scientific knowledge that is predicated upon the assumption that the human can, through what is ultimately macroscopic knowledge about the human organism, build tools to control its own fate, including at the level of the microscopic. Genomics, on this view, is a project of and for homo faber: the human understood as master of its own fate. This places the question at hand in sharper terms: will genomic health information, operating fundamentally as it does at a macro level, help you know how to care for *your* child?

To answer that question, consider the following example. Since 2010, the American College of Medical Genetics has supported chromosomal microarray as a first-tier test for individuals with several types of suspected genetic diseases.[13] These screenings can determine whether or not someone has a copy-number-variant (CNV), and here is the sort of information a parent, presented with the option or suggestion to agree to such a test for their child, might encounter:

> CNVs are a type of structural variant involving alterations in the number of copies of specific regions of DNA, which can either be deleted or duplicated. These chromosomal deletions and duplications involve fairly large stretches of DNA (that is, thousands of nucleotides [>1 kb], which may span many different genes) but can range considerably in size as well as prevalence. As is the case for other types of genetic mutations, some CNVs are inherited whereas others spontaneously arise de novo . . . There are several well-characterized rare developmental phenotypes caused by CNVs of known pathogenicity, such as Velocardiofacial, Prader-Willi, and Smith-Magenis syndromes. Although the role of most CNVs is far less clear, there is now growing evidence that the genetic architecture of more common psychiatric and neurodevelopmental conditions includes different types of both common and rare genetic variation. An increased burden of rare CNVs has been observed and replicated in several conditions. These include autism spectrum disorder (ASD), attention-deficit/hyperactivity disorder (ADHD), and intellectual disability (ID), as well as schizophrenia. CNVs also contribute to risk of idiopathic epilepsy.[14]

Werner-Lin and colleagues detail the case of a mother who underwent chromosomal microarray screening. Her baby tested positive for a copy-number-variant with a highly variable phenotype. The mother reports that her provider reactions ran the gamut from: "Doom and gloom" to "this baby's perfectly fine, why are they putting you through this?" As her daughter reached six months, she said: "I'm constantly questioning 'is this because of her disorder?' For example, she's a really bad sleeper so for the longest time I thought 'wow, is this her deletion or is it just that she's five months old and she sucks at sleeping like most babies?'"[15] Another parent said:

> Once or twice it's crept into my head where I've been like, "what if this microarray result . . . like there's something wrong with her and we don't know and one day she just has SIDS [sudden infant death syndrome] and stops breathing." She's got such a strangely mellow temperament, so I think, "is there something wrong with her that she's just so lovely"—which makes no sense.[16]

Geneticists study evolution from the point of view of homo faber, yet parents, these studies suggest, seek out and interpret genomic information from the point of view of homo curare. I coin this term to refer to the human understood from the point of view of a being oriented and defined by care, i.e., a being instituted and constituted through relations of concern.[17] These parents are not interpreting genetic information qua homo faber, but qua homo curare. That is to say, these parents report micro-level concerns—specifically ones concerning the possibility of their child becoming "abnormal," which, tellingly, always acts in these studies as a synonym for "disabled."[18] They struggle to reconcile macro, genomic information understood from the view of homo faber with its micro, lived meaning understood from the view of homo curare.

By characterizing the issues and scenes at hand in this way, I do not merely aim to invoke the architectonic role of care (*Sorge*) in Heidegger's *Being and Time*. As important as that analysis is, it offers little understanding of the role of embodiment for the institution, determination, and provision of care. Instead, I primarily aim to highlight the way that our reasons, actions, judgments, perceptions, and cognitions are all shaped by *Einfühlung*, which is to say, shaped by a *fleshly* body that feels above and beyond any of those "feelings" that rise to the level of consciousness and thereby earn the name. "Before trying," Merleau-Ponty writes, "we notice that the body as corporal schema, the esthesiological body, the flesh (*le corps, comme schéma corporel, le corps esthésiologique, la chair*) have already given us the *Einfühlung* [typically translated as "empathy"] of the body with perceived being (*l'être perçu*) and with other bodies. That is, the body as the power (*pouvoir*) of *Einfühlung* is already desire, libido, projection-introjection, identification."[19] The body, for Merleau-Ponty, is always already a scene of *em-pathy* understood in this expansive sense, a scene of what I understand in terms of and as defined by care. And the meaningfulness of bodily actions and bodily styles—from being a "really bad sleeper" as the first parent worries to having a "strangely mellow temperament" as the second parent worries—are interpreted in the light of enfleshed *Einfühlung*. In these cases that translates to a desire for normality, the fear of "becoming disabled," and the preemptive identification of their "true" child—the child they were supposed to have and/or the child who was supposed to develop—as "normal" and "healthy."

To appreciate this point, a more careful discussion of the meaning of the flesh (*la chair*) is in order. For Merleau-Ponty, the flesh names that texture in and through which the body and world touch—the origin point of all horizons in which things become possible phenomena of concern. He writes, "This magical relation, this pact between them [things] and me . . . this fold, this central cavity of the visible which is my vision, these two mirror arrangements of the seeing and the visible, the touching and the touched, form a close-bound system that I count on . . . the flesh (of the world or my own) is not contingency, chaos, but a *texture* that returns to itself and conforms to itself."[20] To understand the flesh as a texture indicates that it neither exists in pure space (the geometer's formulae cannot, e.g., render the "red shaggy carpet"), nor in pure time (there is no quantifiable time in which the run of one's hand over the carpet "grasps" its shagginess, specific texture, or its redness). The flesh, in short, is that medium through which things become meaningful.[21] The flesh, one could say, is a turgid or tumescent concept, which is to say, part of what the concept picks out is precisely a conceptual excess beyond the binary couplings so easily birthed and latched onto by beings like us. The "really bad sleeper" and the "strangely mellow temperament" are not the results, potential or actual, of genomic differences. They are moments of apprehension of our fleshly being in the unending project to understand its meaningfulness.

Understood as flesh, the body is the ground of the possibilities of the human as homo curare, and it is so through a complex interaction of the body as the power (*pouvoir*) of *Einfühlung*, as a texture already shot through with specific desires, libidos, projection-introjections, and identifications. To be a fleshly being, then, just is to be a being defined by care. As I explain in more detail below, both homo curare and homo faber are modalities of beings of flesh; both are responses to and ways in which such a form of existence is taken up as a project.

Homo Curare, Homo Faber, and Flesh

You agree to whole genome sequencing, just as those parents did. You do so because you think it is the best way, and perhaps also the last way, to figure out what is going on in order for you to know how to care for your child. However, during the appointment to receive the results of this test, you are told the sequencing revealed a piece of information about your child's future that has nothing to do with either your present concerns or that of your doctors. Hence the name incidental or secondary variants. Among other things, these findings could suggest that your child will succumb to Huntington's disease, a fatal genetic disorder that causes the progressive breakdown of nerve cells in the brain. "Symptoms usually appear between the ages of 30 to 50 and worsen over a 10- to 25-year period. Ultimately, someone with Huntington's succumbs to pneumonia, heart failure, or other complications" due to the progression of the disease.[22] It is possible, however, that the variants portend a condition far less severe, or maybe they end up meaning nothing at all.

But your medical provider can't explain any details until you first agree to hear the information. And even if the variant does suggest something as momentous as Huntington's, the data could be wrong or ambiguous. Because, it always bears repeating, these tests do not tell you what will happen. They do not and cannot predict the future with absolute certainty. Your genome does not, all on its own, fully decide your future. One's environment affects which genes are expressed over time, and also how they are expressed. Even in the case of monogenic diseases—diseases originating from a mutation in a single gene present on one or both chromosomes—the story and timeline of their phenotypic expression is complicated and diverse.

Even if genes did have this magical power, these tests can provide false positives. They are, of course, limited both to the current state of medical knowledge about genomics and also to the information sequencing and analysis on the computer science side,

> *which is to say, all the many technological devices and programming algorithms that make possible in the first place the sequencing and analysis of genomes on the way to their diagnostic-prognostic interpretation.*

To address this situation, let us return to the tension discussed above between the micro and the macro. Merleau-Ponty continues, "there is a complementarity that forbids the simultaneous fixing on the micro and the macro."[23] The term "complementarity" is here deployed in the sense used by physicists to describe how "the capacity of the wave and particle theories of light" are complementary insofar as they together "explain all phenomena of a certain type, although each separately accounts for only some of the phenomena."[24] Complementarity, in this sense, does not suggest that one of two (or more) ways of understanding, perceiving, judging, or conceiving of a phenomenon is necessarily better or more accurate than another; it is only to say that (a) those ways are distinct in determinate respects, (b) it is only through bringing both explanatory modes together that one will end up with a more holistic understanding of the phenomenon in question, and (c) one cannot hold both ways together at the same time. Indeed, how would one bring together the explanatory modes at the macro-level of genomics with the micro-level of a singular life? How would one bring together information, knowledge, and understanding fashioned in the light of homo faber with that of homo curare?

The role of the flesh—and, thereby, the distinct modalities of homo curare and homo faber—is difficult to see on the dominant macro-level understanding of the meaning of genomics. David Morris, working to correct the dominant interpretation, writes:

> [Genomic] information has standing as such only by virtue of ongoing and historical material and energetic dynamic flows that are part and parcel of what it takes to inherit genetic material and grow a body. These flows move through the medium of growing bodies in environments. We think the genetic information is there, right in and reducible to genetic material. But what we are really seeing when we (rightly) grasp genetic material as having an informative role is an effect of ongoing biochemical histories and dynamics washing through a body growing in this-here place.[25]

Although Morris does not use the language of the flesh at this point in his argument, I understand "a body growing in this-here place" as a gloss on that concept. A properly "enfleshed" understanding of genomics sees the way in which it neither presents us with definitive control over populations or individuals, nor does it tell us how to care. It is, instead, but one slice of ongoing and historical material and energetic dynamic flows—one slice of an organism understood in terms of what Merleau-Ponty calls an "envelopment-phenomenon":

> [The] organism is not only its local-instantaneous reality, neither for a proximal thinking, nor moreover another reality. It is the macroscopic "envelopment-phenomenon" [*phénomène-enveloppe*] that we do not engender from elements, that invests the local-instantaneity, that is not to be sought *behind*, but rather *between* the elements . . . instead of a science of the world by relations contemplated from the outside (relations of space, for example), the body is the measurement of the world [*le corps est le mesurant du monde*].[26]

To say that the body—again, understood here as flesh—is the measurement of the world is to say that the meaningfulness of the world emerges against the horizon of our cares. The tension of the micro and the macro is that span in which we measure our cares. The tension at play in the scenes of care analyzed above for parents seeking out genomic information is a tension between such measurement understood as a tool for control and such measurement understood as a tool for care. Our imbrication with the world, our fleshly being-in-the-world, is the stuff out of which and by which measurements like these can be taken.

Recall the central question at stake in GSTs: what does it mean, today, to care for one's child—and not just their present, but as modern biomedical technologies increasingly promise, their future? More specifically, what does the twentieth-century project of genetics all the way from Watson and Crick's (and Franklin's) discovery of the double-helix to the contemporary promises of the Human Genome Project indicate about the evolution of the flesh? About the human as a being shot-through not merely with senses trained by the social and scientific, not merely causes and determinates, but also cares—the weight of an ever-unique texture that both conditions us and opens us up to what makes our condition *our own*? What does this evolution portend for the epistemic space and intentional reach of our care for others, especially, in this case, intimate others? Concerning such questions, homo faber, just as homo curare, is condemned to uncertainty. Heeding Merleau-Ponty's concept of the flesh, the difference between homo faber and homo curare is, then, not one of kind, but degree. Cares borne in the body qua flesh already span the hermeneutic distance between homo faber and homo curare, for it is as flesh that the micro and the macro come together at the level of lived experience.[27]

At this point, the following claim can be offered: the meaning-making relationship between homo faber and homo curare is one of modes of fleshly care. The human as creator of a world and of its fashioning is one modality of the human who explicitly measures the world in terms of its cares; cares that are always indexed to its institution and constitution as a fleshly, embodied being. Cares envelop all phenomena within one's world—that is, within the totality of meaningful relations of one's experience—and the meaningfulness of caring as well as any of our particular cares emerges out of the envelopment-phenomenon that is the flesh in its irreducible relationship with its environment. It is in this sense that care operates at the interstices of inside/outside, first- and third-person, micro and macro views. Care is determinate for meaning, for *sens*, by fundamentally mediating the phenomenality of phenomena.

Existential Homeostasis and Existential Support

While I have explained the relationship between homo faber and homo curare in some depth, I have not yet addressed the problem of how we care or how we conceive of care. It is through this question that the differences between homo faber and homo curare emerge at their starkest. For homo faber, what is ultimately at stake in scenes of genetic and genomic sequencing technologies is *care conducted as control over fate*—a control fashioned through the creation and use of tools. For homo curare, what is ultimately at stake in scenes of genetic and genomic sequencing technologies is *care conducted as provisioning of support*—a control fashioned through working with others and community and acting upon the social conditions that make caring possible in the first place.

For homo faber, care conducted as control over fate aims at *existential homeostasis*: the experience of feeling that the meaning of one's life will stay the same. Existential homeostasis is underwritten by a desire for normality; it is an experience of the continuity or trapping of ability relations and the linking of that experience with the meaning and maintenance of health.[28] If that account is right, then health as a reverie of homo faber is a project to extend the trap of fluctuation that constitutes the organism to the experiential field of that organism. Health becomes a forgetting of both fluctuation and the traps that hold it. That is to say, there is a way in which the desire to establish normality—in this sense of the trapping of what is taken to be "one's own" abilities as the only way to establish health—is an act taken in defiance of both the life course and bodily difference. As long as human cares are shaped by a demand for health as longevity and health as normality, a fundamentally ableist demand, that vision of health will orient the measurement of the world. It will become a phenomenon through which the world is enveloped and, thus, against which it is measured. In this light and based upon the qualitative sociological work analyzed above that one can see why scenes of care driven primarily by homo faber are destructive, for this way of being-toward-health seeks not to create the conditions of support for the health of all, but instead to conduct control over the fate of solely one's own, in this case, one's own child.

For homo curare, care conducted as provisioning of support aims not merely for existential support, but social support: the provisioning of assistance for the care of those around one. Insofar as the orbit of concern of homo curare extends beyond oneself and one's kin, social support is a project of justice. Scenes of care like those involving GSTs are not simply about the meaning of one's child's life but about the world in which one and one's child lives. Homo curare is actively attuned to the ways in which one is always already in relation with others and with their wellbeing. The demand for health as individual longevity and health as normality, paradigmatic of homo faber, transforms into a demand for health for *all of us* for homo curare.

To better appreciate the distinction between homo faber and homo curare, take another study of parental responses to receiving information from GSTs concerning their children. J.A. Anderson and colleagues write that

> Of 83 invited, 23 parents from 18 families participated [in the study]. These parents supported WGS [a form of GSTs] as a diagnostic test, perceiving clear intrinsic and instrumental value. However, many parents were ambivalent about receiving

> SVs [secondary variants], conveying a sense of self-imposed obligation to take on the 'weight' of knowing [this information], however unpleasant.²⁹

They found themselves in the thralls of duty, undergoing a deep normative pull, to take on the weight of this knowledge. Would you take on this weight?

> *After being told that there is secondary variant information, you, after much deliberation, decide to decline the information. Yet, if something happens down the road, how will you deal with knowing you might have mitigated it? If you accept it, won't that information affect how you treat your child? When and in what way will you tell them? How old is old enough to learn you might suffer an early death or will soon be living with some kind of illness or disease? Fifteen? Twenty-one? Forty? There are no easy answers and no easy way out of this dilemma once you're in it.*³⁰

Anderson and colleagues suggest the term *inflicted oughts* to refer to the obligation to take on the weight of knowing secondary variant information. What does it mean to inflict an ought? To inflict a responsibility or duty as one would a wound? What is the relationship between control and care, between homo faber and homo curare offered here? Most imagine the knowledge provided by secondary variants of GSTs to be a good—a good even if the specific information they proffer portend something bad—a good we seek and simultaneously hate to find. Is it, though? Even if research concerning the psychosocial impacts of genomic testing found it to not cause empirically demonstrable harm, would that mean this information thereby contributes to individual or familial well-being or—just as, if not far more importantly—contributes to a more just and equitable society?³¹ What reveries are at play here?

Justice and the Realization of Care

If, for homo faber, care is conducted as control over fate, conducted as a desire for existential homeostasis, then the scenes of care and the use of GSTs discussed above turn on the conversion of the fear of death as linked to abnormality into a knowledge that allows one to regulate or control that fear, the course of one's life, and the eventualities of one's ability transitions and ultimate death—and/or, by extension, that of one's loved ones. As Attic tragedy works to make clear, such knowledge always comes with a cost. And, as contemporary scholarship in critical theory, feminist theory, critical philosophy of race, disability studies, and queer theory, among multiple other fields, makes clear, such knowledge is also always a product of power—of one's place, historical context, social position, and other elements. Knowledge such as this is haunted by epistemologies of ignorance.[32]

For example, there are harrowing racial dimensions embedded in the value and interpretation of genomic knowledge. That a middle-class white couple—demographically those most likely to have access to and use such genetic screening technologies—would be aghast at the thought that their child might die at age thirty-five of, say, Huntington's disease, is in part an existential effect of white privilege.[33] It evidences an ignorance that too many Black or Latinx parents, for example, must face this prospect as an everyday social-political reality rather than as a rare genetic circumstance. It must be faced by such parents due to factors ranging from police violence, to hate crimes, to inequalities of health, housing, employment, and other systemic problems perpetuated at state and federal levels across the United States—as well as many other parts of the globe, to invoke the global colonial and imperial conditions supporting such practices.[34]

With respect to the experience, interpretation, and ensuing psychosocial and existential impacts of receiving results from pediatric genome sequencing, what is ultimately at stake here for homo faber is the desire to establish that the meaning of one's child's life will stay the same. This involves a core, operative assumption that this meaning will include a *long*, *able-bodied* life indexed to white, settler colonial privilege. Within these cases, at least, homo faber figures concern over controlling the fate and facts of one's child's life and death as a question of the meaning of one's child's life as a particular, hegemonic figure of the *normal*. And normality is always already shot through with problematic frameworks based on race, gender, sexuality, nationality, ethnicity, class, and so on.

In *The Phenomenology of Perception*, Merleau-Ponty writes, "I can only encompass a certain duration of my life by once again unfolding it according to its own *tempo* . . . the 'synthesis' of time is a 'transition synthesis' and the movement of a life that unfolds, and the only way to actualize this life is to live it [*et il n'y a pas d'autre manière de l'effectuer que de vivre cette vie*]; time has no place, rather time carries itself along and launches itself forward."[35] In order to function as a reverie, health for homo faber must act in ignorance of the very dimensions of living it seeks to uphold. For example, it must ignore aging,[36] adaptation, and the profound necessity of ability transitions and their many bearings and sendoffs; it must focus on the micro at the expense of the macro—taking the macro as having meaning only insofar as it affords the micro its desires; it must overlook and forget all the fluctuations, deprivations, and assaults on health that are not simply inevitable but which condition the possibility of life and any form of "health" within and along its course. And, ultimately, it must take on the form of a dogmatic idea that suppresses homo curare. Finally, to function as a reverie, health for homo faber must occlude the fact that we are beings of flesh.

In Defense of Reveries of Egalitarian Health

The desire to know one's own or one's loved one's future, I have argued, is underwritten by two foundational ways in which we live in and as beings of flesh: homo faber and homo curare. I have argued that whereas homo faber leads to the desire for existential homeostasis, a feeling of surety that the meaning of one's life will stay the same, homo curare leads to the desire for existential support, the provisioning of assistance for the care of those around one. Both homo faber and homo curare are integral modalities of fleshly beings like us. I have devoted a significant amount of the chapter to criticizing the dominance of homo faber because it is, regrettably, the default and dominant modality at play in these scenes of care. Insofar as homo faber is not balanced with homo curare, it creates a serious problem—especially if one keeps larger concerns of social justice and equitable health care in mind. On the other hand, the modality of homo curare is certainly problematic, morally and otherwise, insofar as it alone is dominant. A generalized care for all that fails to attend to particular others, including loved ones and close friends, is a failure of care and can lead to harms against individuals in all sorts of ways.[37] But that is not the chief problem genomic medical sciences and what I have discussed in terms of the reverie of modern health presents us with; it is instead the dominance and hegemony of homo faber.

I have further suggested that insofar as modern ideas of health are based solely or unevenly on a conception of the human as homo faber, health functions not simply as any reverie but as a dangerous reverie that maintains unjust and inequitable systems of care. Health is not and never has been individual. It is a question of the reach of one's entire community and society—including the reach of oneself into and with all those other beings, human and nonhuman, that make up one's flesh:

> If we can show that the flesh is an ultimate notion, that it is not the union or compound of two substances, but thinkable by itself, if there is a relation of the visible with itself that traverses me and constitutes me as a seer, this circle which I do not form, which forms me, this coiling over of the visible upon the visible, can traverse, animate other bodies as well as my own . . . [then] I can understand a fortiori that elsewhere it also closes over upon itself and that there are other landscapes besides my own.[38]

Just as the most minute change in one's position can alter not simply the "qualities" of any given object in the visual field but the entire tenor of that field as flesh, we are caught up, captivated, and yet in cahoots with others and the world in profoundly intricate ways.

Yet, that is not how most think about or experience health. There is an argument to be made that the reverie of health, as sustained by the dominance of homo faber, has become a paradigm of the times, metastasizing, as it were, off of an individualism at the foundation of the larger neoliberal geopolitical economy of the twentieth century.[39] Let us not forget that much of biomedicine has historically operated with a "research takes all" approach. That is to say, the bodies, minds, and well-being of those under the auspices of medical care have too often come second or been entirely disregarded for the ends of knowledge-building. This is especially so with respect to bodies considered socially or politically disposable. The Tuskegee and Guatemala Syphilis Experiments.[40] Forced institutionalization and sterilization.[41] Henrietta Lacks, the Havasupai people, and biological theft.[42] Jim Crow medical care.[43] On the other side of this Mobius strip of the value of health is the pervasive individual desire for health and the demands we place—as citizens and consumers, patients and practitioners, and workers and employers—to assure and insure it.

In order to understand a range of pressing ethical, social, political, and philosophical implications of GSTs in general and the problem of secondary variants in particular, I have suggested that one must, at minimum, ask (a) the phenomenological question of *what it is like* for parents and children in this situation, (b) the evolutionary biological question of *what it means* for an organism to have discovered the genetic basis of its existence, and (c) the sociopolitical and normative question of *whether these practices contribute to justice* given the larger health concerns of everyone and especially historically oppressed groups. I have further suggested that Merleau-Ponty's concept of the flesh and his claims concerning the fundamental tension between macro and micro views (a) help us appreciate the complexity of this problematic and formulate responses to it and (b) that by linking his work to a further elaboration of the concepts of homo faber and homo curare, we get some traction in analyzing how this problematic relates to much larger existential issues.

To combat health as a reverie, to combat health as solely figured by homo faber, we (and who precisely constitutes this "we" must always be called into question) would need to prioritize care and community.[44] We would need to articulate and realize the values of a future for health driven more equally by homo curare—a future that is truly egalitarian, by and for all. We would need, in other words, to replace health as individual reverie with health as social justice reality.

Notes

1. Rosemarie Garland-Thomson, "Human Biodiversity Conservation: A Consensual Ethical Principle," *The American Journal of Bioethics* 15, no. 6 (2015): 14.

2. Maurice Merleau-Ponty, *The Visible and the Invisible*, trans. Claude Lefort (Evanston, IL: Northwestern University Press, 1968), 116; *Le Visible et L'invisible: Suivi De Notes De Travail*, Collection Tel 36 (Paris: Gallimard, 1979), 153.

3. My thanks to the participants of the 2018 International Merleau-Ponty Circle as well as Susan Bredlau and Talia Welsh for constructive feedback on earlier versions of this chapter. In the introductory paragraph to the chapter and in a few other spots, I have reused or modified a small amount of materials from Joel Michael Reynolds, "The Healtholocene," *Syndicate*, published November 12, 2018. https://syndicate.network/symposia/ philosophy/kierkegaard-after-the-genome. Reynolds's piece was an essay response to Ada S. Jaarsma, *Kierkegaard after the Genome: Science, Existence, and Belief in This World* (Cham, Switzerland: Palgrave Macmillan, 2017).

4. Jason W. Moore, ed. *Anthropocene or Capitalocene? Nature, History, and the Crisis of Capitalism* (Oakland, CA: PM Press/Kairos, 2016); Axelle Karera, "Blackness and the Pitfalls of Anthropocene Ethics," *Critical Philosophy of Race* 7, no. 1 (2019).

5. Colin Koopman, *How We Became Our Data: A Genealogy of the Informational Person* (Chicago: University of Chicago Press, 2019).

6. Rosemarie Garland-Thomson, "Misfits: A Feminist Materialist Disability Concept," *Hypatia* 26, no. 3 (2011).

7. Maurice Merleau-Ponty, *The Visible and the Invisible*, 116; *Le Visible et L'invisible*, 153.

8. To be fair, the narrative medicine approach/movement is one area of medical education trying to counter this trend. See Rita Charon, *Narrative Medicine: Honoring the Stories of Illness* (New York: Oxford University Press, 2006).

9. Aristotle, *Nicomachean Ethics*, trans. Terence Irwin, 2nd ed. (Indianapolis, IN: Hackett Pub. Co., 1999), 1.6.

10. Charon, *Narrative Medicine: Honoring the Stories of Illness*; Mila Petrova, Jeremy Dale, and Bill Fulford, "Values-Based Practice in Primary Care: Easing the Tensions between Individual Values, Ethical Principles and Best Evidence," *British Journal of General Practice* (2006): 7.

11. Maurice Merleau-Ponty, *Nature: Course Notes from the Collège De France*, trans. Robert Vallier (Evanston, IL: Northwestern University Press, 2003), 211. *La Nature. Notes. Cours Du Collège De France. Suivi De: Résumés De Cours Correspondants* (Paris: Le Seuil, 1968), 272.

12. A rich and fascinating literature has taken up the concept of homo faber in various ways across the last few decades. Due to considerations of space and the specific aims at hand, I do not engage that literature here, but I plan to in a future project.

13. David T. Miller et al., "Consensus Statement: Chromosomal Microarray Is a First-Tier Clinical Diagnostic Test for Individuals with Developmental Disabilities or Congenital Anomalies," *American Journal of Human Genetics* 86, no. 5 (2010): 749–764. https://doi.org/10/ckmnsx

14. Anita Thapar and Miriam Cooper, "Copy Number Variation: What Is It and What Has It Told Us About Child Psychiatric Disorders?," *Journal of the American Academy of Child and Adolescent Psychiatry* 52, no. 8 (August 2013): 772–774. https://doi.org/10/f2xj89

15. Allison Werner-Lin et al., "'They Can't Find Anything Wrong with Him, Yet': Mothers' Experiences of Parenting an Infant with a Prenatally Diagnosed Copy Number Variant (CNV)," *American Journal of Medical Genetics* 173, no. 2 (2016): 446. https://doi.org/10/f9ptcp

16. Werner-Lin et al., 447.

17. Merleau-Ponty, *Nature: Course Notes from the Collège De France*, 211. *La Nature. Notes. Cours Du Collège De France. Suivi De: Résumés De Cours Correspondants*, 272. Due to space constraints, I am bracketing the question of how genetic counselors and other medical providers tasked with the delivery of such information interpret this scene.

18. I explore many of the same studies analyzed here with respect to larger questions of epistemic injustice and the specific issue of ableism in Joel Michael Reynolds, "'What if There's Something Wrong With Her?': How Biomedical

Technologies Harm Patients as Knowers," *Southern Journal of Philosophy* 58, no. 1 (2020): 161–185. I also reuse some small portions of the language from that article here, and my thanks to the editor for permission to do so. I am grateful to Allison Werner-Lin for first bringing my attention to qualitative work on these issues.

19. *Nature: Course Notes from the Collège De France*, 211. *La Nature. Notes. Cours Du Collège De France. Suivi De: Résumés De Cours Correspondants*, 272.

20. Maurice Merleau-Ponty, *The Visible and the Invisible*, 146; my emphasis.

21. Maurice Merleau-Ponty, *The Visible and the Invisible*, 139–140.

22. "What is Huntington's Disease?" Huntington's Disease Society of America. http://hdsa.org/what-is-hd

23. *Nature: Course Notes from the Collège De France*, 263. *La Nature. Notes. Cours Du Collège De France. Suivi De: Résumés De Cours Correspondants*, 330.

24. "Complementarity, n." in OED, "Oxford English Dictionary," in *Oxford English Dictionary* (Oxford, England: Oxford University Press, 2002).

25. David Morris, *Merleau-Ponty's Developmental Ontology* (Evanston, IL: Northwestern University Press, 2018), 181.

26. Maurice Merleau-Ponty, *Nature: Course Notes from the Collège De France*, 213, 217. Merleau-Ponty, *La Nature. Notes. Cours Du Collège De France. Suivi De: Résumés De Cours Correspondants*, 275, 279.

27. I am grateful to Erik Parens for the insight and insistence that binaries emerge from the failure to think their respective purchases on experience. The framework I present here of homo faber as a contrast with homo curare, creator versus carer—each as dimensions or modes of a greater whole—is directly inspired by Parens's work. See Erik Parens, *Shaping Our Selves: On Technology, Flourishing, and a Habit of Thinking* (Oxford & New York: Oxford University Press, 2015).

28. I am thinking here especially of when Merleau-Ponty writes, expounding upon Edgar Dacqué, "the living being, reduction of fluctuation, sum of instabilities . . . the organism shows itself as a trap of fluctuation [*L'organisme monte lui-même un piège à fluctuation*]." Merleau-Ponty, *Nature: Course Notes from the Collège De France*, 263. *La Nature. Notes. Cours Du Collège De France. Suivi De: Résumés De Cours Correspondants*, 331.

29. J.A. Anderson et al., "Parents Perspectives on Whole Genome Sequencing for Their Children: Qualified Enthusiasm?" *Journal of Medical Ethics*, no. 43 (2016). There is a large and ever-growing body of research surrounding this context. I have consciously avoided wading through that research in this chapter in order to instead focus on what I take to be its central existential concerns.

30. Note that this is not just a question of what to do *as a parent*. Providers responsible for delivering and/or counseling about genomic findings report moral distress when parents decline it. Bernhardt et al., "Distress and Burnout among Genetic Service Providers," *Genetics in Medicine* 11, no. 7 (July 2009): 527–535. There is also the question of the lived experience of the technicians and numerous, different labs who help decide the diagnostic line between variants of significance and unknown significance. We live in a political context where parental

obligations include compiling and acting upon as much medical information as possible. Indeed, we jail those who fail in particularly egregious ways. Despite uncertainty over the meaning of such information and its existential impact, the perception of increased control over a child's future seems, for many, to warrant overriding other concerns. While, as I've noted, genetic information is just one factor determining phenotypic expression and, furthermore, well-being, it certainly doesn't seem to feel that way for many parents today. This situation raises harrowing ethical questions: what are the conditions under which parents are presented with this choice? Which are the determinate factors—the differences that make a difference? And, perhaps most troubling of all for loving parents, whose welfare is ultimately at stake? What form does—and should—care take here?

31. Erik Parens and Paul S. Appelbaum, "On What We Have Learned and Still Need to Learn about the Psychosocial Impacts of Genetic Testing," *Hastings Center Report* 49, no. S1 (2019).

32. Linda Alcoff, "Epistemologies of Ignorance: Three Types," in *Race and Epistemologies of Ignorance*, ed. Shannon Sullivan and Nancy Tuana (Albany, NY: SUNY Press, 2007); Gaile Pohlhaus, "Relational Knowing and Epistemic Injustice: Toward a Theory of Willful Hermeneutical Ignorance," *Hypatia* 27, no. 4 (2012); Kristie Dotson, "A Cautionary Tale. On Limiting Epistemic Oppression," *Frontiers: A Journal of Women Studies* 33, no. 1 (2012); Joel Michael Reynolds and David Peña-Guzmán, "The Harm of Ableism: Medical Error and Epistemic Injustice," *Kennedy Institute of Ethics Journal* 29, no. 3 (2019): 205–242.

33. My thanks to Andrea Pitts for this point.

34. Among the many studies detailing these phenomenon in relation to health, see Jonathan Metzl, *Dying of Whiteness: How the Politics of Racial Resentment Is Killing America's Heartland* (New York: Basic Books, 2019). In section one, I focused on the question: will genomic health information, operating fundamentally as it does at a macro level, help you *know* how to care for *your* child? The problem with this framing should now be apparent: the myopic focus on genomic information concerning one's child misses the equitable health forest for the individualized health trees. It further misunderstands the social nature of health. As more than one study has shown, with respect to overall health outcomes, your zip code matters more than your genetic code. See Garth N. Graham, "Why Your ZIP Code Matters More Than Your Genetic Code: Promoting Healthy Outcomes from Mother to Child," *Breastfeeding Medicine: The Official Journal of the Academy of Breastfeeding Medicine* 11 (2016): 396–397, https://doi.org/10/gf9sfx. See also Harvard Medical School's study, "CaTCH: Claims Analysis of Twins Correlations and Heritability," http://apps.chiragjpgroup.org/catch. To help care for your child, you will need knowledge that spans the macro and micro—you will need local, community-based knowledge.

35. Maurice Merleau-Ponty, *Phenomenology of Perception*, trans. Donald A. Landes (Oxford & New York: Routledge, 2011), 446; *Phénoménologie De La Perception* (Paris: Gallimard, 1945), 483–484.

36. See Gail Weiss, "The 'Normal Abnormalities' of Disability and Aging: Merleau-Ponty and Beauvoir" in *Feminist Phenomenology Futures*, eds. Helen Fielding and Dorothea Olkowski (Bloomington: Indiana University Press, 2017). I am thankful to Gail Weiss for noting that this raises very complex questions about enhancement.

37. Eva Feder Kittay, "The Ethics of Care, Dependence, and Disability," *Ratio Juris: An International Journal of Jurisprudence and Philosophy of Law* 24, no. 1 (2011): 49–58. https://doi.org/10/ffnrp2

38. Maurice Merleau-Ponty, *The Visible and the Invisible*, 140–141; *Le Visible et L'invisible*, 183.

39. Martha Fineman, *The Autonomy Myth: A Theory of Dependency* (New York: New Press, 2004); David T. Mitchell and Sharon L. Snyder, *Biopolitics of Disability: Neoliberalism, Ablenationalism, and Peripheral Embodiment*, ed. Sharon L. Snyder (Ann Arbor: University of Michigan Press, 2015); Joshua Alan Ramey, *Politics of Divination: Neoliberal Endgame and the Religion of Contingency* (London: Rowman & Littlefield International, 2016); Jennifer Scuro, "The Ableist Affections of a Neoliberal Politics," *APA Newsletter on Philosophy and Medicine* 16, no. 1 (2016).

40. Britt Rusert, "'A Study in Nature': The Tuskegee Experiments and The New South Plantation," *Journal of Medical Humanities* 30, no. 3 (2009): 155–171. https://doi.org/10/b6qhkp; Michael A. Rodriguez and Robert García, "First, Do No Harm: The US Sexually Transmitted Disease Experiments in Guatemala," *American Journal of Public Health* 103, no. 12 (2013): 2122–2126. https://doi.org/10/gf9gdr

41. Nancy Ordover, *American Eugenics: Race, Queer Anatomy, and the Science of Nationalism* (Minneapolis: University of Minnesota Press, 2003).

42. Jessica L. Stump, "Henrietta Lacks and the HeLa Cell: Rights of Patients and Responsibilities of Medical Researchers," *The History Teacher* 48, no. 1 (2014): 127. Robyn L. Sterling, "Genetic Research among the Havasupai—a Cautionary Tale," *The Virtual Mentor* 13, no. 2 (2011): 113–117. https://doi.org/10/gf9gdv

43. Harriet A. Washington, *Medical Apartheid: The Dark History of Medical Experimentation on Black Americans from Colonial Times to the Present* (New York: Anchor Books, 2008).

44. Cf. Carolyn Neuhaus, "Does Solidarity Require 'All of Us' to Participate in Genomics Research?," *The Hastings Center Report* 50, no. S1 (2020): S62–S69.

Chapter 11

The Desexualization of Disabled People as Existential Harm and the Importance of Ambiguity

CHRISTINE WIESELER

... to speak of disability *ontologically*, as a way of being, rather than *pathologically*, as a way of being medically out of whack, is to replace a well-charted set of questions with less-familiar ones.

—Jackie Leach Scully[1]

Introduction

People with visibly identifiable impairments[2] are often not perceived to be sexual.[3] It is assumed not only that they do not have sexual desires or relations but also that they are *incapable* of having sexual desires or being sexually desired. I contend that the failure to recognize disabled people as sexual beings is an existential harm insofar as it limits the possibilities they can take up and denies them the ambiguity that is fundamental to human existence. This lack of recognition has further implications for disabled men and women alike, but I focus here primarily on the effects on disabled women. As a result of the assumption that disabled women are not in romantic and/or sexual relationships, there are often insufficient resources for disabled women attempting to leave abusive partners,[4] and health care providers may not attend to concerns related to reproductive health.[5] Yet even aside from these consequences, being desexualized is harmful, as will become clear in my account of the relationship between sexuality and existence.

In the first section, I discuss the relationship between Merleau-Ponty's approach to phenomenology and contemporary disability theory. I argue that, in spite of differences in assumptions about disability made by contemporary disability theory and Merleau-Ponty, he provides a useful framework for theorizing the lived experiences of disabled people. In section 2, I describe Merleau-Ponty's account of the relationship between sexuality and human existence. I recount his analysis of Schneider in order to bring out both the ambiguity that Schneider lacks as well as the ambiguity that Merleau-Ponty posits as characteristic of "normal" sexuality.[6] I then characterize the phenomenon of desexualization of people with visually identifiable impairments.[7] In section 3, I explain and apply Ann Cahill's account of the desexualization of disabled women, which she characterizes as a lack of objectification. I consider two examples in which disabled women are objectified in order to further distinguish objectification that reinforces ableism from sexual and other types of desirable social recognition of disabled people. I then return to Merleau-Ponty's account of sexuality, in section 4, in order to describe the harm of desexualization and to connect it with other ways that failure to recognize the ambiguity of human existence can be harmful.

Merleau-Ponty, Embodiment, and Social Identity

In the *Phenomenology of Perception*, Merleau-Ponty contends that developing an account of embodied being in the world is central to phenomenology. In light of the embodied nature of intersubjectivity, the ways one's body is given meaning by others influence an individual's ability to take up possibilities. Social categories—such as race, gender, and disability—play a role in how we perceive others and ourselves.[8] Numerous philosophers have criticized Merleau-Ponty for failing to consider the ways that gender and race impact lived experience, yet they have adapted his approach to phenomenology for their own projects that do take these categories of social identity into account.[9]

Some may wonder how useful Merleau-Ponty's ideas are for philosophy of disability given that he uses case studies as well as hypothetical examples centered on disabled people in order to construct an account of the "normal" subject. As I have argued elsewhere:

> Merleau-Ponty seeks to clarify the characteristics of the "normal" subject, locating normality at the level of the individual. This is opposed to what many disability activists and theorists hold to be a central tenet: normality and disability are not traits of individual bodies but are instead the results of social values, attitudes, and practices that enable some types of bodies and disable others.[10]

His approach assumes that disability is a trait of an individual's body without acknowledgment that what is counted as "normal" or "pathological" is value-laden. He focuses on the functional limitations of individuals, paying little attention to the ways that social attitudes and practices matter for lived experiences of disability. For example, when he mentions a man who is blind and uses a cane, Merleau-Ponty does not consider how aspects of the built environment and other people's ways of interacting with him enable or disable him.[11] These aspects of his approach are in tension with the ways that disability activists and theorists conceptualize disability insofar as their accounts attend to ways that social practices shape how we think about bodies and create disadvantages for disabled people. Merleau-Ponty does not address these aspects of disability, but his approach to phenomenology allows for their inclusion. Importantly, he does not consider disabled people's lived experiences to be deficient in relation to those of nondisabled people. In addition, Merleau-Ponty contends that it is philosophically interesting and worthwhile to explore the question of what it is like to be disabled—a position philosophers of disability are still called to defend.[12]

Although Merleau-Ponty does not explore in a sustained way the impacts of intersubjectivity on the experiences of disabled people, his approach to phenomenology contains rich conceptual resources for philosophy of disability.[13] Lisa Guenther suggests distinguishing critical phenomenology from classical phenomenology, stating "by critical phenomenology I mean a method that is rooted in first-person accounts of experience but also critical of classical phenomenology's claim that the first-person singular is absolutely prior to intersubjectivity and to the complex textures of social life."[14] Guenther claims that engagement with the work of Merleau-Ponty, among others, provides the "critical edge" of philosophical projects that take social identity and context into account.[15] Although she does not reference Merleau-Ponty specifically, Sandra Bartky advocates "setting aside 'normal' phenomenology, i.e., the search for the a priori, necessary structures of any embodied consciousness whatsoever in favor of an analysis of the structures of meaning embedded in the experience of an historically, culturally, and sexually specific subject."[16] Bartky describes ways that normative femininity structures nondisabled women's experiences, whether they are attempting to conform to its demands or defining themselves in opposition to it in the context of Western consumer society. Most existing work in what might be called critical phenomenology is concerned with the experiences of nondisabled people. Recently, theorists have begun to recognize Merleau-Ponty's existential phenomenology as a productive framework for theorizing embodied subjectivity in relation to disability.[17] I believe this developing area shows great promise.

The current chapter takes the approach of using Merleau-Ponty's account of sexuality and intersubjectivity in order to consider how shared assumptions about sexuality and disability can impact the self-perceptions and experiences of disabled women. My primary focus in the following section is on the ambiguity that is essential for existence and the sexuality that pervades it. Related to this theme, I develop the relationship between the body and existence in sexual desire and Merleau-Ponty's notion of situatedness.

Sexuality and Human Existence

If subjectivity is thought of as embodied, then the body cannot be considered separable or opposed to one's self. Merleau-Ponty states, "Thus, I am my body . . . and reciprocally my body is something like a natural subject, or a provisional sketch of my total being."[18] The body provides the possibility of a genuine presence. To build on Merleau-Ponty's comparison between the body and a sketch, the existence one expresses through the body would then be the next stage of the art-making process. Its lack of completeness allows for new possibilities to be taken up. In adopting this formulation, he commits himself to the view that the relation between existence and the body is characterized by ambiguity in experience. The body is ambiguous in a number of ways: it is both an actual and a habitual body, it is in and toward the world, and the body and soul fuse in action.[19]

In order to explore how bodily change impacts being in the world, Merleau-Ponty focuses on the case of Johann Schneider, who sustained a brain injury as a soldier during World War I and was subsequently a patient of Gelb and Goldstein. Schneider was diagnosed with "psychic blindness."[20] While retaining the ability to complete tasks familiar to him, he demonstrates difficulty engaging with others and the world in certain ways, such as thinking abstractly or acting spontaneously. Merleau-Ponty asserts, "Beneath intelligence, understood as an anonymous function or as a categorial operation, we must acknowledge a personal core that is the patient's being and his power of existing. Here is where the disorder resides."[21] Rather than focusing on what medical practitioners might consider isolated functional "deficits," Merleau-Ponty is interested in how the structure of Schneider's "world" has been leveled out.[22] He applies the method of existential analysis in order to provide an account of the shift Schneider has undergone as a result of his brain injury, which impacts how he relates to objects and other humans in experimental as well as everyday situations.

According to Merleau-Ponty, understanding the origin of "being for us" requires an examination of our "affective milieu" because it "has sense and reality only for us," and does not exist for the rest of the natural world.[23] He claims that understanding how objects or beings begin to exist for us through desire or love will elucidate how objects and beings exist for us in general.[24] Thus, sexuality is a privileged domain in terms of understanding our relationship with the world, temporality, and others.

Schneider's lack of ambiguity is a significant factor in his lack of sexual desire. Let us consider temporal ambiguity and how the lack of temporal ambiguity manifests in Schneider's case. Typically, the ability to imagine a possible situation is enabled by one's capacity to actively assume time.[25] However, for Schneider, the flow of time has been broken up into points, thereby making it impossible for him to construct a narrative connecting his history with his present and future. Regarding Schneider's involvement in sexual acts, Merleau-Ponty remarks, "Things happen at each moment as if the subject did not know what to do."[26] Schneider's experience seems to be an aggregate of events taking place at distinct moments rather than a fluid experience in which past, present, and future are integrally connected. For this reason, he cannot imagine possible situations; he is tied to the actual situation and can no longer engage in spontaneous acts. Merleau-Ponty asserts, "Schneider is 'bound' to the actual, and he 'lacks freedom,' he lacks the concrete freedom that consists in the general power of placing oneself in a situation."[27] One of the ways this is made manifest is in Schneider's inability to situate himself sexually.

Merleau-Ponty uses an analysis of Schneider's lack of sexual desire and ability to engage with others in sexual situations in order to develop an account of "normal" sexuality. For example, he suggests that for "normal" subjects, erotic perception imbues aspects of the world with a sexual signification for the body and the possibility of "adapting sexual behavior to it."[28] In contrast, he claims that for Schneider, "close bodily contact only produces a 'vague' feeling or the 'knowledge of something indeterminate,' which is never enough 'to launch' sexual behavior or to create a situation calling for a definite mode of resolution."[29] It should be noted that Merleau-Ponty reports that Schneider responds when another person initiates sexual activity with him, but due to his lack of erotic perception he does not seek out sexual activity.

Merleau-Ponty contends that sexuality should not be conceived of as an autonomous cycle; rather, it is integral to being.[30] He states, "Sexuality, no more than the body in general, must not be taken for a fortuitous content of our experience."[31] Just as we must recognize the necessity and centrality of embodiment for human existence, so too we need to recognize that sexuality permeates human life. Furthermore, Merleau-Ponty maintains, "If the sexual history of a man gives the key to his life, this is because his manner of being toward the world—that is, toward time and toward others—is projected in his sexuality."[32] Indeed, we see that Schneider's difficulties in his relation to temporality and others characterize his sexuality as well as his ability to have long-lasting friendships. Lack of spontaneity characterizes all aspects of Schneider's life.

Schneider's impairment clearly inhibits his sexuality insofar as he no longer has sexual desires. In addition, the specific nature of his impairment is relevant insofar as it impacts how he relates to others and the world. His experience lacks temporal and other types of ambiguity, and this limits his possibilities. Many types of impairment do not impact sexual desire or ability in the ways that Schneider's does; yet the general public, the media, and medical professionals often assume that disabled people are uniformly asexual or "unsexed."[33] In *Sex and Disability*, disability theorists Anna Mollow and Robert McRuer state, "Rarely are disabled people regarded as either desiring subjects or subjects of desire . . . pleasurable sexual sensations are generally dissociated from disabled bodies and lives."[34] This passage helps to clarify the phenomenon with which I am concerned here.[35]

In the following section, I turn to Cahill's discussion of desexualization of disabled women and what she considers the harms and benefits of objectification. She contests the position that objectification is always undesirable, and she proposes the concept of derivatization to refer to the features of harmful objectification. I examine two types of objectification that specifically affect disabled people.[36] Drawing on these examples in conjunction with Cahill's account, I characterize sexual recognition as a remedy to desexualization. I conclude the chapter by returning to Merleau-Ponty in order to develop further the connections between sexual recognition and broader social recognition of disabled people.

Theorizing the Harm of Desexualization of Disabled People

Cahill's Account of Desexualization of Disabled Women

In *Overcoming Objectification: A Carnal Ethics*, Cahill asserts that to be "unsexed" is to be deemed "profoundly outside the bounds of appropriate sexuality."[37] She focuses on two categories of women in her analysis: mothers and disabled women, groups that are, of course, not mutually exclusive.[38] To desexualize someone, that is, to perceive a person as being unsexed, goes beyond not being sexually attracted to that person. Rather, it involves assuming that the person is incapable of having sexual desires and that they are fundamentally undesirable—that is, no one could desire that person. Conversely, being recognized as sexual does not require being found sexually attractive by another, much less being engaged in sexual acts. This is an important distinction for the purposes of the present discussion. Desexualization is also likely to have the normative implication that no one *should* desire people in unsexed categories.

Cahill considers sexuality to be an important aspect of selfhood. Like Merleau-Ponty, she contends that it is necessary to consider subjectivity as inherently bodily and shaped by bodily experiences.[39] Indeed, she explicitly draws on his insights. However, rather than limiting the focus to an individual's sexuality in order to understand their life and relations with others as Merleau-Ponty does, she is also interested by what we can learn about a society from how it objectifies or fails to objectify certain categories of people.[40] She examines the harm women with visibly noticeable impairments[41] may experience through not being perceived as sexual and suggests that some types of objectification may be not only morally permissible but even desirable insofar as they contribute to one's sense of self. It is important to clarify her assumptions regarding objectification in order to understand why she claims it can be beneficial.

Cahill contends that the framework of objectification relies on a split between "body-as-thing and person-as-subject" that makes "the body-as-subject incomprehensible."[42] The notion of objectification depends on the claim that the wrongness of some kinds of sexist actions stems from treating women as bodies rather than rational agents. According to Cahill, this explanation fails to account for either the possibility of bodily pleasure or the embodied nature of subjectivity, generally. For example, philosopher Martha Nussbaum attempts to account for morally permissible sexual encounters while maintaining the distinction between persons and objects by claiming that if instrumentalization occurs within the context of a relationship that generally includes mutual respect for autonomy, this subsequently renders it morally permissible.[43] Cahill expresses dissatisfaction with this approach, suggesting that the notion of objectification is premised on a problematic distinction between personhood and embodiment.

Cahill suggests that if we reject the opposition between personhood and embodiment, then to be objectified, that is, treated as a thing, cannot be an affront to one's self. In her words, "No longer can it be said that it is obviously harmful to treat women, or men for that matter, as mere bodies—in fact the qualifier 'mere' or 'just' no longer makes sense in relation to embodiment."[44] On her account, "thing-ness and object-ness are not contradictory to embodied intersubjectivity."[45] To treat someone as an object is simply to treat them as an embodied subject, and this can have harmful or beneficial effects. Cahill further claims that theories of objectification fail to allow for the pleasure that can result from "being treated as a body," which she asserts can contribute to "a flourishing sense of self."[46] Treating someone as a body is compatible with treating them as a person and is not automatically morally problematic.

To illustrate the difference between positive and negative types of objectification, Cahill provides an example of each. In the first, after looking her "up and down," a man remarks to a woman, "Not too bad."[47] Cahill asserts, "I would argue that the actual offense consists in his reducing her value to the degree to which she does or does not meet his own standard of physical beauty."[48] To understand the harm of a comment like this, Cahill encourages us to consider this incident in the context of a power asymmetry—"a moment in a larger pattern of inequity."[49] In her second example, a person says to a woman "I just love the way you've combined those colors—I've never seen anything like it."[50] Cahill states that this second instance is not offensive, even though it focuses on the woman's appearance. Thus, a more nuanced account is needed than the term "objectification" can provide.

Cahill introduces the concept of *derivatization* to refer to the harms that others have associated with objectification, while retaining the concept of objectification to refer to positive experiences of being treated as a body. She explains, "to derivatize is to portray, render, understand, or approach a being solely or primarily as the reflection, projection, or expression of another being's identity, desires, fears, etc."[51] Derivatization involves an emphasis on the perceiver's wants and needs at the expense of the one who is perceived—leading to a failure to take into account that person in their particularity. This term provides a more specific description than the term "objectification" of what makes certain ways of treating an embodied subject morally impermissible and avoids making the blanket claim that it is always wrong to treat a person as a body. It is possible to objectify someone without derivatizing them. Furthermore, Cahill contends, "the sexually derivatized subject is not quite a non-person."[52] On her account, being derivatized does not prevent someone from expressing "desires, emotions, and preferences."[53] However, derivatization does entail that the derivatizer fails to adequately respond to those desires, emotions, and preferences.

Cahill suggests that *not* being the object of a desirous gaze can threaten one's personhood. She states:

> Because sexuality necessarily entails intersubjectivity and because sexuality is a crucial element of selfhood, to be on the receiving end of a sexualizing gaze can enhance one's sense of self. To have that gaze skip over you, to be rendered sexually invisible by society at large, is to have your personhood denied.[54]

Since she views being the object of a sexualizing gaze as an experience that can affirm one's sense of self, Cahill asserts that women who are treated as unsexed are harmed through nonobjectification. She goes so far as to claim that it is possible to judge a society as "oppressive and unjust" if it is "incapable of sexually objectifying them [women with visible impairments]."[55] Individual selves, including sexual aspects of these selves, develop within the "context of cultural, political, and social relationships."[56] Cahill contends that disabled women may have difficulties seeing themselves as sexual and expressing their sexuality in the context of a society that persistently desexualizes them.

In "Playing the Online Dating Game, in a Wheelchair" disability activist Emily Ladau reports that within the context of an exchange of messages on a dating site, one man replied: "Sorry. The wheelchair's a deal-breaker for me."[57] While not everyone expresses this sentiment so blatantly, many men refuse to consider a woman who uses a wheelchair to be a prospective date. Ladau says that she edited her dating profile to omit the fact that she uses a wheelchair and decided instead to convey this information after interacting with a potential match. She reports that, "after dropping the "wheelchair bomb," I'd have to brace myself for their reactions, which were always a mixed bag, often ranging from indifference to ghosting."[58] Ladau goes on to say, "It is part of my identity, shaping everything I do and everything I value. But in the online dating world, my disability was my secret shame."[59] Disabled women are faced with numerous double binds in regard to dating due, in part, to the assumptions that they are not sexual and it is inappropriate to be attracted to them.

Disabled people may have ambivalent responses to being desexualized. Disability activist Eli Clare states:

> On the one hand, disabled people mostly escape the sexual objectification and harassment many nondisabled women face every day at their jobs and on the streets. It is an escape that has given me a bit of space. Amidst all the staring I absorb and deflect, I am grateful not to have to deal with sexual leering. On the other hand in the absence of sexual gaze of any kind directed at us—wanted or unwanted—we lose ourselves as sexual beings.[60]

Clare describes not being sexually objectified as having both beneficial and harmful aspects. In addition, he intimates another sort of clearly unwanted objectification—in which people stare at those whose bodies depart from socially established norms.

Jennifer Bartlett, a disabled woman, expresses sentiments in "Longing for the Male Gaze" similar to those of Clare. She describes creating an online dating profile that allows her to pass as nondisabled in order to "explore the sexual world as an able-bodied woman, if only online, and see what all the fuss was about."[61] She describes how men stopped responding to her messages after she disclosed her impairment. "I know that I am 'lucky' not to be sexually harassed as I navigate the New York City streets. [. . .] But I still would much rather have a man make an inappropriate sexual comment than be referred to in the third person or have someone express surprise over the fact that I have a career."[62] While recognizing the harm of sexual harassment, Bartlett contends that the harm she experiences through being made to feel invisible is worse.[63]

Even if we maintain that objectification is not always harmful, there are two forms of objectification that specifically impact disabled people and reinforce ableism: inspiration porn and devoteeism. While individual disabled people may not experience these types of objectification as harmful—indeed some may derive benefit in the context of a society that devalues and desexualizes disabled people—they contribute to maintaining the status quo. In what follows, I examine the examples of inspiration porn and devoteeism and apply the concept of derivatization in order to highlight the harm in each case.

Inspiration Porn, Devoteeism, and Derivatization

In a 2014 TED Talk, disability activist Stella Young discusses what she calls "inspiration porn." This term refers to the pairing of images of disabled people along with motivational quotations in an attempt to inspire viewers. *Prima facie*, this practice may seem benign; it may even seem to be portraying disabled people in a positive way. Indeed, Young anticipates this objection; taking on the voice of an imagined interlocutor, she asks "But, Stella, aren't you sometimes inspired by disabled people?"[64] She admits that she is, but she locates the source of inspiration in particular disabled people finding innovative ways of accomplishing tasks (e.g., charging a cell phone using the battery of a motorized wheelchair). Young notes that in using the term "porn" she intends to convey that this practice is objectifying—it uses disabled people in the service of nondisabled people. Inspiration porn serves to assuage the fears of nondisabled people and individualizes disability rather than drawing attention to the ways that structural factors create obstacles for disabled people.

Inspiration porn encourages nondisabled people to be grateful; after all, no matter how bad their lives are, at least they aren't disabled. It sends the message that success is solely the result of one's attitude with the implicit assumption that failure stems from having the wrong attitude. This is an incredibly distorted narrative that ignores the disability rights movement and the real needs of disabled people such as adequate health care, education, employment, and transportation—none of which will be addressed with a positive attitude. Thus, it encourages quietism rather than an acknowledgment that society has a responsibility to work for justice for disabled people. In addition, inspiration porn serves to other disabled people by suggesting that doing ordinary things makes them extraordinary, whereas Young states that disabled people are simply using their bodies to the best of their abilities just like nondisabled people do. Disabled people do not exist in order to help nondisabled people feel grateful or inspired.

Philosopher Havi Carel reports "Once you are ill, I realise, you become fair game. You slide down an implicit social ladder. Others begin to perceive you as weak and unimportant, an object of pity and fascination."[65] Notice that Carel, like Young, uses the language of being treated as an "object." Cahill's concept of derivatization helps to hone in on the problem with inspiration porn and daily interactions between disabled and nondisabled people—they are based upon the desires and fears of nondisabled people and do not take disabled people's perspectives into account.

The second example I want to consider is devoteeism. Devotees are solely or especially sexually attracted to people with impairments. The following discussion centers on the most apparent subset of this population: heterosexual white nondisabled men who are attracted to women who are amputees.[66] In "Desire and Disgust: My Ambivalent Adventures in Devoteeism," disability theorist Alison Kafer reflects upon her own interactions with devotees as well as on the phenomenon of nondisabled heterosexual male devoteeism more generally. She describes the typical reaction of friends and family members when she explains this phenomenon: "'Ewww, that's weird. What's wrong with those people?' Although I confess to following this train of thought myself, wondering what's 'wrong' with devotees, hearing it with such consistency troubled me."⁶⁷ Kafer explores the complex dynamics between devotees and amputees, situating them within broader narratives regarding gender, sexuality, and disability.

We might wonder if being attracted to a woman due to her status as an amputee is that different from having a preference for women with another sort of physical trait: hair color, eye color, or height, for example. Either type of attraction, I would argue, can be problematic if it overemphasizes the importance of this characteristic, especially if it becomes the only relevant criterion. Kafer includes excerpts of an email she received from a devotee using the pseudonym "Steve" that details the excitement he feels when catching a glimpse of an amputee. Regarding this message, she asserts, "For Steve, my 'beautiful looks' are the result of my two above-the-knee amputations; the fact that he knows nothing else about my appearance, or my life in general, does nothing to dampen his desire."⁶⁸ It seems clear that, indeed, there is one factor alone that elicits Steve's desire.

Kafer expresses discomfort with devoteeism, not only with receiving messages from strangers detailing their attraction to her but also with reports that some devotees take photos of amputees without permission and post them online, stalk amputees, and share their personal information with other devotees. Yet, she admits "as someone who is routinely met with hostile stares because of the oddness of my body, I can't help but be intrigued by the notion of finding eroticism in bodies typically marked as undesirable."⁶⁹ Kafer also acknowledges that other amputee women have had affirming experiences through involvement with devotees.

While it may be tempting to consider devoteeism to be an important exception to the otherwise pervasive desexualization of disabled women, this phenomenon is informed by problematic assumptions about gender and disability. For example, Kafer notes that "devotee discourses present disability as an individual problem" rather than a social or political one.⁷⁰ She also contends that devotee discourses are harmful insofar as they send the message to amputees that no one else will find them attractive or worthy of a relationship, making devoteeism "an amputee's only path out of disgust."⁷¹ Kafer advocates instead "contextualizing 'dating obstacles' within a larger analysis of ableism and political oppression, recognizing that sexual marginalization is deeply connected to political and social marginalization."⁷² This approach considers desexualization along with other ways that society limits the ability of disabled people to flourish.

The examples of inspiration porn and devoteeism demonstrate that the remedy to desexualization is not just any type of objectification. Cahill likens nonderivatizing sexual recognition to Marilyn Frye's notion of the "loving eye."[73] In Frye's words:

> It is the eye of one who knows that to know the seen, one must consult something other than one's own will and interests and fears and imagination. [. . .] In particular, it is a matter of being able to tell one's own interests from those of others and of knowing where one's self leaves off and another begins."[74]

One of the significant problems with derivatization is that it excludes the perceived subject's perspective—their interests, desires, and fears. It fails to recognize their "ontological distinctiveness."[75] Thus, the corrective involves approaching the other with self-awareness as well as openness to the other person as an individual. Cahill adds to Frye's account that nonderivatizing objectification should also entail "willingness to be transformed by the encounter."[76] This implies not only being prepared to revise claims to knowledge and expectations but also how one experiences their very self in relation to another.

Cahill advises that "to avoid derivatization, one must look with wonder. One must take bodies on their own terms, without imposing a pre-existing standard upon them."[77] Bodies that differ from social norms of what a body "should" be like can be disruptive and unpredictable, but this provides an opportunity to rethink assumptions and to experience embodied intersubjectivity in new ways. Clare writes: "I've had lovers tell me how good my shaky touch feels, tremors likened to extra caresses or driving over a gravel road, their words an antidote to shame. But until now I had never felt the pleasure they describe. Your twitches spread across my skin—tingle, dance, echo."[78] Centering disabled people's experiences makes clear that divergences from social norms cannot be reduced to lack. Indeed, Clare provides an example of a pleasure specifically experienced between embodied subjects who diverge from social norms.

I agree with Cahill that the starting point of any account of sexuality that strives to be true to experience must start with embodied intersubjectivity and that desexualization can be harmful. Indeed, I agree with most of the points she makes in her discussion of the desexualization of disabled women. She advocates changing how we understand objectification so it can include harmful as well as self-affirming experiences of being perceived as a body. I think, however, that it would be preferable to use a term other than "objectification." Cahill's critique of the notion of objectification as assuming a split between personhood and embodiment, as well as the fact that this term is generally used to articulate negative experiences, pose serious obstacles to changing its meaning. In addition, Cahill sometimes conflates perceiving disabled women as sexual with finding them sexually desirable. While it is certainly necessary to consider someone to be sexual in order to desire them, recognizing that a woman is sexual is not the same as finding her sexually attractive. I propose, therefore, the term "sexual recognition" as an alternative that seems to better articulate positive acknowledgment of another embodied subject as a sexual being.

Merleau-Ponty and Desexualization of Disabled People

Merleau-Ponty considers embodiment and social context to be central for theorization of human existence and suggests that sexuality permeates existence rather than being a separate, peripheral realm. Earlier, I highlighted the centrality of ambiguity for sexuality and human existence in general. Now, I will demonstrate how Merleau-Ponty's notion of ambiguity can be used to describe the phenomenon of desexualization and the obstacles desexualization presents to situating oneself sexually within a social context that largely denies one's ambiguity.

According to Merleau-Ponty, freedom requires the power to situate oneself. Ambiguity enables one to situate oneself in several aspects of life. So, ambiguity is necessary for freedom. Let us briefly review his conceptualization of situation before turning to the role of ambiguity. He claims that Schneider is bound to the actual insofar as he is unable to place himself in a situation; this prevents him from envisioning and taking up possibilities—Schneider "lacks freedom."[79] Merleau-Ponty asserts:

> . . . the life of consciousness—epistemic life, the life of desire, or perceptual life—is underpinned by an "intentional arc" that projects around us our past, our future, our human milieu, our physical situation, our ideological situation, our moral situation, or rather, that ensures that we are situated within all of these relationships.[80]

Merleau-Ponty contends that the intentional arc allows for knowledge, desire, and perception to occur within the multiple ways that one is situated. Though my primary focus is on Schneider's difficulties in regard to sexuality, the change to his intentional arc impacts all aspects of his existence.

In the case of people with visible identifiable impairments, the ability to situate oneself may be impaired by a lack of ambiguity imposed by others. The impact of desexualization for disabled people can be clarified by considering what is required for sexual situatedness and taking up possibilities. Disabled people are assumed to lack temporal ambiguity insofar as others behave as if one's status as disabled precludes future possibilities—including those that are not actually prevented by impairment itself.

In the context of discussing temporality and trauma, Merleau-Ponty states that "one present among all of them thus acquires an exceptional value. It displaces the others and relieves them of their value as authentic present moments."[81] He is referring to the first-person experience of trauma here. However, I think that this description is helpful for understanding one way that people with visibly identifiable impairments—perhaps those acquired through traumatic injury in particular—are perceived by others. When one's impairment is noted, this aspect of existence is often privileged over all others. Temporality is rendered unambiguous insofar as the perceiver cannot imagine a disabled person being able to assume temporality in order to express existence through their body.

Regarding the remarks nondisabled people have made to her regarding her life possibilities, Alison Kafer asserts:

> They can apparently see into my immediate future, forecasting an inability to perform specific tasks and predicting the accidents and additional injuries that will result. Or, taking a longer view, they imagine a future that is both banal and pathetic: rather than involving dramatic falls from my wheelchair, their visions assume a future of relentless pain, isolation, and bitterness, a representation that leads them to bless me, pity me, or refuse to see me altogether.[82]

Though others cannot completely arrest the flow of temporality for disabled people, being approached as if one no longer has the ability to create a genuine existence does serve to curtail one's subjectivity and limit possibilities.

The perception that disabled people are unsexed serves as a prime example of how common perceptions serve to limit the possibilities for expressing existence. Realizing that one is seen as incapable of sexual desire or being desired can severely impinge upon the ways that one attempts to express their sexuality. As noted previously, Merleau-Ponty suggests that if we can conceive of "the sexual history of a man" as providing the key to his life, this is because sexuality projects being toward time and toward others.[83] Expressions of sexuality are also greatly impacted by how others behave toward an individual. When one is not recognized as sexual, this seems to be a manifestation of an even broader harm, which impacts most, if not all, areas of life.

We are not immune from the meanings others assign to the existence we embody. In fact, it is impossible to construct meaning apart from a social context. Though we may attempt to shut out others, this is never entirely possible. As Merleau-Ponty states, ". . . we are literally what others think of us and we are our world."[84] This is not to say that we are completely determined by others; he points out that for that to be possible we would need to be reduced to the status of a thing.[85] On his account, one cannot be reduced to a thing insofar as one *is* a body rather than *having* a body. Insofar as human existence is characterized by incompleteness, people can have possible situations and not only actual situations. However, I think that disabled people can be perceived as lacking bodily as well as temporal ambiguity, and this places limitations on their capacity to take up possibilities.

Merleau-Ponty often returns to the comparison of human existence to an artwork. He asserts that "bodily existence, which streams forth through me without my complicity, is but a sketch of a genuine presence in the world."[86] Bodily existence is a necessary condition for the creative acts through which one constitutes a genuine existence. To perceive another as lacking the capacity to take up possible situations when they actually possess this ability is to mistake a preparatory sketch for the artwork it will become. When disabled people are thought to be unable to assume possibilities, an artificial completeness is imposed upon them. While disabled people cannot be completely precluded from situating themselves, failure to recognize their ambiguity impinges upon their ability to assume meanings and possibilities, which are intersubjectively constituted.

Conclusion

I developed Merleau-Ponty's account of sexuality prior to showing some of the ways that his notions of ambiguity, embodied intersubjectivity, and situation can be used to describe the desexualization experienced by disabled people. I have examined the relationship between sexuality and existence in an attempt to clarify the harm of desexualization of disabled people. I considered Cahill's account of the harms of desexualization of women with impairments premised upon embodied intersubjectivity. I advocated sexual recognition, rather than objectification, as the alternative concept for understanding the desexualization of disabled people. By viewing sexuality as coextensive with life, it becomes possible to sketch an account of the harmfulness of the desexualization of disabled people and to develop ideals that instead support the flourishing of disabled people.

Notes

I am grateful to Susan Bredlau, Ann Cahill, Anthony Fernandez, Alex Levine, Joel Michael Reynolds, and Talia Welsh for reading multiple drafts of this chapter and providing generous and helpful feedback. I would also like to thank audiences at meetings for the Association for Feminist Ethics and Social Theory, the Society for Phenomenology and Existential Philosophy, and the Merleau-Ponty Circle for questions and comments that helped me to clarify my position.

    1. Jackie Leach Scully, *Disability Bioethics: Moral Bodies, Moral Differences* (Lanham, MD: Rowman & Littlefield, 2008), 3.

    2. The social model of disability distinguishes between "impairment" and "disability." The former refers to characteristics of an individual considered to be atypical and the latter refers to oppression individuals with impairments face. "Ableism" is used to name this type of oppression. See Ron Amundson, "Disability, Ideology, and Quality of Life: A Bias in Biomedical Ethics" in *Quality of Life and Human Difference*, eds. David Wasserman, Jerome Bickenbach, and Robert Wachbroit (Cambridge: Cambridge University Press, 2005), 101–124; Colin Barnes, "Understanding the Social Model of Disability: Past, Present, and Future," in *Routledge Handbook for Disability Studies*, ed. Nick Watson, Alan Roulstone, and Carol Thomas, 12–29 (New York: Routledge 2012); Michael Oliver, *The Politics of Disablement: A Sociological Approach* (London: Macmillan, 1990).

    3. My discussion does not address considerations regarding sexuality that are specific to people with cognitive impairments. See Michel Desjardins, "The Sexualized Body of the Child," in *Sex and Disability*, eds. Anna Mollow and Robert McRuer (Durham, NC: Duke University Press, 2012), 69–88; Alison Kafer, *Feminist, Queer, Crip* (Bloomington: Indiana University Press, 2013). I also do not attend to how the position that sexuality is central to existence accounts for people who identify as asexual. These are important concerns but beyond the scope of the current project.

4. Karen Yoshinda, Fran Odette, Susan Hardie, Heather Willis, and Mary Bunch. "Women Living with Disabilities and Their Experiences and Issues Related to the Context and Complexities of Leaving Abusive Situations," *Disability and Rehabilitation* 31, no. 22 (2009): 1843–1852.

5. Lisa Iezzoni and Bonnie O'Day. *More than Ramps: Improving the Accessibility and Quality of Health Care for People with Disabilities* (Oxford: Oxford University Press, 2011).

6. The notion of "normal sexuality" itself is in need of interrogation. This is beyond the scope of my chapter. See Abby Wilkerson "Normate Sex and Its Discontents," in *Sex and Disability*, ed. Anna Mollow and Robert McRuer (Durham, NC: Duke University Press, 2012), 183–207.

7. I use the term "impairment" to make clear that I am referring to characteristics of bodies that are categorized as atypical or "abnormal."

8. Linda Alcoff, *Visible Identities: Race, Gender, and the Self* (Oxford: Oxford University Press, 2006); Havi Carel, *Phenomenology of Illness* (Oxford: Oxford University Press, 2016). Emily Lee, "The Meaning of Visible Differences of the Body" *APA Newsletter Asian and Asian-American Philosophers and Philosophies* 2, no. 2 (2003): 633–638; Shannon Sullivan, "Ontological Expansiveness," in *50 Concepts for a Critical Phenomenology*, edited by Gail Weiss, Ann Murphy, and Gayle Salamon (Evanston, IL: Northwestern University Press, 2019), 249–254; George Yancy "White Gazes: What It Feels Like to Be an Essence," in *Living Alterities: Phenomenology, Embodiment, and Race*, ed. Emily Lee (Albany, NY: SUNY Press, 2014), 43–64.

9. See Sara Ahmed, *Queer Phenomenology: Orientations, Objects, Others* (Durham, NC: Duke University Press, 2006); Linda Alcoff, "Merleau-Ponty and Feminist Theory on Experience" in *Chiasms: Merleau-Ponty's Notion of the Flesh*, ed. Fred Evans (Albany, NY: SUNY Press, 2000); Simone de Beauvoir, *The Second Sex*, translated by H.M. Parshely (New York: Random House, 2010); Frantz Fanon, *Black Skin, White Masks*, translated by Richard Philcox (New York: Grove Press, 2008); Emily Lee, "The Meaning of Visible Differences of the Body" 2003; Emily Lee, "Introduction," in *Living Alterities: Phenomenology, Embodiment, and Race*, ed. Emily Lee (Albany, NY: SUNY Press, 2014), 43–64; Sara C. Shabot and Christina Landry, *Rethinking Feminist Phenomenology* (Durham, NC: Duke University Press, 2018); Yancy, "White Gazes: What It Feels Like to Be an Essence," 43–64; George Yancy, *Black Bodies, White Gazes: The Continuing Significance of Race in America*, 2nd ed. (Lanham, MD: Rowman & Littlefield, 2017); Iris Marion Young, *"Throwing Like a Girl" and Other Essays* (Oxford: Oxford University Press, 2005).

10. Christine Wieseler, "Challenging Conceptions of the 'Normal' Subject of Phenomenology," in *Race as Phenomena: Between Phenomenology and Philosophy of Race*, ed. Emily Lee (Lanham, MD: Rowman & Littlefield, 2019), 69.

11. Maurice Merleau-Ponty, *Phenomenology of Perception*, trans. Donald Landes (New York: Routledge, 2012), 153.

12. Shelley Tremain, *Foucault and Feminist Philosophy of Disability* (Ann Arbor: University of Michigan Press, 2017).

13. The following is one of the few places in the *Phenomenology of Perception* in which he considers instances in which a disabled person's self-perception might be shaped by others' perceptions as well as how disabled people resist incorporating others' perceptions into their own.

> We are often amazed that the disabled person or the person suffering from a disease can bear their situation. But in their own eyes they are not disabled or dying. Until the moment he slips into a coma, the dying person is inhabited by a consciousness; he is everything that he sees, he has this means of escape. Consciousness can never objectify itself as sick-consciousness or disabled consciousness; and even if the elderly man complains of his old age or the disabled person of his disability, they can only do so when they see themselves through the eyes of others, that is, when they adopt a statistical or an objective view of themselves; and these complaints are never wholly made in good faith: in returning to the core of his consciousness, everyone feels himself to be beyond his particular characteristics and so resigns himself to them. (458–459)

Although he describes the potential relationship between observers and a disabled or dying person's experience, he appeals to "escape" and feeling "beyond . . . particular characteristics" in order to explain the discrepancy between their perspectives.

14. Lisa Guenther, *Solitary Confinement: Social Death and Its Afterlives* (Minneapolis: University of Minnesota Press, 2013), viii.

15. Guenther, *Solitary Confinement*, viii.

16. Sandra Bartky, *Suffering to Be Beautiful*. Lanham, MD: Rowman & Littlefield, 2002. 15–16.

17. See Jessica Cadwallader "Stirring up the Sediment: The Corporeal Pedagogies of Disabilities," *Discourse: Studies in the Cultural Politics of Education* 31(2010): 513–526; Miho Iwakuma, "The Body as Embodiment: An Investigation of the Body by Merleau-Ponty," in *Disability/Postmodernity*, eds. Mairian Corker and Tom Shakespeare (New York: Continuum, 2002); Corinne Lajoie, "Being at Home: A Feminist Phenomenology of Disorientation in Illness," *Hypatia* 34, no. 3 (2019): 546–569; Joel Reynolds "The Normate," in *50 Concepts for a Critical Phenomenology*, eds. Gail Weiss, Ann Murphy, and Gayle Salamon, 243–248. (Evanston, IL: Northwestern University Press, 2019); Scully, *Disability Bioethics*, 2008; Gayle Salamon, "The Phenomenology of Rheumatology: Disability,

Merleau-Ponty, and the Fallacy of Maximal Grip," *Hypatia* 27, no. 2 (2012): 243–260; Margrit Shildrick, *Dangerous Discourses of Disability, Subjectivity and Sexuality* (New York: Palgrave McMillan, 2009); Gail Weiss, "The Normal, the Natural, and the Normative: A Merleau-Pontian Legacy to Feminist Theory, Critical Race Theory, and Disability Studies," *Continental Philosophy Review* 48 (2015): 77–93.

    18. Merleau-Ponty, *Phenomenology of Perception*, 205.
    19. Merleau-Ponty, *Phenomenology of Perception*, 86–87.
    20. Merleau-Ponty, *Phenomenology of Perception*, 105. For additional discussion of Johann Schneider and his place in Merlau-Ponty's thinking, see Susan Bredlau and Talia Welsh's Introduction to this volume, Jenny Slatman, chapter 1 of this volume, and Gabrielle Jackson, chapter 2 of this volume.
    21. Merleau-Ponty, *Phenomenology of Perception*, 136.
    22. Merleau-Ponty, *Phenomenology of Perception*, 132.
    23. Merleau-Ponty, *Phenomenology of Perception*, 156.
    24. Merleau-Ponty, *Phenomenology of Perception*, 127.
    25. Merleau-Ponty, *Phenomenology of Perception*, 105.
    26. Merleau-Ponty, *Phenomenology of Perception*, 157.
    27. Merleau-Ponty, *Phenomenology of Perception*, 137.
    28. Merleau-Ponty, *Phenomenology of Perception*, 159.
    29. Merleau-Ponty, *Phenomenology of Perception*, 158.
    30. Merleau-Ponty, *Phenomenology of Perception*, 160.
    31. Merleau-Ponty, *Phenomenology of Perception*, 173.
    32. Merleau-Ponty, *Phenomenology of Perception*, 161.
    33. See also Fiona Kumari Campbell, *Contours of Ableism: The Production of Disability and Abledness* (London: Palgrave Macmillan, 2009); Shildrick, *Dangerous Discourses of Disability*, 2009.
    34. Anna Mollow and Robert McRuer, *Sex and Disability* (New York: Routledge, 2012), 1.
    35. Tobin Siebers discusses the lack of privacy afforded to people with disabilities who reside in long-term care facilities, hospitals, and group homes. He states: "Medical authorities make decisions about access to erotic literature, masturbation, and sexual partners." See "A Sexual Culture for Disabled People," in *Sex and Disability*, ed. Anna Mollow and Robert McRuer (Durham, NC: Duke University Press, 2002), 45. While I think it is important to consider the ways that institutions impinge upon disabled people's expressions of sexuality, my primary focus will be on the harm resulting from the (mis)perception that disabled people are not sexual.
    36. Although race is seldom mentioned in discussion of these examples, I suspect that they are, in fact, centered on the experiences of white disabled women.
    37. See Ann Cahill, *Overcoming Objectification* (New York: Routledge, 2011), 84. I find inclusion of the word "appropriate" interesting here. Cahill draws atten-

tion to the notion that attraction to people with disabilities is a perversion. She notes that unsexed women, including those with visually identifiable disabilities "show up in pornographic subgenres as fetishes" (104). Margrit Shildrick notes that public representations of disabled people "veer between the asexual and the hypersexual" (*Dangerous Discourses of Disability*, 84).

38. Cahill, *Overcoming Objectification*, 85.
39. Cahill, *Overcoming Objectification*, 22.
40. Cahill, *Overcoming Objectification*, 97.
41. Regarding the choice to focus on this subset of disabled women, Cahill remarks, "given the emphasis on sexual objectification (or lack of the same), my analysis will focus on those disabled women whose disability is *visibly obvious*" (*Overcoming Objectification*, 87). My discussion focuses on this group for the same reason. I expect that disabled women with less obvious impairments are desexualized as well but that their experiences are likely to differ from those of women who are readily identifiable as disabled.
42. Cahill, *Overcoming Objectification*, 25.
43. Cahill, *Overcoming Objectification*, 15.
44. Cahill, *Overcoming Objectification*, 25.
45. Cahill, *Overcoming Objectification*, 84.
46. Cahill, *Overcoming Objectification*, 32.
47. Cahill, *Overcoming Objectification*, 48.
48. Cahill, *Overcoming Objectification*, 48.
49. Cahill, *Overcoming Objectification*, 49.
50. Cahill, *Overcoming Objectification*, 49.
51. Cahill, *Overcoming Objectification*, 32.
52. Cahill, *Overcoming Objectification*, 33.
53. Cahill, *Overcoming Objectification*, 32.
54. Cahill, *Overcoming Objectification*, 84.
55. Cahill, *Overcoming Objectification*, 93.
56. Cahill, *Overcoming Objectification*, 90.
57. Emily Ladau. "Playing the Online Dating Game, in a Wheelchair." *New York Times*. September 27, 2017. www.nytimes.com/2017/09/27/opinion/online-dating-disability.html?searchResultPosition=4
58. Ladau, "Playing the Online Dating Game, in a Wheelchair."
59. Ladau, "Playing the Online Dating Game, in a Wheelchair."
60. Eli Clare, *Pride and Exile* (Boston: South End Press, 1999), 113–114, quoted in Cahill, *Overcoming Objectification*, 93.
61. Jennifer Bartlett. "Longing for the Male Gaze." *New York Times*. September 21, 2016. www.nytimes.com/2016/09/21/opinion/longing-for-the-male-gaze.html
62. Bartlett, "Longing for the Male Gaze."
63. Bartlett, "Longing for the Male Gaze."

64. Stella Young, "I'm Not Your Inspiration, www.ted.com/talks/stella_young_i_m_not_your_inspiration_thank_you_very_much?language=en

65. Havi Carel, "My 10-year Death Sentence." www.independent.co.uk/news/people/profiles/havi-carel-my-10-year-death-sentence-5332425.html

66. Kafer states:

Demographic analyses of devotees are rare and reliant on small sample sizes, but they suggest that devotees in the United States tend to be white, middle to upper-middle class, well-educated men between the ages of twenty-five and sixty-five [. . .] Most devotees are nondisabled men interested in disabled women, but, judging from the numerous websites catering to gay male devotees, there seems also to be a significant population of gay men involved in the attraction. (*My Ambivalent Adventures in Devoteeism*, 335)

67. Kafer, *My Ambivalent Adventures in Devoteeism*, 332.
68. Kafer, *My Ambivalent Adventures in Devoteeism*, 332.
69. Kafer, *My Ambivalent Adventures in Devoteeism*, 334.
70. Kafer, *My Ambivalent Adventures in Devoteeism*, 338.
71. Kafer, *My Ambivalent Adventures in Devoteeism*, 339.
72. Kafer, *My Ambivalent Adventures in Devoteeism*, 338.
73. Cahill, *Overcoming Objectification*, 46.
74. Marilyn Frye, *The Politics of Reality* (Berkeley, CA: Crossing Press, 1983), 75; quoted in Cahill 2011, *Overcoming Objectification*, 46.
75. Cahill, *Overcoming Objectification*, 49.
76. Cahill, *Overcoming Objectification*, 47.
77. Cahill, *Overcoming Objectification*, 103.
78. Eli Clare, *Brilliant Imperfection* (Durham, NC: Duke University Press, 2017), 19.
79. Merleau-Ponty, *Phenomenology of Perception*, 137.
80. Merleau-Ponty, *Phenomenology of Perception*, 137.
81. Merleau-Ponty, *Phenomenology of Perception*, 85.
82. Alison Kafer, *Feminist, Queer, Crip* (Bloomington: Indiana University Press, 2013), 2.
83. Merleau-Ponty, *Phenomenology of Perception*, 161.
84. Merleau-Ponty, *Phenomenology of Perception*, 109; Jenny Slatman builds on Merleau-Ponty's insight in her chapter in this volume: "When you are average or normal in a certain population, you do not stand out and you do not attract attention. However, if you are not average, then you stand out and are confronted with comparative views of others who may hinder you."
85. Merleau-Ponty, *Phenomenology of Perception*, 459.
86. Merleau-Ponty, *Phenomenology of Perception*, 168.

Works Cited

Ahmed, Sara. *Queer Phenomenology: Orientations, Objects, Others*. London: Duke University Press, 2006.
Alcoff, Linda. "Epistemologies of Ignorance: Three Types." In *Race and Epistemologies of Ignorance*, edited by Shannon Sullivan and Nancy Tuana. Albany, NY: SUNY Press, 2007. 39–56.
Alcoff, Linda. "Merleau-Ponty and Feminist Theory on Experience." In *Chiasms: Merleau-Ponty's Notion of the Flesh*, edited by Fred Evans. Albany, NY: SUNY Press, 2000.
Alcoff, Linda. *Visible Identities: Race, Gender, and the Self*. Oxford: Oxford University Press, 2006.
Allatt, Kate, and Alison Stokes. *Running Free*. Bedlinog, Wales: Accent Press, 2011.
Alper, Meryl. "Inclusive Sensory Ethnography: Studying New Media and Neurodiversity in Everyday Life." *New Media and Society* 20, no. 10 (2018): 3560–3579.
Alvis, Jason. "Making Sense of Heidegger's 'Phenomenology of the Inconspicuous' or Inapparent." *Continental Philosophy Review* 51 (2018): 211–238.
Amundson, Ron. "Disability, Ideology, and Quality of Life: A Bias in Biomedical Ethics." In *Quality of Life and Human Difference*, edited by David Wasserman, Jerome Bickenbach, and Robert Wachbroit. Cambridge: Cambridge University Press, 2005. 101–124.
Anderson, Elijah. *The Cosmopolitan Canopy: Race and Civility in Everyday Life*. New York: W. W. Norton & Co., 2011.
Anderson, J.A., M.S. Meyn, C. Shuman, R. Zlotnik Shaul, L.E. Mantella, M. J. Szego, S. Bowdin, N. Monfared, and R.Z. Hayeems. "Parents' Perspectives on Whole Genome Sequencing for Their Children: Qualified Enthusiasm?" *Journal of Medical Ethics* 43 (2016): 535–539.
Aristotle. *Nicomachean Ethics*. 2nd edition. Translated by Terence Irwin. Indianapolis: Hackett, 1999.

Assari, Shervin. "Unequal Gain of Equal Resources across Racial Groups." *International Journal of Health Policy and Management* 7, no. 1 (2018): 1–9.

Assari, Shervin, and Maryam Moghani Lankarani. "Poverty Status and Childhood Asthma in White and Black Families: National Survey of Children's Health." *Healthcare* 6, no. 62 (2018). doi:10.3390/healthcare602002

Bakris, George, and Matthew Sorrentino. "Redefining Hypertension—Assessing the New Blood-Pressure Guidelines." *New England Journal of Medicine* 378, no. 6 (2018): 497–499.

Barbaras, Renaud. *The Being of the Phenomenon: Merleau-Ponty's Ontology*. Translated by Ted Toadvine. Bloomington: Indiana University Press, 2004.

Barham, Peter. "Foucault and the Psychiatric Practitioner." In *Rewriting the History of Madness: Studies in Foucault's* "Histoire de la folie," edited by Arthur Still and Irving Velody. London: Routledge, 1992. 45–50.

Barnes, Colin. "Understanding the Social Model of Disability: Past, Present, and Future." In *Routledge Handbook for Disability Studies*, edited by Nick Watson, Alan Roulstone, and Carol Thomas. New York: Routledge 2012. 12–29.

Bartky, Sandra. *Suffering to Be Beautiful*. Lanham, MD: Rowman & Littlefield, 2002.

Bartlett, Jennifer. "Longing for the Male Gaze." *The New York Times*. September 21, 2016. www.nytimes.com/2016/09/21/opinion/longing-for-the-male-gaze.html

Bateson, Gregory. *Steps to an Ecology of Mind*. Chicago: University of Chicago Press, 1990.

Bauby, Jean-Dominique. *The Diving-Bell and the Butterfly*. Translated by Jeremy Leggatt. London: Harper Perennial, 2004.

Bausch, Pina. "Vollmond." Dance Performance. Online video. Daily Motion. https://dai.ly/x11kljy

Beauvoir, Simone de. *The Second Sex*. Translated by H.M. Parshley. New York: Random House, 2010.

Behrman, M., and J.J. Marotta. "Patient Schn: Has Goldstein and Gelb's Case Withstood the Test of Time?" *Neuropsychologia* 42 (2004): 633–638.

Beith, Don. *The Birth of Sense: Generative Passivity in Merleau-Ponty's Philosophy*. Athens: Ohio University Press, 2018.

Belanger, E.A., B.L. Leonhardt, S.E. George, R.L. Firmin, and P.H. Lysaker. "Negative Symptoms and Therapeutic Connection: A Qualitative Analysis in a Single Case Study with a Patient with First Episode Psychosis." *Journal of Psychotherapy Integration* 28, no. 2 (2018): 171–187.

Bernhardt, Barbara A., Cynda H. Rushton, Joseph Carrese, Reed E. Pyeritz, Ken Kolodner, and Gail Geller. "Distress and Burnout among Genetic Service Providers." *Genetic Medicine* 11, no. 7 (2009): 527–535.

Bert, Jean-François. "Retour à Münsterlingen." In *Foucault à Münsterlingen. À l'origine de l'Histoire de la folie*, edited by Jean-François Bert and Elisabetta Basso. Paris: Éditions EHESS, 2015. 9–47.

Bogdashina, Olga. *Sensory Perceptual Issues in Autism and Asperger Syndrome: Different Sensory Experiences—Different Perceptual Worlds.* London: Jessica Kingsley Publishers, 2003.
Bottini, Gabriella, Eraldo Paulesu, Martina Gandola, Lorenzo Pia, Paola Invernizzi, and Anna Berti. "Anosognosia for Hemiplegia and Models of Motor Control: Insights from Lesional Data." In *The Study of Anosognosia*, edited by George P. Prigatano. New York: Oxford University Press, 2010. 17–38.
Bredlau, Susan M. "A Respectful World: Merleau-Ponty and the Experience of Depth." *Human Studies* 33, no. 4 (December 1, 2010): 411–423. doi.org/10.1007/s10746-011-9173-1
Bredlau, Susan M. "Monstrous Faces and a World Transformed: Merleau-Ponty, Dolezal, and the Enactive Approach on Vision without Inversion of the Retinal Image." *Phenomenology and the Cognitive Sciences* 10 (2011): 481–498.
Bredlau, Susan M. *The Other in Perception*. Albany, NY: SUNY Press, 2018.
Brody, Jane E. "Interventions to Prevent Psychosis." *The New York Times*. September 2, 2019.
Broome, Matthew, Robert Harland, Gareth S. Owen and Argyris Stringaris. *The Maudsley Reader in Phenomenological Psychiatry*. Cambridge: Cambridge University Press, 2012.
Bruno, Marie-Aurélie, Marie-Christine Nizzi, Steven Laureys, and Olivia Gosseries. "Consciousness in the Locked-in Syndrome." In *The Neurology of Consciousness*, 2nd edition, edited by Steven Laureys, Olivia Gosseries, and Giulio Tononi. San Diego, London, & Waltham: Academic Press, 2016. 187–202.
Butler, Judith. *Gender Trouble*. New York: Routledge, 1990.
Cadwallader, Jessica. "Stirring up the Sediment: The Corporeal Pedagogies of Disabilities." *Discourse: Studies in the Cultural Politics of Education* 31 (2010): 513–526.
Cahill, Ann. *Overcoming Objectification*. New York: Routledge, 2011.
Call, Nathan, Mindy C. Scheithauer, and Joanna Lomas Mevers. "Functional Behavioral Assessments." In *Applied Behavior Analysis Advanced Guidebook: A Manual for Professional Practice*, edited by James K. Luiselli. San Diego: Elsevier Academic Press, 2017. 41–71.
Campbell, Fiona Kumari. *Contours of Ableism: The Production of Disability and Abledness*. London: Palgrave Macmillan, 2009.
Canguilhem, Georges. *The Normal and the Pathological*. Translated by Carolyn R. Fawcett and Robert S. Cohen. New York: Zone Books, 1991.
Carel, Havi. "My 10-year Death Sentence." www.independent.co.uk/news/people/profiles/havi-carel-my-10-year-death-sentence-5332425.html
Carel, Havi. *Phenomenology of Illness*. Oxford: Oxford University Press, 2016.
Carman, Taylor. *Merleau-Ponty*. New York: Routledge, 2008.
Carvahlo, John. "Folds in the Flesh: Merleau-Ponty/Foucault." In *Rereading Merleau-Ponty: Essays beyond the Continental-Analytic Divide*, edited by Lawrence Hass and Dorothea Olkowski. Amherst, NY: Humanity Books, 2000.

Cascio, Ariel. "Cross-Cultural Autism Studies, Neurodiversity, and Conceptualizations of Autism." *Culture, Medicine, and Psychiatry: An International Journal of Cross-Cultural Health Research* 39, no. 2 (2015): 207–212.

Cassirer, Ernst. "Two Letters to Kurt Goldstein." *Science in Context* 12, no. 4 (1999/1925): 661–667.

"CaTCH: Claims Analysis of Twins Correlations and Heritability." Harvard Medical School. http://apps.chiragjpgroup.org/catch

Charon, Rita. *Narrative Medicine: Honoring the Stories of Illness*. Oxford & New York: Oxford University Press, 2006.

Churchill, Scott D., and Frederick J. Wertz. "An Introduction to Phenomenological Research in Psychology: Historical, Conceptual, and Methodological Foundations." In *The Handbook of Humanistic Psychology: Theory, Research and Practice*, 2nd edition, edited by Kirk J. Schneider, J. Fraser Pierson, and James F.T. Bugental. Los Angeles: Sage Publications, 2015. 275–296.

Clare, Eli. *Brilliant Imperfection: Grappling with Cure*. Durham, NC & London: Duke University Press, 2017.

Clare, Eli. *Pride and Exile*. Boston: South End Press, 1999.

Craig, Megan. "Locked In." *Journal of Speculative Philosophy* 22, no. 3 (2008): 145–158.

Crossley, Nick. *The Politics of Subjectivity: Between Foucault and Merleau-Ponty*. Aldershot: Avebury, 1994.

Davis, Kathy. *Reshaping the Female Body: The Dilemma of Cosmetic Surgery*. London: Routledge, 1995.

Davis, Lennard. *Enforcing Normalcy: Disability, Deafness, and the Body*. New York: Verso, 1995.

Dennett, Daniel. *Consciousness Explained*. Boston: Bay Books, 1991.

DeRoo, Neal. *Futurity in Phenomenology: Promise and Method in Husserl, Levinas and Derrida*. New York: Fordham University Press, 2013.

DeRoo, Neal. "Spiritual Expression and the Promise of Phenomenology." In *The Subject(s) of Phenomenology: Re-Reading Husserl*, edited by Iulian Apostelescu. Springer, 2019. 245–269.

Desjardins, Michel. "The Sexualized Body of the Child." In *Sex and Disability*, edited by Anna Mollow and Robert McRuer. Durham, NC: Duke University Press, 2012. 69–88.

Diagnostic and Statistical Manual of Mental Disorders: DSM-5. Arlington, VA: American Psychiatric Association, 2013.

Diedrich, Lisa. "Breaking Down: A Phenomenology of Disability." *Literature and Medicine* 20, no. 2 (2001): 209–230.

Dillon, M.C. *Merleau-Ponty's Ontology*. Bloomington: Indiana Press University, 1988.

Donnellan, Ann., David Hill, and Martha Leary. "Rethinking Autism: Implications of Sensory and Movement Differences for Understanding and Support." *Frontiers in Integrative Neuroscience*, no. 28 (2013): 1–11.

Dotson, Kristie. "A Cautionary Tale: On Limiting Epistemic Oppression, *Frontiers: A Journal of Women Studies* 33, no. 1 (2012): 24–47.

Dreyfus, Hubert L., and Paul Rabinow. *Beyond Structuralism and Hermeneutics*, 2nd edition, with an Afterword by and an Interview with Michel Foucault. Chicago: University of Chicago Press, 1983.

Dumas, Alexandre. *The Count of Monte Cristo*. London: Wordsworth Editions, 1997.

Eribon, Didier. *Michel Foucault*. Translated by Betsy Wing. Boston: Harvard University Press, 1992.

Evangelou, Angelos. *Philosophizing Madness from Nietzsche to Derrida*. London: Palgrave Macmillan, 2017.

Fanon, Frantz. *Black Skin, White Masks*. Translated by Richard Philcox. New York: Grove Press, 2008.

Fanon, Frantz. *Peau Noire, Masques Blancs*. Paris: Seuil, 1952.

Farah, Martha. *Visual Agnosia*. Cambridge, MA: MIT Press., 2004.

Fein, Elizabeth. "Making Meaningful Worlds: Role-Playing Subcultures and the Autism Spectrum." *Culture, Medicine, and Psychiatry: An International Journal of Cross-Cultural Health Research* 39, no. 2 (2015): 299–321.

Felder, Andrew J., and Brent Dean Robbins. "A Cultural-Existential Approach to Therapy: Merleau-Ponty's Phenomenology of Embodiment and Its Implications for Practice." *Theory & Psychology* 21, no. 3 (2011): 355–376.

Ferrari, Martina. "Poietic Transpatiality: Merleau-Ponty and the Sense of Nature." *Chiasmi International* 20 (2018): 385–401.

Fineman, Martha. *The Autonomy Myth: A Theory of Dependency*. New York: New Press, 2004.

Fisher, Max. "Why Coronavirus Conspiracy Theories Flourish. And Why It Matters." *The New York Times*. April 8, 2020. www.nytimes.com/2020/04/08/world/europe/coronavirus-conspiracy-theories.html

Fitzmaurice, Simon. *It's Not Yet Dark*. Boston & New York: Houghton Mifflin Harcourt, 2017.

Foucault, Michel. *Abnormal: Lectures at the Collège de France 1974–1975*. Edited by Valerio Marchetti, Antonella Salomoni and Arnold I. Davidson. Translated by Graham Burchell. New York: Picador, 2003.

Foucault, Michel. *Birth of the Clinic*. Translated by A.M. Sheridan. London: Routledge, 1973.

Foucault, Michel. *Discipline and Punish: The Birth of the Prison*. Translated by Alan Sheridan. New York: Vintage Books, 1995.

Foucault, Michel. *History of Madness*. Translated by Jonathan Murphy and Jean Khalfa. London: Routledge, 2006.

Frankenberg, Ruth. *White Women, Race Matters: The Social Construction of Whiteness*. Minneapolis: University of Minnesota Press, 1993.

Frenkel-Brunswik, Else. "Intolerance of Ambiguity as an Emotional and Perceptual Personality Variable." *Journal of Personality* 18 (1949): 108–143.

Frith, C.D., S.J. Blakemore, and D.M. Wolpert. "Abnormalities in the Awareness and Control of Action." *Philosophical Transactions of the Royal Society of London; Biological Sciences* 355, no. 1404 (2000): 1771–1778.

Frye, Marilyn. *The Politics of Reality*. Berkeley, CA: Crossing Press, 1983.

Funk, Cary, and Meg Hefferon. "U.S. Public Views of Climate and Energy." *Pew Research Center: Science & Society*. November 25, 2019. www.pewresearch.org/science/2019/11/25/u-s-public-views-on-climate-and-energy

Gallagher, Shaun. *How the Body Shapes the Mind*. Oxford: Oxford University Press, 2005.

Gardner, Murphy. "Personal Impressions of Kurt Goldstein." In *The Reach of Mind*, edited by Marianne Simmel. New York: Springer, 1968. 31–35.

Garfinkel, Harold. *Studies in Ethnomethodology*. Englewood Cliffs: Prentice-Hall, Inc., 1967.

Garland-Thomson, Rosemarie. "Human Biodiversity Conservation: A Consensual Ethical Principle." *The American Journal of Bioethics* 15, no. 6 (2015): 13–15.

Garland-Thomson, Rosemarie. "Misfits: A Feminist Materialist Disability Concept." *Hypatia* 26, no. 3 (2011): 591–609.

Gelb, Adhémar, and Kurt Goldstein. "Psychologische Analysen Hirnpathologischer Fälle Auf Grund von Untersuchungen Hirnverletzer." *Zeitschrift Für Die Gesamte Neurologie Und Psychiatrie* 41, no. 1 (1917): 1–142.

Gelb, Adhémar, and Kurt Goldstein. *Psychologische Analysen Hirnpathologischer Fälle*. Leipzig: Barth, 1920.

Geraets, Theodore. *Vers Une Nouvelle Philosophie Transcendantale: La Genèse de La Philosophie de Maurice Merleau-Ponty Jusqu' à La Phénoménologie de La Perception*. La Haye: Springer, 1971.

Gérard, Marie. "Canguilhem, Erwin Straus et la phénoménologie: la question de l'organisme vivant." *Bulletin D'Analyse* 6, no. 2 (2010): 118–145.

Geroulanos, Stefanos, and Todd Meyers. *The Human Body in the Age of Catastrophe: Brittleness, Integration, Science and the Great War*. Chicago: University of Chicago Press, 2018.

Goffman, Erwin. *Stigma: Notes on the Management of Spoiled Identity*. London: Penguin, 1963.

Goldenberg, G. "Goldstein and Gelb's Case Schn: A classic case in neuropsychology?" In *Classic Cases in Neuropsychology, Vol. II*, edited by C. Code, C.W. Wallesch, Y. Joanette, and A.R. Lecours. Hove: Psychology Press, 2003. 281–300.

Goldstein, Kurt. *Human Nature in the Light of Psychopathology*. Cambridge, MA: Harvard University Press, 1951.

Goldstein, Kurt. "Kurt Goldstein." In *A History of Psychology in Autobiography*, edited by Walther Riese. New York: Appleton-Century-Crofts, 1967. 147–166.
Goldstein, Kurt. "L'analyse de l'aphasia et l'étude de l'essence Du Langage." In *Selected Papers/Ausgewählte Schriften.*, edited by Aaron Gurwitsch, Else Goldstein, and William Haudek. The Hague: Martinus Nijhoff, 1971. 282–344.
Goldstein, Kurt. "Notes on the Development of My Concepts." In *Selected Papers/ Ausgewählte Schriften*, edited by Aaron Gurwitsch, Else Goldstein, and William Haudek. The Hague: Martinus Nijhoff, 1971. 1–12.
Goldstein, Kurt. "Remarks on Localisation." *Stereotactic and Functional Neurosurgery* no. 7 (1946): 25–34.
Goldstein, Kurt. *The Organism: A Holistic Approach to Biology Derived from Pathological Data in Man*. New York: Zone Books, 1995.
Gordon, Colin. "Rewriting the History of Misreading," in *Rewriting the History of Madness: Studies in Foucault's* "Histoire de la folie," edited by Arthur Still and Irving Velody. London: Routledge, 1992. 167–184.
Graham, Garth N. "Why Your ZIP Code Matters More Than Your Genetic Code: Promoting Healthy Outcomes from Mother to Child." *Breastfeeding Medicine: The Official Journal of the Academy of Breastfeeding Medicine* 11 (2016): 396–397. https://doi.org/10/gf9sfx
Grandin, Temple. *Thinking in Pictures: And Other Reports from My Life with Autism*. New York: Vintage, 1997.
Gros, Frédéric. *Foucault et la folie*. Paris: Presses Universitaires de France, 1997.
Guenther, Lisa. *Solitary Confinement: Social Death and Its Afterlives*. Minneapolis: University of Minnesota Press, 2013.
Gurwitsch, Aaron. "Gelb-Goldstein's Concept of 'Concrete' and 'Categorical' Attitude and the Phenomenology of Ideation." *Philosophy and Phenomenological Research* 10 (1949): 172–196.
Haan, Joost. "Locked-in: The Syndrome as Depicted in Literature." In *Literature, Neurology and Neuroscience: Neurological and Psychiatric Disordersi*, edited by Stanley Finger, François Boller, and Anne Stiles. Amsterdam: Elsevier, 2013. 19–34.
Hacking, Ian. *The Taming of Chance*. Cambridge: Cambridge University Press, 1990.
Hamrick, William. "Language and Abnormal Behavior: Merleau-Ponty, Hart and Laing." In *Merleau-Ponty and Psychology, A Special Issue from the Review of Existential Psychology and Psychiatry*" 18, nos. 1, 2 & 3 (1982–1983): 181–203.
Harrington, Anne. "Kurt Goldstein's Neurology of Healing and Wholeness." In *Greater Than the Parts*, edited by Christopher Lawrence and George Weisz. New York: Oxford University Press, 1998. 25–45.
Hasemyer, David, and Neela Banerjee. "Decades of Science Denial Related to Climate Change Has Led to Denial of the Coronavirus Pandemic." *Inside Climate News*. April 9, 2020. https://insideclimatenews.org/news/09042020/science-denial-coronavirus-covid-climate-change

Head, Henry. "Disorders of Symbolic Thinking and Expression." *British Journal of Psychology* 11, no. 2 (1921): 179–193.
Heidegger, Martin. "Seminar in Zahringen." In *Seminare*, edited by Curd Ochwadt. Frankfurt am Main: Klostermann, 1986.
Heilman, K.M. "Anosognosia: Possible Neuropsychological Mechanisms." In *Awareness of Deficit after Brain Injury: Clinical and Theoretic Issues*, edited by George P. Prigatano and Daniel L. Schacter. New York: Oxford University Press, 1991. 53–62.
Heinämaa, Sara. "Transcendental Intersubjectivity and Normality: Constitution by Mortals." In *The Phenomenology of Embodied Subjectivity*, edited by Rasmus Thybo Jensen and Dermot Moran. New York: Springer International Publishing, 2013. 83–103.
Heinämaa, Sara, and Joona Taipale. "Normality." In *The Oxford Handbook of Phenomenological Psychopathology*, edited by Giovanni Stanghellini, Matthew Broome, Andrea Raballo, Anthony Vincent Fernandez, Paolo Fusar-Poli, and René Rosfort. New York: Oxford University Press, 2019. 284–298.
Hill, Elizabeth L., and Uta Frith. "Understanding Autism: Insights from Mind and Brain." *Philosophical Transactions: Biological Sciences* 358, no. 1430 (2003): 281–289.
Howell, Whitney. "Learning and the Development of Meaning: Husserl and Merleau-Ponty on the Temporality of Perception and Habit." *The Southern Journal of Philosophy* 53, no. 3 (September 2015): 311–337.
Husserl, Edmund. *Analyses Concerning Active and Passive Synthesis: Lectures on Transcendental Logic*. Translated by A.J. Steinbock. Dordrecht, Boston, & London: Kluwer Academic, 2001.
Husserl, Edmund. "Husserl Archives." Manuscript D 13, XII and XIV. Leuven, 1910.
Husserl, Edmund. *The Crisis of European Sciences and Transcendental Phenomenology*. Translated by David Carr. Evanston, IL: Northwestern University Press, 1970.
Husserl, Edmund. *Die Lebenswelt. Auslegungen der vorgegebenen Welt und ihrer Konstitution. Texte aus dem Nachlass (1916–1937)*, Husserliana Band XXXIX. Dordrecht: Springer, 2008.
Husserl, Edmund. *Erfahrung und Urteil. Untersuchungen zur Genealogie der Logik*, edited by Ludwig Landgrebe. Hamburg: Meiner, 1948.
Husserl, Edmund. *Erste Philosophie. Zweiter Teil: Theorie der phänomenologischen Reduktion*, Husserliana Band VIII. The Hague: Martinus Nijhoff, 1959.
Husserl, Edmund. *Experience and Judgment: Investigations in a genealogy of logic*. Edited by Ludwig Landgrebe. Translated by James S. Churchill and Karl Ameriks. Evanston, IL: Northwestern University Press, 1973.
Husserl, Edmund. *Ideen zu einer reinen Phänomenologie und Phänomenologischen Philosophie. Zweites Buch: Phänomenologische Untersuchungen zur Konstitution*, Husserliana Band IV. The Hague: Martinus Nijhoff, 1952.

Husserl, Edmund. *Logical Investigations*. Translated by J.N. Findlay. London & New York: Routledge, 2001.
Husserl, Edmund. *Phänomenologische Psychologie. Vorlesungen Sommersemester 1925*, Husserliana Band IX. The Hague: Martinus Nijhoff, 1962.
Iezzoni, Lisa, and Bonnie O'Day. *More than Ramps: Improving the Accessibility and Quality of Health Care for People with Disabilities*. Oxford: Oxford University Press, 2011.
Iwakuma, Miho. "The Body as Embodiment: An Investigation of the Body by Merleau-Ponty." In *Disability/Postmodernity*, edited by Mairian Corker and Tom Shakespeare. New York: Continuum, 2002. 75–87.
Jaarsma, Ada S. *Kierkegaard after the Genome: Science, Existence, and Belief in This World*. Cham, Switzerland: Palgrave Macmillan, 2017.
Jackson, Gabrielle. "Maurice Merleau-Ponty's Concept of Motor Intentionality: Unifying Two Kinds of Bodily Agency." *European Journal of Philosophy* 26, no. 2 (2018): 763–779.
Jacobson, Kirsten. "A Developed Nature: A Phenomenological Account of the Experience of Home." *Continental Philosophy Review* 42 (2009): 355–373.
Jacobson, Kristen. "Neglecting Space: Making Sense of a Partial Loss of One's World through a Phenomenological Account of the Spatiality of Embodiment." In *Perception and Its Development in Merleau-Ponty's Phenomenology*, edited by Kirsten Jacobson and John Russon. Toronto: University of Toronto Press, 2017. 101–122.
Jacobson, Kirsten. "The Body as Family Narrative: Russon and the Education of the Soul." *Anekaant: A Journal of Polysemic Thought* 3 (2015): 49–57.
Janicaud, Dominique. "The Theological Turn of French Phenomenology." In *Phenomenology and the "Theological Turn": The French Debate*. Translated by Bernard G. Prusak. New York: Fordham University Press, 2000. 16–103.
Jensen, Rasmus. "Motor Intentionality and the case of Schneider." *Phenomenology and the Cognitive Sciences* 8 (2009): 371–388.
Johnson, Galen A. "The Invisible and the Unrepresentable: Barnett Newman's Abstract Expressionism and the Aesthetics of Merleau-Ponty." *Analecta Husserliana* 75 (2002): 179–189.
Jonas, Hans. "In Memoriam: Kurt Goldstein, 1878–1965." *Social Research* 32, no. 4 (1965): 351–356.
Jonas, Hans. "Kurt Goldstein and Philosophy." *American Journal of Psychoanalysis* 19 (1959): 161–164.
Jonathan, Metzl. *Dying of Whiteness: How the Politics of Racial Resentment Is Killing America's Heartland*. New York: Basic Books, 2019.
Kafer, Alison. *Feminist, Queer, Crip*. Bloomington: Indiana University Press, 2013.
Kafer, Alison. *My Ambivalent Adventures in Devoteeism*. Durham, NC: Duke University Press, 2012.

Karera, Axelle. "Blackness and the Pitfalls of Anthropocene Ethics." *Critical Philosophy of Race* 7, no. 1 (2019): 32–56.
Kearney, P.J. "Autopathography and Humane Medicine: *The Diving Bell and the Butterfly*—an Interpretation." *Medical Humanities* 32 (2006): 111–113.
Kelly, Michael. *Phenomenology and the Problem of Time*. New York: Palgrave MacMillan, 2016.
Kelly, Michael. "The Subject as Time: Merleau-Ponty's Transition from Phenomenology to Ontology." In *Time, Memory, Institution: Merleau-Ponty's New Ontology of the Self*, edited by David Morris and Kym Maclaren. Athens: Ohio University Press, 2015. 199–215.
Kittay, Eva Feder. *Love's Labor: Essays on Women, Equality, and Dependency*. New York: Routledge, 1999.
Kittay, Eva Feder. "The Ethics of Care, Dependence, and Disability." *Ratio Juris: An International Journal of Jurisprudence and Philosophy of Law* 24, no. 1 (2011): 49–58. https://doi.org/10/ffnrp2
Koopman, Colin. *How We Became Our Data: A Genealogy of the Informational Person*. University of Chicago Press, 2019.
Kyselo, Miriam, and Ezequiel Di Paolo. "Locked-in Syndrome: A Challenge for Embodied Cognitive Science." *Phenomenology and Cognitive Science* 14 (2015): 517–542
Kyselo, Miriam. "More Than Our Body: Minimal and Enactive Selfhood in Global Paralysis." *Neuroethics* (2019): 1–18. https://doi.org/10.1007/s12152-019-09404-9
Ladau, Emily. "Playing the Online Dating Game, in a Wheelchair." *The New York Times*. September 27, 2017. www.nytimes.com/2017/09/27/opinion/online-dating-disability.html?searchResultPosition=4
Laing, R.D. *The Divided Self*. New York: Penguin Books, 1990.
Lajoie, Corinne. "Being at Home: A Feminist Phenomenology of Disorientation in Illness." *Hypatia* 34, no. 3 (2019): 546–569.
Landes, Donald. *Merleau-Ponty and the Paradoxes of Expression*. London & New York: Continuum, 2013.
Langlois, Judith H., and Loria A. Roggman. "Attractive Faces Are Only Average" *Psychological Science* 1, no. 2 (1990): 115–121.
Larøi, Frank, Tanya Marie Luhrmann, Vaughan Bell, William A. Christian Jr., Smita Deshpande, Charles Fernyhough, Janis Jenkins, and Angela Woods. "Culture and Hallucinations: Overview and Future Directions." *Schizophrenia Bulletin* 40 (Suppl. 4) (July 2014): S213–S220. doi:10.1093/schbul/sbu012
Lashley, Karl. "Foreword." In Kurt Goldstein's *The Organism*. Boston: Back Bay Books, 1963. xii–xiii.
Lawlor, Leonard. *Thinking through French Philosophy: The Being of the Question*. Bloomington: Indiana University Press, 2003.

Leder, Drew. "A Tale of Two Bodies: The Cartesian Corpse and the Lived Body." In *The Body in Medical Thought and Practice*, edited by Drew Leder. Dordrecht: Kluwer Academic Publishers, 1992. 17–35.

Lee, Emily. "The Meaning of Visible Differences of the Body" *APA Newsletter Asian and Asian-American Philosophers and Philosophies* 2, no. 2 (2003): 633–638.

Lee, Emily. "Introduction." In *Living Alterities: Phenomenology, Embodiment, and Race*, edited by Emily Lee. Albany, NY: SUNY Press, 2014. 43–64.

Linton, Simi. *Claiming Disability: Knowledge and Identity*. New York: New York University Press, 1998.

Lugones, María. "Playfulness, 'World'-Traveling, and Loving Perception." In *Pilgrimages/Peregrinajes: Theorizing Coalition against Multiple Oppressions*. New York: Rowman & Littlefield, 2003. 77–100.

Lysaker, Paul Henry, Jason K. Johannesen, and John Timothy Lysaker. "Schizophrenia and the Experience of Intersubjectivity as Threat." *Phenomenology and the Cognitive Sciences* 4 (2005): 335–352.

Mallon, Thomas. "In the Blink of an Eye." *The New York Times*. June 15, 1997. www.nytimes.com/1997/06/15/books/in-the-blink-of-an-eye.html?mtrref=www.google.com&gwh=544F2E74E44F33E3C3AD24E37873F4C3&gwt=pay

Marion, Jean-Luc. *Reduction and Givenness: Investigations of Husserl, Heidegger and Phenomenology*. Translated by T.A. Carlson. Evanston, IL: Northwestern University Press, 1998.

Marotta, J.J., and M. Behrmann. "Patient Schn: Has Goldstein and Gelb's Case Withstood the Test of Time?" *Neuropsychologia* 42 (2004): 633–638.

Maslow, Abraham. "A Theory of Human Motivation." *Psychological Review* 50 (1943): 370–396.

Matthews, Eric. *Body-Subjects and Disordered Minds: Treating the "Whole" Person in Psychiatry*. New York: Oxford University Press, 2007.

May, Todd. "Foucault's Relation to Phenomenology." In *The Cambridge Companion to Foucault*, edited by Gary Gutting. Cambridge: Cambridge University Press, 2005. 284–311.

McRuer, Robert. *Crip Theory: Cultural Signs of Queerness and Disability*. Edited by Michael Bérubé. New York: New York University Press, 2006.

Merleau-Pony, Maurice. *Adventures of the Dialectic*. Translated by Joseph Bien. Evanston, IL: Northwestern University Press, 1973.

Merleau-Ponty, Maurice. "An Unpublished Text by Maurice Merleau-Ponty: A Prospectus of his Work." In *The Primacy of Perception*, edited by J.M. Edie. Translated by A.B. Dallery. Evanston, IL: Northwestern University Press, 1964. 3–11.

Merleau-Ponty, Maurice. "Eye and Mind." In *The Merleau-Ponty Aesthetics Reader: Philosophy and Painting*, edited by Galen A. Johnson. Evanston, IL: Northwestern University Press, 1993. 121–150.

Merleau-Ponty, Maurice. "Hegel's Existentialism." In *Sense and Non-Sense*. Translated by Hubert L. Dreyfus and Patricia Allen Dreyfus. Evanston, IL: Northwestern University Press, 1964. 63–70

Merleau-Ponty, Maurice. *L'institution/ la passivité: Notes de cours au Collège de France (1954–1955)*. Paris: Editions Belin, 2003.

Merleau-Ponty, Maurice. *Nature: Course notes from the College de France*. Edited by Dominique Seglard. Translated by Robert Vallier. Evanston, IL: Northwestern University Press, 2003.

Merleau-Ponty, Maurice. *La Nature. Notes. Cours Du Collège De France. Suivi De: Résumés De Cours Correspondants*. Paris: Le Seuil, 1968.

Merleau-Ponty, Maurice. *Phenomenology of Perception*. Translated by Colin Smith. London: Routledge and Kegan Paul, 1981.

Merleau-Ponty, Maurice. *Phenomenology of Perception*. Translated by Donald A. Landes. New York: Routledge, 2012.

Merleau-Ponty, Maurice. *The Structure of Behavior*. Translated by Alden Fischer. Boston: Beacon Press, 1942.

Merleau-Ponty, Maurice. "The Child's Relations with Others." Translated by William Cobb. In *The Primacy of Perception*, edited by James M. Edie. Evanston, IL: Northwestern University Press, 1964. 96–158.

Merleau-Ponty, Maurice. "Themes from the Lectures at the College de France, 1952–1960." In *In Praise of Philosophy and Other Essays*. Translated by John O'Neill. Evanston, IL: Northwestern University Press, 1988. 71–201.

Merleau-Ponty, Maurice. *The Visible and the Invisible*. Edited by Claude Lefort. Translated by Alphonso Lingis. Evanston, IL: Northwestern University Press, 1968.

Metzl, Jonathan. *Dying of Whiteness: How the Politics of Racial Resentment Is Killing America's Heartland*. New York: Basic Books, 2019.

Miéville, China. *The City & the City*. New York: Random House, 2010.

Miller, David T., Margaret P. Adam, Swaroop Aradhya, Leslie G. Biesecker, Arthur R. Brothman, Nigel P. Carter, Deanna M. Church, John A. Crolla, Evan E. Eichler, Charles J. Epstein, W. Andrew Faucett, Lars Feuk, Jan M. Friedman, Ada Hamosh, Laird Jackson, Erin B. Kaminsky, Klaas Kok, Ian D. Krantz, Robert M. Kuhn, Charles Lee, James M. Ostell, Carla Rosenberg, Stephen W. Scherer, Nancy B. Spinner, Dimitri J. Stavropoulos, James H. Tepperberg, Erik C. Thorland, Joris R. Vermeesch, Darrel J. Waggoner, Michael S. Watson, Christa Lese Martin, and David H. Ledbetter. "Consensus Statement: Chromosomal Microarray Is a First-Tier Clinical Diagnostic Test for Individuals with Developmental Disabilities or Congenital Anomalies." *American Journal of Human Genetics* 86, no. 5 (2010): 749–764. https://doi.org/10/ckmnsx

Mitchell, David T., and Sharon L. Snyder. *Biopolitics of Disability: Neoliberalism, Ablenationalism, and Peripheral Embodiment*. Edited by Sharon L. Snyder. Ann Arbor: University of Michigan Press, 2015.

Mollow, Anna, and Robert McRuer *Sex and Disability*. New York: Routledge, 2012
Moore, Jason W. *Anthropocene and Capitalocene? Nature, History, and the Crisis of Capitalism*. Oakland, CA: PM Press/Kairos, 2016.
Morris, David. *Merleau-Ponty's Developmental Ontology*. Evanston, IL: Northwestern University Press, 2018.
Morris, David. "The Chirality of Being: Exploring a Merleau-Pontian Ontology of Sense." *Chiasmi International* 12 (2011): 165–182.
Morris, David. "The Enigma of Reversibility and the Genesis of Sense in Merleau-Ponty." *Continental Philosophy Review* 43, no. 2 (May 2010): 141–165. https://doi.org/10.1007/s11007-010-9144-7
Morris, David. *The Sense of Space*. Albany, NY: SUNY Press, 2013.
Morris, Katherine J. *Starting with Merleau-Ponty*. London & New York: Continuum Books, 2012.
Muhle, Maria. "From the Vital to the Social: Canguilhem and Foucualt—Reflections on Vital and Social Norms." *Republics of Letters: A Journal for the Study of Knowledge, Politics, and the Arts* 3, no. 2 (2014): 1–12.
Murphy, Robert F. *The Body Silent*. New York & London: W. W. Norton, 1990.
Nancy, Jean-Luc. *Listening*. Translated by Charlotte Mendell. New York: Fordham University Press, 2007.
Neuhaus, Carolyn. "Does Solidarity Require 'All of Us' to Participate in Genomics Research?" *The Hastings Center Report* 50 (2020).
Nizzi, Marie-Christine. Veronique Blandin, and Athena Demertzi. "Attitudes towards Personhood in the Locked-in Syndrome: From Third- to First-Person Perspective and to Interpersonal Significance." *Neuroethics* 8 (2018): 1–9. https://doi.org/10.1007/s12152-018-9375-6
Nizzi, Marie-Christine, Athena Demertzi, Olivia Gosseries, Marie-Aurélie Bruno, François Jouen, and Steven Laureys. "From Armchair to Wheelchair: How Patients with a Locked-in Syndrome Integrate Bodily Changes in Experienced Identity." *Consciousness and Cognition* 21 (2012): 431–437.
Ngo, Helen. "Racist Habits: A Phenomenological Analysis of Racism and the Habitual Body." *Philosophy and Social Criticism* 42, no. 9 (2016): 847–872.
Ochs, Elinor, Tamar Kremer-Sadlik, Karen Gainer Sirota, and Olga Solomon. "Autism and the Social World: An Anthropological Perspective." *Discourse Studies* 6, no. 2 (2004), 147–183.
Oliver, Michael. *The Politics of Disablement: A Sociological Approach*. London: Macmillan, 1990.
Ordover, Nancy. *American Eugenics: Race, Queer Anatomy, and the Science of Nationalism*. Minneapolis: University of Minnesota Press, 2003.
Ostrum, Andrea E. "Brain Injury: A Personal View." *Journal of Clinical and Experimental Neuropsychology* 15, no. 4 (1993): 623–624.
Ostrum, Andrea E. "The 'Locked-in' Syndrome—Comments from a Survivor." *Brain Injury* 8, no. 1 (1994): 95–98.

Parens, Erik, and Paul S. Appelbaum. "On What We Have Learned and Still Need to Learn about the Psychosocial Impacts of Genetic Testing." *Hastings Center Report* 49, no. S1 (2019).

Parens, Erik. *Shaping Our Selves: On Technology, Flourishing, and a Habit of Thinking.* Oxford & New York: Oxford University Press, 2015.

Petrova, Mila, Jeremy Dale, and Bill Fulford. "Values-Based Practice in Primary Care: Easing the Tensions between Individual Values, Ethical Principles and Best Evidence." *British Journal of General Practice* 7 (2006): 703–709.

Phillips, Louise. *Mental Illness and the Body: Beyond Diagnosis.* New York: Routledge, 2006.

Plato, *Theatetus*, in *The Dialogues of Plato*, 4th ed., vol. 3. Translated by B. Jowett. Oxford: Clarendon Press, 1953.

Pohlhaus, Gaile. "Relational Knowing and Epistemic Injustice: Toward a Theory of Willful Hermeneutical Ignorance." *Hypatia* 27, no. 4 (2012): 715–735.

Porter, Theodore M. *The Rise of Statistical Thinking, 1820–1900.* Princeton, NJ: Princeton University Press, 1986.

Posner, Jerome B., Clifford B. Saper, Nicholas D. Schiff, and Fred Plum. *Plum and Posner's Diagnosis of Stupor and Coma*, 4th edition. Oxford & New York: Oxford University Press, 2007.

Pulkinnen, Simo. "Lifeworld as an Embodiment of Spiritual Meaning: The Constitutive Dynamics of Activity and Passivity in Husserl." In *The Phenomenology of Embodied Subjectivity*. Contributions to Phenomenology 71. Edited by R.T. Jensen and Dermot Moran. Cham: Springer, 2013. 121–141.

Raffoul, Francois. "Phenomenology of the Inapparent." In *Unconsciousness between Phenomenology and Psychoanalysis*. Contributions to Phenomenology. In Cooperation with the Center for Advanced Research in Phenomenology, 88. Edited by Dorothée Legrand and Dylan Trigg. Cham: Springer, 2017. 113–131.

Ramey, Joshua Alan. *Politics of Divination: Neoliberal Endgame and Religion of Contingency.* London: Rowman & Littlefield International, 2016.

Redlener, Irwin, Jeffrey D. Sachs, Sean Hansen, and Nathaniel Hupert. "130,000–210,000 Avoidable COVID-19 Deaths and Counting in the U.S." October 21, 2020. https://ncdp.columbia.edu/custom-content/uploads/2020/10/Avoidable-COVID-19-Deaths-US-NCDP.pdf

Reeve, Christopher. *Still Me.* London: Century, 1998.

Revel, Judith. *Foucault avec Merleau-Ponty.* Paris: Vrin, 2015.

Reynolds, Joel Michael, and David Peña-Guzmán. "The Harm of Ableism: Medical Error and Epistemic Injustice." *Kennedy Institute of Ethics Journal* 29, no. 3 (2019): 205–242.

Reynolds, Joel Michael. "The Healtholocene." *Syndicate.* November 12, 2018. https://syndicate.network/symposia/ philosophy/kierkegaard-after-the-genome

Reynolds, Joel Michael. "How Biomedical Technologies Harm Patients as Knowers." *Southern Journal of Philosophy* 58, no. 1 (2020): 161–185.
Reynolds, Joel Michael. "The Normate." In *50 Concepts for a Critical Phenomenology*, edited by Gail Weiss, Ann Murphy, and Gayle Salamon. Evanston, IL: Northwestern University Press, 2019. 243–248.
Riese, Walther. "Kurt Goldstein—The Man and His Work." In *The Reach of Mind*, edited by Marianne Simmel. New York: Springer, 1968. 17–30.
Robillard, Albert. Albert Robillard, *Meaning of a Disability: The Lived Experience of Paralysis*. Philadelphia: Temple University Press, 1999.
Rodriguez, Michael A., and Robert Garcia. "First, Do No Harm: The US Sexually Transmitted Disease Experiments in Guatemala." *American Journal of Public Health* 103, no. 12 (October 17, 2013): 2122–2126. https://doi.org/10/gf9gdr
Rusert, Britt. "'A Study In Nature': The Tuskegee Experiments and The New South Plantation." *Journal of Medical Humanities* 30, no. 3 (2009): 155–171. https://doi.org/10/b6qhkp
Russon, John. *Bearing Witness to Epiphany*. Albany, NY: SUNY Press, 2009.
Russon, John. *Human Experience*. Albany, NY: SUNY Press, 2003.
Russon, John. *Sites of Exposure*, Albany, NY: SUNY Press, 2017.
Sabot, Philippe. "Entre psychologie et philosophie. Foucault à Lille, 1952–1955." In *Foucault à Münsterlingen. À l'origine de l'Histoire de la folie*, edited by Jean-Françoise Bert and Elisabetta Basso. Paris: EHESS, 2015. 110.
Sacks, Oliver. "Foreword." In Kurt Goldstein's *The Organism*. Cambridge: MIT Press, 1995. 7–14.
Salamon, Gayle. "The Phenomenology of Rheumatology: Disability, Merleau-Ponty, and the Fallacy of Maximal Grip" *Hypatia* 27, no. 2 (2012): 243–260.
Sarrett, Jennifer C. "Custodial Homes, Therapeutic Homes, and Parental Acceptance: Parental Experiences of Autism in Kerala, India and Atlanta, GA USA." *Culture, Medicine and Psychiatry* 39, no. 2 (2015): 254–276.
Sartre, Jean-Paul. *Being and Nothingness*. Translated by Hazel E. Barnes. New York: Washington Square Press, 1992.
Sass, Louis A., Jennifer Whiting, and Josef Parnas. "Mind, Self and Psychopathology: Reflections on Philosophy, Theory and the Study of Mental Illness." *Theory & Psychology* 10, no. 1 (2000): 87–98.
Schreyach, Michael. "Pre-objective Depth in Merleau-Ponty and Jackson Pollock." *Research in Phenomenology* 43, 1 (2013): 49–70. doi: https://doi-org.proxy.library.stonybrook.edu/10.1163/15691640-12341243
Schirato, Tony, Geoff Danaher, and Jen Webb. *Understanding Foucault: A Critical Introduction*, 2nd edition. London: Sage Publications, 2012.
Scully, Jackie Leach. *Disability Bioethics: Moral Bodies, Moral Differences*. Lanham, MD: Rowman & Littlefield, 2008.

Scully, Jackie Leach. "What Is a Disease? Disease, Disability and their Definitions." *EMBO Reports* 5, no. 7 (2004): 650–653.

Scuro, Jennifer. "The Ableist Affections of a Neoliberal Politics." *APA Newsletter on Philosophy and Medicine* 16, no. 1 (2016): 50–56.

Shabot, Sara C., and Christina Landry. *Rethinking Feminist Phenomenology*. Durham, NC: Duke University Press, 2018.

Shakespeare, Thomas. *Disability Rights and Wrongs Revisited*. New York: Routledge, 2013.

Shakespeare, Thomas. "Review of Oliver Sacks' *An Anthropologist on Mars*." *Disability & Society* 11 (1996): 137–139.

Shakow, David. "Kurt Goldstein: 1878–1965." *American Journal of Psychology* 79, no. 1 (1966): 150–154.

Sheets-Johnstone, Maxine. "Emotion and Movement: A Beginning Empirical-Phenomenological Analysis of Their Relationship." *Journal of Consciousness Studies* 6, no. 11–12 (1999): 259–277.

Sheets-Johnstone, Maxine. "Moving in Concert." *Choros International Dance Journal* 6 (Spring 2017): 1–19.

Sheets-Johnstone, Maxine. *Phenomenology of Dance*, 50th anniversary edition. Philadelphia: Temple University Press, 2015.

Shildrick, Margrit. *Dangerous Discourses of Disability, Subjectivity and Sexuality*. New York: Palgrave McMillan, 2009.

Siebers, Tobin. *Disability Aesthetics*. Ann Arbor: University of Michigan Press, 2010.

Silverman, Chloe. "Fieldwork on Another Planet: Social Science Perspectives on the Autism Spectrum." *BioSocieties* no. 3 (2008): 325–341.

Simmel, Marianne. "Foreword" to *The Reach of Mind*, edited by Marianne Simmel. New York: Springer, 1968. v–x.

Simmel, Marianne. "Kurt Goldstein 1878–1965." In *The Reach of Mind*, edited by Marianne Simmel. New York: Springer, 1968. 3–12.

Slatman, Jenny. "Multiple Dimensions of Embodiment in Medical Practices." *Medicine, Health Care and Philosophy* 17, no. 4 (2014): 549–557.

Smith, Jane Case, Lindy L., Weaver, and Mary A. Fristad. "A Systematic Review of Sensory Processing Interventions for Children with Autism Spectrum Disorders." *Autism: The International Journal of Research and Practice* 19, no. 2 (2015): 133–158.

Solmon, Olga. "Sense and the Senses: Anthropology and the Study of Autism." *Annual Review of Anthropology* 39 (2010): 241–259.

Soylu, Tulay G., Eman Elashkar, Fatemah Aloudah, Munir Ahmed, and Panagiota Kitsantas "Racial/Ethnic Differences in Health Insurance Adequacy and Consistency among children: Evidence from the 2011/12 National Survey of Children's Health." *Journal of Public Health Research* 7, no. 1280 (2018): 56–62.

Stahnisch, Frank, and Thomas Hoffman. "Kurt Goldstein and the Neurology of Movement during the Interwar Years." In *Was Bewegt Uns?*, edited by

Christian Hoffstadt, Andreas Schulz-Buchta, and Franz Peschke. Freiburg: Verlag, 2010. 283–312.

Steinbock, Anthony. "Phenomenological Concepts of Normality and Abnormality." *Man and World* 28, no. 3 (1995): 241–260.

Sterling, Robyn L. "Genetic Research among the Havasupai—a Cautionary Tale." *The Virtual Mentor* 13, no. 2 (2011): 113–17. https://doi.org/10/gf9gdv

Strominger, Mitchell B. "Morning Glory Syndrome." *American Academy of Ophthalmology*. November 9, 2017. www.aao.org/disease-review/neuro-ophthalmology-morning-glory-syndrome

Stump, Jessica L. "Henrietta Lacks and The HeLa Cell: Rights of Patients and Responsibilities of Medical Researchers." *The History Teacher* 48, no. 1 (2014): 127–180.

Sullivan, Shannon. "Ontological Expansiveness." In *50 Concepts for a Critical Phenomenology*, edited by Gail Weiss, Ann Murphy, and Gayle Salamon. Evanston, IL: Northwestern University Press, 2019. 249–254.

Sullivan, Shannon. *Revealing Whiteness: The Unconscious Habits of Racial Privilege*. Bloomington: Indiana University Press, 2006.

Taipale, Joona. "Twofold Normality: Husserl and the Normative Relevance of Primordial Constitution." *Husserl Studies* 28, no. 1 (2012): 49–60.

Talero, Maria. "Perception, Normativity, and Selfhood in Merleau-Ponty: The Spatial 'Level' and Existential Space." *The Southern Journal of Philosophy* 43, no. 3 (2005): 443–461. https://doi.org/10.1111/j.2041-6962.2005.tb01962.x

Teuber, Hans. "Kurt Goldstein's Role in the Development of Neuropsychology." *Neuropsychologia* 4, no. 4 (1966): 299–310.

Thapar, Anita, and Miriam Cooper. "Copy Number Variation: What Is It and What Has It Told Us about Child Psychiatric Disorders?" *Journal of the American Academy of Child and Adolescent Psychiatry* 52, no. 8 (August 2013): 772–774. https://doi.org/10/f2xj89

Tremain, Shelley. *Foucault and Feminist Philosophy of Disability*. Ann Arbor: University of Michigan Press, 2017.

Twaddle, Andrew C. "Illness and Deviance." *Social Science & Medicine (1967)* 7, no. 10 (1973): 751–762.

Ulrich, Robert. "Personal Impressions of Kurt Goldstein." In *The Reach of Mind*, edited by Marianne Simmel. New York: Springer, 1968. 13–16.

Venable, Hannah Lyn. "At the Opening of Madness: An Exploration of the Nonrational with Merleau-Ponty, Foucault, and Kierkegaard." *Journal of Speculative Philosophy* 33, no. 3 (2019): 475–488.

Vidal, Fernando. "Phenomenology of the Locked-in Syndrome: An Overview and Some Suggestions." *Neuroethics* (2018): 1–25. https://doi.org/10.1007/s12152-018-9388-1

Waldenfels, Bernhard. "Normalité et normativité." *Revue de métaphysique et de morale* 45, no. 1 (2005): 57–67.

Walker, Nick. "Neurodiversity: Some Basic Terms & Definitions." Neurocosmopolitanism [blog]. September 27, 2014. http://neurocosmopolitanism.com/neurodiversity-some-basic-terms-definitions

Washington, Harriet A. *Medical Apartheid: The Dark History of Medical Experimentation on Black Americans from Colonial Times to the Present.* New York: Anchor Books, 2008.

Wehrle, Maren. "'There Is a Crack in Everything.' Fragile Normality: Husserl's Account of Normality Re-Visited." *Phaenomenon* 28 (2019): 49–75.

Weil, Simone. "Reflections on the Right Use of School Studies with a View to the Love of God." In *Waiting for God.* Translated by Emma Craufurd. New York: Harper Perennial Modern Classics, 2009. 57–65.

Weiss, Gail. *Body Images: Embodiment as Intercorporeality.* New York & London: Routledge, 1999.

Weiss, Gail. "The 'Normal Abnormalities' of Disability and Aging: Merleau-Ponty and Beauvoir." In *Feminist Phenomenology Futures*, edited by Helen Fielding and Dorothea Olkowski. Bloomington: Indiana University Press, 2017. 203–217.

Weiss, Gail. "The Normal, the Natural, and the Normative: A Merleau-Pontian Legacy to Feminist Theory, Critical Race Theory, and Disability Studies." *Continental Philosophy Review* 48 (2015): 77–93.

Welsh, Talia. "Many Healths: Nietzsche and Phenomenologies of Illness." *Frontiers of Philosophy in China* 11, no. 3 (2016): 338–357.

Welsh, Talia. *The Child as Natural Phenomenologist.* Evanston, IL: Northwestern University Press, 2013. ix–xix.

Welsh, Talia. "Translator's Introduction." In Maurice Merleau-Ponty, *Child Psychology and Pedagogy: The Sorbonne Lectures 1949–1952.* Translated by Talia Welsh. Evanston, IL: Northwestern University Press, 2010.

Werner-Lin, Allison, Sarah Walser, Frances K. Barg, and Barbara A. Bernhardt. "'They Can't Find Anything Wrong With Him, Yet': Mothers' Experiences of Parenting an Infant with a Prenatally Diagnosed Copy Number Variant (CNV)." *American Journal of Medical Genetics* 173, no. 2 (2016): 444–451. https://doi.org/10/f9ptcp

"What Is Huntington's Disease?" Huntington's Disease Society of America. http://hdsa.org/what-is-hd

Wieseler, Christine. "Challenging Conceptions of the 'Normal' Subject of Phenomenology." In *Race as Phenomena: Between Phenomenology and Philosophy of Race*, edited by Emily Lee. Lanham, MD: Rowman & Littlefield, 2019. 69–85.

Wilkerson, Abby. "Normate Sex and Its Discontents." In *Sex and Disability*, edited by Anna Mollow and Robert McRuer. Durham, NC: Duke University Press, 2012. 183–207.

Wiskus, Jessica. *The Rhythm of Thought: Art, Literature, and Music After Merleau-Ponty.* Chicago: University of Chicago Press, 2013.
Woerkom, Willem van. "Sur La Notion de l'espace (Le Sense Géométrique), Sur La Notion Du Temps et Du Nombre." *Revue Neurologique* 35 (1919): 113–119.
Wolfe, Julia. "Stronghold." The Hartt School, 2008. https://juliawolfemusic.com/music/stronghold
Yancy, George. *Black Bodies, White Gazes: The Continuing Significance of Race in America.* 2nd edition. Lanham, MD: Rowman & Littlefield, 2017
Yancy, George. "White Gazes: What It Feels Like to Be an Essence." In *Living Alterities: Phenomenology, Embodiment, and Race*, edited by Emily Lee. Albany, NY: SUNY Press, 2014. 43–64.
Yoshinda, Karen, Fran Odette, Susan Hardie, Heather Willis, and Mary Bunch. "Women Living with Disabilities and Their Experiences and Issues Related to the Context and Complexities of Leaving Abusive Situations." *Disability and Rehabilitation* 31, no. 22 (2009): 1843–1852.
Young, Iris Marion. *"Throwing Like a Girl" and Other Essays.* Oxford: Oxford University Press, 2005.
Young, Stella. "I'm Not Your Inspiration." www.ted.com/talks/stella_young_i_m_not_your_inspiration_thank_you_very_much?language=en
Zahavi, Dan. "Locked-In Syndrome: A Challenge to Standard Accounts of Selfhood and Personhood?" *Neuroethics* 4 (2019): 1–8. https://doi.org/10.1007/s12152-019-09405-8
Zahavi, Dan. "Merleau-Ponty on Husserl." In *Merleau-Ponty's Reading of Husserl*, edited by Ted Toadvine and Lester Embree. Boston: Springer, 2002. 3–29.
Zaner, Richard M. "Sisyphus without Knees: Exploring Self–Other Relationships through Illness and Disability." *Literature and Medicine* 22, no. 2 (2003): 188–207.
Zola, Émile. *Thérèse Raquin.* Translated by Andrew Rothwell. Oxford: Oxford University Press, 1992.

Notes on Contributors

Adam Blair is a doctoral student in philosophy at SUNY Stony Brook. His research currently centers around the structure of creativity and how to motivate *creative spectatorship*. His interests include the descriptive practice of phenomenology, art education (especially in the pedagogies of Josef Albers, Black Mountain College, and the Bauhaus), jazz performance and composition, and synesthetic perception. He has published and presented work on Merleau-Ponty's concepts of generality and indeterminacy, the emplaced poetics of Bachelard and Proust, disability and universal design in museum curation, the phenomenology of humor, and the working process of Joan Mitchell. He seeks to practice phenomenology and creativity just as much as he theorizes about them through photography, descriptive poetry, jazz piano, drawing, and cross-sensory experimentation with other artists and thinkers. AdamBlair.me

Jennifer E. Bradley is a PhD Candidate in Clinical Psychology at Duquesne University, Pittsburgh, PA. and is currently completing her doctoral residency at the Centre for Interpersonal Relationships in Ottawa, Canada where she practices psychotherapy with individuals across the lifespan. After graduating with honors from the University of Prince Edward Island in 2012 with a Bachelor of Arts in Psychology, Jennifer worked as an educational assistant and an intensive behavioral intervention tutor for two years. This work experience inspired her to pursue a PhD in Clinical Psychology with a clinical and research interest working with children with exceptional needs and their families.

Susan Bredlau is Affiliated Faculty in the Philosophy Department at the University of Maine. Her work is grounded in the phenomenological tradition and focuses on the critical role of other people within our lived experience. She is the author of *The Other in Perception: A Phenomenological Account of Our Experience of Other Persons* (SUNY Press, 2018) and has published articles in *Continental Philosophy of Review*, *Medical Humanities*, and *Phenomenology and the Cognitive Sciences*.

Neal DeRoo is Canada Research Chair in Phenomenology and Philosophy of Religion and Professor of Philosophy at The King's University (Edmonton, Canada). He is the author of *Futurity in Phenomenology: Promise and Method in Husserl Levinas and Derrida* (Fordham UP, 2013) and has co-edited several books, including *Merleau-Ponty at the Limits of Art, Religion and Perception* (Continuum, 2010). He has just finished writing a book *The Political Logic of Experience: On Expression in Phenomenology*.

Whitney Howell is Associate Professor of Philosophy at La Salle University in Philadelphia. Her research draws on the phenomenological tradition to consider how environments facilitate the development of bodily and moral capacities. Her recent work has focused urban environments and the distinctive material and social resources they offer their inhabitants.

Gabrielle Jackson is a Visiting Assistant Professor at Stanford University, and formerly Assistant Professor at SUNY Stony Brook. She works in the areas of phenomenology, philosophy of mind, and feminist philosophy. Her research concerns the relationship between mind and body, specifically how our mental capacities are shaped by our motor abilities. Her articles have appeared in *Phenomenology and the Cognitive Sciences*, *European Journal of Philosophy*, and *British Journal for the History of Philosophy*, and she is finishing a book manuscript that addresses the question of what lesion studies tell us about normal life entitled *What Can We Learn about the Normal from the Pathological?*

James Rakoczi is a researcher and writer affiliated with the Centre for the Humanities and Health at King's College London. He earned his doctorate in 2020 for a thesis on Merleau-Ponty and contemporary literatures of the brain and nervous system. He has published and presented on topics such as the poetry of neuropathic pain, disability activism, epilepsy in colonial imaginaries, and the politics of narcolepsy. His current book project, *The Making of Disorder: Neural Politics and Critical Therapeutics in Contemporary Illness Life Writing*, addresses the significance of compositional difficulty in neurological memoir.

Joel Michael Reynolds is an Assistant Professor of Philosophy and Disability Studies at Georgetown University, Senior Research Scholar in the Kennedy Institute of Ethics, Senior Advisor to The Hastings Center, and core faculty in Georgetown's Disability Studies Program. He is also the founder of *The Journal of Philosophy of Disability*, which he edits with Teresa Blankmeyer Burke. He is the author or co-author of over thirty peer-reviewed articles and chapters as well as the books *The Life Worth Living: Disability, Pain, and the History of Morality* (forthcoming with The University of Minnesota Press), *The Meaning of Disability* (under contract with Oxford University Press), *Philosophy of Disability: An Introduction* (under contract with Polity), and *The Disability Bioethics Reader* (forthcoming with Routledge and co-edited with Christine Wieseler).

Jenny Slatman is Professor of Medical Humanities in the department of Culture Studies at Tilburg University, the Netherlands. She has published widely on issues of embodiment in art, expression and contemporary medical practices. Her publications include a book-length philosophical study on the meaning of expression in the work of Merleau-Ponty: *L'expression au-delà de la représentation. Sur l'aisthêsis et l'esthétique chez Merleau-Ponty* (Paris, 2003), and the monograph *Our Strange Body: Philosophical Reflections on Identity and Medical Interventions* (Amsterdam-Chicago, 2014). In 2017 Slatman was awarded a 1.5 million euro grant from the Dutch Research Council (NWO) for her research project *Mind the Body: Rethinking embodiment in healthcare* (2017–2022). www.jennyslatman.nl; www.mindthebody.eu

Hannah Lyn Venable works in ethics and continental philosophy, especially existentialism, phenomenology and post-structuralism. Her publications include an upcoming book, *Madness in Experience and History: Merleau-Ponty's Phenomenology and Foucault's Archaeology*, and articles in the *Journal of Speculative Philosophy* and *Philosophy & Theology*. She has taught at the University of Dallas, Texas State University and Trinity University and is currently a Visiting Scholar at Texas State University.

Talia Welsh is a UC Foundation Professor of Philosophy and Women, Gender, and Sexuality Studies at the University of Tennessee at Chattanooga. She researches Maurice Merleau-Ponty's work in child psychology and philosophy and has published extensively in feminist theory, particularly on parenting, pregnancy, and how bodies are normalized in health care. Her books include the translation of Merleau-Ponty's lectures in child psychology and pedagogy in the volume *Child Psychology & Pedagogy: Maurice Merleau-Ponty at the Sorbonne* (Northwestern University Press, 2010) and the monograph on Merleau-Ponty entitled *The Child as Natural Phenomenologist: Primal and Primary Experience in Merleau-Ponty's Psychology* (Northwestern University Press, 2013). Her current book is *Feminist Existentialism, and Biopolitics, and Critical Phenomenology in a Time of Bad Health* (Routledge, 2022).

Christine Wieseler is Assistant Professor in the Department of Philosophy at California State Polytechnic University, Pomona. She is an advisory board member for Philosophy in a Key Summer Institute (PIKSI) and associate editor for *The Journal of Philosophy of Disability*. Her areas of specialization are biomedical ethics, feminist philosophy, and philosophy of disability. She has published numerous articles at the intersection of these areas as well as phenomenology in journals including *Hypatia*, *IJFAB: International Journal of Feminist Approaches to Bioethics*, *American Association of Philosophy Teachers Studies in Pedagogy*, and *Social Philosophy Today*. She is co-editing *The Disability Bioethics Reader* (under contract with Routledge) with Joel Michael Reynolds. www.christinewieseler.com

Index

ability, 7, 10, 53, 87, 92, 121–122, 172–173, 177; to choose, 84, 86, 92; linguistic, 177; loss of, 4; normal, 50, 81; in relation to disability, 8, 42, 215, 217–218, 226, 229–230, 237, 240–241. *See also* disability

abnormal/abnormality, 2–3, 5–6, 8–13, 39n38, 48, 72, 91, 97–100, 103–111, 111n7, 113n30, 120–121, 141–142, 153, 155, 158, 209, 216; behavior, 105–106; embodiment, 31–37; as equated with illness or injury, 19–21, 26–31, 48, 59n16; individual, 101, 106; perception/vision, 124, 129–130; phenomenology, 34–35, 72; physiological, 90

adaptation, 25, 43, 52–53, 151, 181, 218

Ahmed, Sara, 11, 35–36, 156–158

Alper, Meryl, 187, 188

ambiguity, 12, 66, 87, 89, 120–121, 131, 133, 174, 176, 204, 225–226, 228; in relation to ambivalence, 89; as temporal, 229–230, 240–241

anatomy, 23, 27–28, 129–130

anosognosia, 52, 166, 173–175

aphasia, 41, 47; motor, 136; as paraphasia, 12

apraxia, 41, 56, 180

atmosphere, 122, 129, 136n6, 151

Autism Spectrum Disorder, 11–12, 187–196, 208; as neurodiversity/neurodivergence, 188–189, 199–200; as social and cultural phenomenon, 199–200

average, 21, 29–30, 32–37, 59n16, 133, 203, 247n84

Barbaras, Renaud, 64
Bartky, Sandra, 228
Bartlett, Jennifer, 235
Bauby, Jean-Dominique, 166, 171–178, 181

behavior, 1–2, 7, 10, 41–42, 45–46, 50–51, 53–56, 57n2, 57n4, 58n11, 59n14, 60n19, 63, 80–83, 87–90, 93–94, 96n65, 106–110, 114n46, 163, 167, 180, 185, 190, 192, 196–200, 202n21, 206, 251; as abnormal/disordered, 3, 12, 25, 35, 50, 105–107, 110; clinical assessment of, 47–48, 199; as compulsive, 92; modification of, 84–86, 199–200; as preferred, 25,

273

behavior *(continued)*
  52; as repetitive, 188–190; sexual, 230; stimming, 192, 195
Behrmann, Marlene, 4
being-in-the-world, 5–6, 121, 134, 213
Bichat, Xavier, 27
blindness, 8, 22; mind, 52; psychic, 229
blood pressure, 19–20, 27, 29, 36
body, in action, 195; as dialectic, 19; lived, 29, 36–37, 167, 174, 193; as object, 5–6, 29, 36; as physiological/physical, 5, 20, 25, 28, 37, 193–194; as subject, 5–6, 29, 36; as thing, 31, 129–130, 195, 197–198, 232
body schema, 3, 8, 35, 131, 179, 209
brain, 190, 192, 211; injury, 2–6, 22, 25, 41–45, 48–52, 54, 166, 169, 173, 229
Broussais, François-Joseph-Victor, 28–29, 37
Butler, Judith, 7

Cahill, Ann, 266, 231–234, 236, 238–239, 242
Canguilhem, Georges, 21, 24–31, 35–37, 59n16
Cartesian, 103, 122, 179
catastrophic reaction, 25, 35, 45, 51, 52
Clare, Eli, 234–235, 238
Comte, August, 28–29
control, 12, 23, 41, 81, 127, 133, 135, 192, 196, 205, 208, 213–217, 223n30; self-control, 80, 85
critical phenomenology, 120, 217, 227–228

Davis, Kathy, 34
debility, 42, 50, 51–52

derivatization, 231, 233, 235–236, 238
Descartes, 24, 130
determinacy/indeterminacy, 11, 120, 121, 125, 127–136
devoteeism, 235–238
diagnosis, 10, 20, 195, 262; misdiagnosis, 165
dialectic, 66, 99–101, 104, 193
Diedrich, Lisa, 172, 175–176
Dillon, M.C., 105
disability, 8–9, 20, 59n16, 169, 171, 184n56, 208, 217, 225–226, 228, 230, 234–237, 242n2–3, 243n6, 244n13, 245n35, 246n41; philosophy of, 227. *See also* ability, relation to disability
disease, 4, 8, 20–21, 25–29, 36, 44, 48–50, 52n2, 54, 57, 58n6, 179, 208, 211, 216–217, 244n13
disorientation, 156–157
dissociation, 82–83; double, 54, 62n43
dream, 121–123, 126–127, 129–131, 133–136, 172
dysfunction, 51–52, 114n46, 189, 191–192

eidetic, 22, 75n20
emotion, 10, 42, 80–87, 89–90, 93–94, 109, 161n38, 187, 197, 233
empiricism, 5–6, 73, 90–92
evolution, 100, 204, 207, 209, 213, 219

Fanon, Frantz, 35–36, 181
Farah, Martha, 3
figure-ground 194, 119–120, 124–127, 128, 129–131, 133, 135–136, 137n9, 138n44, 191, 195
first-person perspective, 20, 26–27, 29–31, 37, 62n52
flesh, 13, 104, 107, 110, 114n47, 137n8, 177, 205, 209–214, 218–220; as ontology, 70, 135

Foucault, Michel, 10, 27, 39n46, 59n16, 114n47, 97–115, 206
Frenkel-Brunswik, Else, 87–90
Frye, Marilyn, 238
function/functional, 192, 196, 198–199, 229; basic, 53–56, 62n42; as bodily, 4–5, 24, 42, 44, 103, 121, 128, 143, 180; normal, 5, 20, 22, 47–50, 58, 58, 197; normative, 32, 205, 218; pathological 58n11, 168, 190, 227; primordial, 92, 106

Galton, Francis, 32, 34
Gauss, Carl Friedrich, 32–33
Gelb, Adhémar, 3–5, 14n4, 22, 44–46, 54, 60n19, 61n39, 229
gender, 7–9, 13, 161, 217, 226, 237
genetics/genomics, 206–208, 212–213, 222n30
genome sequencing tests, 12–13, 211
Gestalt, 15n9, 61n32, 194; psychology, 53, 57n4, 124, 127, 193
Goldenberg, Georg, 3, 14n4
Goldstein, Kurt, 2–5, 9, 10, 14n4, 21–37, 43–57, 57n4, 58n5–10, 59n13–16, 60n19–20, 61n25
Grandin, Temple, 190
Guenther, Lisa, 227, 228

habit, 10, 25, 57, 82–84, 86, 90, 92–94, 122–123, 130, 133–135, 136n4, 149, 160n18, 160n20, 162n45, 164n56, 175, 194, 229
habitual/actual body distinction, 175, 181
Hacking, Ian, 21, 28, 31–34, 39n46
hallucination, 6–7, 10, 79–80, 90–94, 104–106, 108–110, 114n44
heterogeneity/homogeneity, 122, 125–126
holism, 45, 49
homeostatic resources, 170

homesickness, 104–105
homo curare, 13, 205, 209–212, 214–216, 218, 220, 222n27
homo faber, 12–13, 205, 207–209, 211–212, 214–220, 221n12, 222n27
horizons, 120, 127, 135, 138n44, 174, 210
hunchback, 30, 35–36
Husserl, Edmund, 10, 22, 59n12, 63–68, 70–71, 73, 74n14, 74n16, 75n19–22, 76n32, 78n54, 129, 160n18

illness/injury, 2, 6, 12, 19, 20, 21–22, 24–30, 35, 43–44, 46–49, 51–52, 56, 85, 108–109, 114n48, 165, 169, 176, 178, 216, 229, 240
immobility, 12, 165–169, 171, 173–174, 176–178, 181
inductive method, 47, 54–56; as revealing the background, 55–57
injustice, 205, 221n18
inspiration porn, 235–236, 238
intellectualism/intellectualist, 5–6, 90–91, 159n4, 193
intentional arc, 23–24, 26, 177–179, 239, 240
intentionality, 7, 23, 36, 42–43, 48, 55–57, 57n3, 67, 132, 172, 178; as "I can," 7, 24, 26, 35–36, 167, 173–179, 181, 217; motor, 54, 62n40, 174, 178, 180
intersubjectivity, 135, 226–227, 228, 232–233, 238, 241–242
irrational, 103–105, 113n29

Jung, Karl, 3
justice, 29, 31, 121, 215–216, 204, 220, 236, 262; social, 205, 218, 220

Kafer, Alison, 236–237, 240, 242n3, 247n66

Kant, 24
Klein, Melanie, 89

Ladau, Emily, 234
Landes, Donald A., 63, 74n12, 77n46
Leder, Drew, 28
Lériche, René, 26
lifeworld, 21, 59n12, 75–76n22
lived body. *See under* body
lived space, 147; political dimensions of, 148–150, 156–157; racial dimensions of, 156, 160–161n24, 162n45, 163n49, 163–164n52. *See also* space

madness, 10–11, 99–104, 107–110, 111n5, 112n13, 112n23
Marotta, Jonathan, 4, 14n4
metaphor, 24, 71, 157, 168
Miéville, China, 11, 148
Morning Glory Syndrome, 11, 121
Morris, David, 212–213
Murphy, Robert, 168, 174

narrative medicine, 207, 221fn8
nature, 21–22, 31, 68–70, 74n16, 81, 103, 111, 132, 136, 149, 160n19, 192, 205, 223n34, 230; embodied, 226, 232; human, 32, 46; phenomenal, 64–65, 67, 73
neurology, 42–44, 46–47, 165, 180
neuropsychology, 3–4, 14n4, 42, 45, 49–50, 52, 54–56, 57n2, 59n16, 62n43
neurosis, 80, 83–85, 87, 89
nonrational, 99–108, 110, 111n5, 113n29
normal/normality, 1–2, 6, 8–14, 24–26, 36–37, 42–44, 47–56, 89, 99–101, 104, 134, 146–147, 167, 204, 217; behavior, 1; distribution, 32–34; experience of space, 151–155, 158; health, 19–21, 25, 28–29, 31, 210, 215; ideal of, 10, 80, 81–85; perception, 11; phenomenology, 10, 63–64, 71–72, 75n20, 228; self/subject, 5, 7, 10, 80–82, 85, 87, 91–92, 106, 227; sensing 192–193; sexuality, 226, 230, 243n6; sight/visual perception, 4, 120–125, 129–130, 132, 141, 143
normalcy, 10, 79–82, 84–85, 90
normative/normativity, 21, 25–26, 29, 32–34, 128, 129, 130–131, 132, 135
norm, 9, 21, 25–26, 29–31, 33, 35, 37

objectification, 104, 226, 231–235, 238–239, 242, 246n41
objective body, 29–30, 36, 172
optimality, 59n12, 120, 129
orientation, 11, 35–36, 57n3, 62, 70, 107, 142, 144, 146–147, 150–153, 159n4, 162n45, 177, 192, 194–196, 198; spatial, 12, 142–143, 158

pathological/pathology, 2, 6–13, 24–28, 35–36, 42–43, 47–56, 57n2, 58n11, 59n12, 59n14, 59n16, 60n22, 62n52, 85–86, 89–90, 92–93, 96n65, 108–109, 111n7, 113n30, 135, 136n5, 178–179, 225, 227; as anatomical, 28; cases, 21–22, 26, 57, 120–121, 129; expressions of, 7; 90; paradigm, 189, 191–192, 199; phenomena, 48–49, 55; defined as rigidity, 87, 89–90; Russon's definition of, 85–86; situation 6, 10, 43, 53, 79–80, 85, 90, 93; states, 9, 29; in relation to perception, 120–121, 129
perception, 22, 63, 173, 192–195, 200; autism, 191, 195–196; distinct from hallucination, 90–93, 106;

determinacy/indeterminacy, 127–136; of disabled people as unsexed, 225–226, 231–232, 234, 240–242, 245n35; erotic, 230; figure-ground structure, 119–128, 135–135; in illness, 179; inverted visual, 11, 141–143; Morning Glory Syndrome, 121–124; of reason and unreason, 99–102, 104–105, 110; as racialized, 162; of self, 69, 228, 244n13; spatial level, 144–145, 147–148, 151–153, 157–158
phantom limb, 41, 174
phenomenal unity, 10, 64–71, 73, 75n22, 174, 214
phenomenological reduction, 22, 31, 56, 62n52, 70, 75n20; the impossibility of, 172
pica, 195–197
plasticity, 49, 171, 181
preferred behavior, 25, 52
psychological rigidity, 80, 87, 89–90

Quetelet, Alphonse, 32–34

racism, 7, 95n33, 162n45, 163n52, 164n56
rational, 90, 99, 101–108, 110, 111n6, 112n13, 113n29, 232
reaction, 48, 51, 55, 59n14, 61n25, 156, 173, 192, 209, 234, 236; catastrophic, 25, 35, 45, 52, 45; modified, 50, 54
real/reality, 68, 88–89, 92, 106, 107–110, 114n47, 130–131, 151, 180, 189, 197, 206, 213, 217, 220, 229; in space, 197
Reeve, Christopher, 169
reflex, 23, 49, 60n20, 93
retinal inversion, 141, 143, 158
Russon, John, 10, 80–85, 87, 89–90, 114n44, 163n47

Sartre, Jean-Paul, 30, 66–67, 150, 179
schizophrenia, 6, 57, 79–80, 90–93, 96n62–65, 104, 106, 108–110, 114n44, 115n52, 208
Schneider, Johann, 2–7, 9, 14n4, 22–26, 31, 35, 43, 45, 47, 52–53, 56, 114n46, 135, 226, 229–230, 239–240
sensation, 11, 29, 119, 124–125, 130, 198, 200, 202n21, 23; as physiological process, 192–196
sense, perceptual 124–127, 131–133; of orientation, 143–148, 158; as phenomenal unity with being, 64–73, 75n20, 76n22, 76n34, 77n35, 77n36, 77n52, 78n59; of self, 81, 169, 232–233; sense-making, 119–120, 126
sensory, 12, 23, 91–92, 146, 148, 153, 177, 187–198, 200; experience, 142–143, 188–190, 192–193, 200; field/milieu 193–194, 196, 198; integration, 191, 193; processing, 187, 191–193; stimulation, 190, 192–193, 195
sexuality, 11, 13, 136n6, 217, 226, 228–231, 233–234, 237–239, 241–242, 243n6, 2454n35
sexual recognition, 231, 238–239, 242
Solomon, Olga, 188
space, 5, 11–12, 104, 110, 129–130, 134, 138n37, 141–142, 145–156, 158–159, 159n4, 160n17, 160n24, 161n24, 162n45, 163n47, 163n49, 164n56, 172, 188–189, 193–196, 200, 210, 213; body in, 145, 194, 197–198; external, 194, 197; nonobjective, 104, 110; objective, 5, 105, 195; public/shared, 170, 172, 188, 200. *See also* lived space
spatial level, 138n31, 142–148, 150–159, 159n10, 160n20, 161n39,

spatial level *(continued)*
162n39, 163n47, 163n52; anchorage points within, 142–143, 145, 152; contingency of, 151, 152–153, 157; as dynamic and flexible, 146–147; as foreclosing other forms of spatial relations, 150, 155; loss of, 151–153, 155, 156–157
statistics, 9, 21, 29–34, 37, 39n46
Stiftung, 69–73
substitution, 47, 50–54, 55–57, 173–174
synesthetic/synesthesia, 131, 269

temporality, 160n18, 229–230, 240
third-person perspective, 20, 30, 35, 37

unreason, 99, 108, 111n6

unsexed, 230–231, 234, 240, 246n37

Vidal, Fernando, 167–168
visual field, 119, 120–126, 129–130, 132–133, 136, 177, 219
vulnerable/vulnerability, 80, 92, 158

Walker, Nick, 189
Weil, Simone, 11, 153–154, 158
Weiss, Gail, 7–8, 224n36
Welsh, Talia, 95n35, 103, 106, 178
Wynter, Sylvia, 181

Young, Iris Marion, 7
Young, Stella, 235

Zahavi, Dan, 55, 170
Zaner, Richard, 171–172, 175

www.ingramcontent.com/pod-product-compliance
Lightning Source LLC
Chambersburg PA
CBHW030529230426
43665CB00010B/818